IMMUNE MECHANISMS AND DISEASE

edited by

D. Bernard Amos

*Division of Immunology
Duke University Medical Center
Durham, North Carolina*

Robert S. Schwartz

*Tufts University School of Medicine
New England Medical Center Hospital
Boston, Massachusetts*

Bernard W. Janicki

*National Institute of Allergy
and Infectious Diseases
National Institutes of Health
Bethesda, Maryland*

ACADEMIC PRESS *New York San Francisco London 1979*

A Subsidiary of Harcourt Brace Jovanovich, Publishers

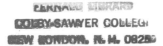

ACADEMIC PRESS, INC.
111 Fifth Avenue, New York, New York 10003

78980

United Kingdom Edition published by
ACADEMIC PRESS, INC. (LONDON) LTD.
24/28 Oval Road, London NW1 7DX

Library of Congress Cataloging in Publication Data
Main entry under title:

Immune mechanisms and disease.

Proceedings of a conference on the interface between
immune mechanisms and disease, which was held at Brook
Lodge, Augusta, Mich., Dec. 12–14, 1977.
    Bibliography: p.
    Includes index.
    1. Immunopathology—Congresses.   I. Amos,
Dennis Bernard, 1923–   II. Schwartz, Robert S.
III. Janicki, Bernard, W. [DNLM: 1. Immunity,
Natural—Congresses.   QW541 C748i 1977]
RC582.2.I44   616.07'9   79-19241
ISBN 0-12-055850-5

IMMUNE MECHANISMS AND DISEASE

Academic Press Rapid Manuscript Reproduction

The Proceeding of a Meeting
Held in Brook Lodge, Michigan
December 1977
Sponsored by
the National Institute of Allergies and Infectious Diseases
and
Hosted by the Upjohn Company

CONTENTS

Session IV
Immunopathology II

Session V
Therapeutic Manipulation

Session VI
Workshop

Collated by Charles H. Kirkpatrick
and Göran Möller

CONTRIBUTORS

Numbers in parentheses indicate pages on which authors' contributions begin.

D. BERNARD AMOS *(ix, 139), Department of Microbiology and Immunology, Division of Immunology, Duke University Medical Center, Durham, North Carolina 27710*

BARRY ARNASON *(179), Department of Neurology, Pritzker School of Medicine, University of Chicago, Chicago, Illinois 60637*

JOSE BARBOSA *(163), University of Minnesota, Minneapolis, Minnesota*

ROBERT E. BAUGHN *(341), Veterans Administration Hospital, Houston, Texas 77211*

SUSAN E. BEAR *(101), Tufts University School of Medicine, New England Medical Center Hospital, Boston, Massachusetts 02111*

HANS BINZ *(13), Department of Medical Microbiology, Zürich University, Zürich, Switzerland*

BARRY R. BLOOM *(69), Department of Microbiology, Immunology, and Cell Biology, Albert Einstein College of Medicine, Bronx, New York 10461*

SVEN BRITTON *(273), Department of Infectious Diseases, Danderyd Hospital, Danderyd, Sweden*

WILLIAM G. CANNADY *(163), Division of Immunogenetics, Sidney Farber Cancer Institute, Boston, Massachusetts 02115*

STANLEY COHEN *(45), Department of Pathology, University of Connecticut Health Center, Farmington, Connecticut 06032*

R. R. P. DE VRIES *(283), Department of Immunohematology, University Hospital, Leiden, The Netherlands*

ERWIN DIENER *(3), Department of Immunology and MRC Group on Immunoregulation, Faculty of Medicine, University of Alberta, Edmonton, Alberta, T6G 2H7 Canada*

DEVENDRA P. DUBEY *(163), Division of Immunogenetics, Sidney Farber Cancer Institute, Boston, Massachusetts 02115*

BO DUPONT *(163), Memorial Sloan-Kettering Cancer Institute, New York, New York 10021*

HAROLD F. DVORAK *(369), Massachusetts General Hospital, Boston, Massachusetts 02114*

KENNETH R. FALCHUK *(163), Peter Bent Brigham Hospital, Boston, Massachusetts*

DONNA FITZPATRICK *(163), Division of Immunogenetics, Sidney Farber Cancer Institute, Boston, Massachusetts 02115*

HANNES FRISCHKNECHT (13), Department of Medical Microbiology, Zürich University, Zürich, Switzerland

ROBERT GOOD (133), Sloan-Kettering Institute for Cancer Research, New York, New York 10021

FRED S. KANTOR (253), Department of Medicine, Yale University School of Medicine, New Haven, Connecticut 06510

CHARLES H. KIRKPATRICK (363), Laboratory of Clinical Investigation, National Institute of Allergy and Infectious Diseases, National Institutes of Health, Bethesda, Maryland 20014

JOHN M. KNOX (341), Department of Dermatology, Texas Medical Center, Baylor College, Houston, Texas 77030

R. F. M. LAI A FAT (283), Dermatological Service, Paramaribo, Surinam

FRANK LILLY (65), Department of Genetics, Albert Einstein College of Medicine of Yeshiva University, Bronx, New York 10461

SHARON MARTIN (163), Division of Immunogenetics, Sidney Farber Cancer Institute, Boston, Massachusetts 02115

N. K. MEHRA (283), Cellular Immunology Laboratory, A.I.I.M.S., New Delhi, India

THOMAS C. MERIGAN (311), Division of Infectious Diseases, Stanford University School of Medicine, Stanford, California 94305

GÖRAN MÖLLER (359), Division of Immunobiology, Karolinska Institute-Wallenberg Laboratory, Lillafreskati, S-104 05, Stockholm 50, Sweden

ROBERT MURGITA (13), Department of Immunology, Biomedicinska Centrum, Uppsala Universitets, Uppsala, Sweden

DANIEL M. MUSHER (341), Veterans Administration Hospital, Houston, Texas 77211

HARRIET NOREEN (163), University of Minnesota, Minneapolis, Minnesota

ERIC A. OTTESEN (215), Laboratory of Parasitic Diseases, National Institute of Allergy and Infectious Diseases, National Institutes of Health, Bethesda, Maryland 20014

AMMON B. PECK (13), Department of Immunology, Biomedicinska Centrum, Uppsala Universitets, Uppsala, Sweden

PER PETERSON (13), Department of Medical Chemistry, Uppsala University Medical School, Uppsala, Sweden

RICHMOND T. PREHN (371), Jackson Laboratories, Bar Harbor, Maine 04609

JAY P. SANFORD (199), School of Medicine, Uniformed Services University, Bethesda, Maryland 20014

ROBERT S. SCHWARTZ (101, 367), Tufts University School of Medicine, New England Medical Center Hospital, Boston, Massachusetts 02111

DR. KARIN SEGE (13), Department of Medical Chemistry, Uppsala University Medical School, Uppsala, Sweden

ALAN SHER (235), Department of Medicine, Robert B. Brigham Hospital, Boston, Massachusetts 02115

GREGORY W. SISKIND *(33), Division of Allergy and Immunology, Department of Medicine, Cornell University Medical College, New York, New York 10021*

HERBERT TANOWITZ *(69), Department of Microbiology, Immunology, and Cell Biology, Albert Einstein College of Medicine, Bronx, New York 10461*

GAIL A. THEIS *(323), Department of Microbiology, Basic Science Building, New York Medical School, Valhalla, New York 10595*

CHARLES TREY *(163), Peter Bent Brigham Hospital, Boston, Massachusetts*

PHILIP N. TSICHLIS *(101), Tufts University School of Medicine, New England Medical Center Hospital, Boston, Massachusetts 02111*

HENRY ST. G. TUCKER *(101), Tufts University School of Medicine, New England Medical Center Hospital, Boston, Massachusetts 02111*

M. C. VAIDYA *(283), Cellular Immunology Laboratory, A.I.I.M.S., New Delhi, India*

J. J. VANROOD *(283), Department of Immunohematology, University Hospital, Leiden, The Netherlands*

THOMAS A. WALDMANN *(303), Metabolism Branch, National Cancer Institute, National Institutes of Health, Bethesda, Maryland 20014*

HANS WIGZELL *(13, 365), Department of Immunology, Biomedicinska Centrum, Uppsala University Medical School, Uppsala, Sweden*

R. MICHAEL WILLIAMS *(163), Division of Tumor Immunology, Sidney Farber Cancer Institute, Boston, Massachusetts 02115*

MURRAY WITTNER *(69), Department of Microbiology, Immunology, and Cell Biology, Albert Einstein College of Medicine, Bronx, New York 10461*

EDMOND J. YUNIS *(139, 163), Division of Immunogenetics, Sidney Farber Cancer Center, Boston, Massachusetts 02115*

PREFACE

Scientists are often accused of allowing a time lapse between the basic discovery and its application. The converse is often equally true. The basic scientist may be unaware of clinical situations where investigation has been slow or the problem neglected for lack of awareness of its existence. One area in which interface has been sporadic and in which progress is urgently needed is in the interface between immunity and infection. Many diseases that should be amenable to immunologic attack are resistant, and the immunity to other diseases that develops, especially some of the parasitic diseases, is still incompletely understood.

In the last decade, immunology has undergone a series of upheavals. Old concepts have been abandoned and new approaches to regulation and functioning of the immune system have been made possible. Many of the most intensive advances have been at the basic and theoretical level, for example, in our understanding of the amplification and suppression of immunity and in the nature of the effector cells in the immune response. A completely new area of knowledge, the immunogenetics of disease, has been developed, and new functions have been found for cell-bound immunoglobulins. The biochemistry of the complement system has been extensively studied, and the role of split products of complement and of lymphokines released from activated lymphocytes in the inflammatory processes has become apparent.

To allow free communication between immunologists, pathologists, and specialists in several areas of infectious disease, a three-day meeting was held in Brook Lodge, Michigan. This volume includes the presentations made during the meeting together with transcripts of the open discussion that followed the papers.

INTRODUCTORY OVERVIEW

D. Bernard Amos

A major discovery in science is often serendipitous. A chance observation leads to a deduction; experiments show if the deduction is valid; and for a period, sometimes for a few weeks but rarely for months or years, logical projections can be made and a series of new findings results. Such "breakthroughs" are rapidly popularized. A fragment of a jawbone in an African ravine, a track on a photographic plate, the disappearance of disease after feeding a trace element, all make interesting headlines for the news media and provide widely read articles in the generalist journals. The expenditure of research funds becomes easily justifiable, more scientists, often in other disciplines, are brought in, and all possible aspects of the discovery are exploited.

After the breakthrough and the rapid progress that follows, further development gradually slows. The obvious questions have all been answered and new problems cannot be solved either because we do not know how to formulate appropriate questions or because the technology is not adequate. After a time another new discovery is made, the formerly "hot" topic is no longer exciting, and attention is focused on the new and exciting development. Usually forgotten is that the old problem had not been completely solved. Sometimes, as in organ transplantation, enough progress has been made so that new treatments can be incorporated into clinical practice. Ethical considerations then question the probity of further clinical experimentation. Not only do the difficult problems remain unsolved, the partial success of the treatment is great enough that any new approach becomes almost unethical.

One of the greatest of the unsolved problems of immunology has remained with us since the 1930s. An earlier era saw the introduction of bacterial and bacterial-product vaccines for the prevention of disease. A series of brilliant discoveries by Pasteur, Koch, Glenny, Lloyd, and others led to the virtual eradication or control of a host of virulent diseases such as plague, cholera, diphtheria, yellow fever, tetanus, and gas gangrene. Progress was being made, although not as rapidly, against other infectious diseases such as pneumonia, meningitis, tuberculosis, and against streptococcal and staphylococcal infections when the introduction of chemotherapeutic drugs and antibiotics for the treatment of an established infection ended much of the hazard from these infectious agents. From being the "white hope," immunology was regarded as having little further to offer in the treatment of infectious disease. Only recently, as an increasing number of organisms become resistant and the pathologic effects of chronic infection with relatively insensitive organisms become apparent and as pharmacologic agents fail to control many viruses, fungi, and parasites, much attention has been drawn to the many opportunities that exist. Some approaches are possible because discoveries made in an earlier era were never adequately followed up; others are now possible because tremendous changes have occurred in the science of immunology.

What then are the challenges? Forty years after the discovery of penicillin, syphilis reemerges as a major disease. A host of "new" veneral diseases are now traced to old but intractable infectious agents such as cytomegalovirus, shigella, or chlamydia. Despite 40 years of pharmacological effort, parasitic diseases affect more than half of mankind. In some areas, schistosomiasis, malaria, amebiasis, filariasis, and even scabiosis gravely affect the quality of life, while endemic bacterial diseases decimate the children in countries too poor to afford therapeutic agents. While sanitation, diet, drugs, and antibiotics all have their role in disease eradication, a better understanding of the host–parasite relationship has much to offer and in some areas has the potential for effective treatment where other agents do not.

The last few years have seen an explosive growth in our understanding of immunologic processes. While much of this new knowledge was initially related to cellular reactions, antibody has reemerged in a dominant role because of our appreciation of the role of antiidiotype antibodies in the regulation of immunity, and because of our better (but still incomplete) understanding of the complex relationship among antibody, complement, and the cells of the immune system. New precision to the study of antibodies has been given by production of "hybridomas," clones derived from the fusion of a myeloma cell line with a specific antibody-producing cell. Methods of coupling antigens to Sephadex beads offer new approaches to enhance immunogenicity. Also offering exciting but clinically unexploited avenues is the marriage between humoral and cellular immunity in those reactions that depend upon the participation of lymphocytes, not themselves immune, but given their specificity by special types of preformed antibody. Natural killing by lymphocytes, the arming of macrophages by antibody, and the activation of macrophages are other exciting fields of study with much potential in disease control. So too is the finding of the involvement of genes of the major histocompatibility systems of mouse and man and monkey in disease susceptibility and resistance, in the regulation of the immune response, and in the production of some components of complement. The possibilities arise of new classifications, through the collaboration of immunologist and clinician, a broad range of diseases including rheumatoid diseases, chronic inflammatory gastrointestinal diseases, some neurologic and psychiatric diseases, and at least some of the collagen diseases.

One very important area that has received little attention is the mode of action of the specific components of the immune system on the initiation, progression, and resolution of infectious diseases. The involvement of immune cells in the resistance to granulomatosis infections such as TB or leprosy is, of course, part of the heritage of microbial immunity. However, in the older studies of these diseases there was no awareness of substances (lymphokines) affecting vascular endothelium and activating and controlling the migration of phagocytic cells, or of the cytolytic potential of lymphocytes against infected cells. Similarly, knowledge of the powerful retrograde effects of immune suppression was not available. The tailoring of new vaccines to stimulate selected subclasses of lymphoid cells or the use of drugs to regulate the activities of other types of lymphocyte are still goals on the horizon and have not been discussed in depth among microbiologists, parasitologists, pharmacologists, and immunologists.

The conference held at Brook Lodge brought together specialists in several fields: parasitology, bacteriology and virology, cellular and humoral immunology, pathology, and immunogenetics. Included in this volume are up-to-date surveys of the various areas and a record of the discussions that were generated between specialists as ideas were exchanged. The topics covered included a survey of immunologic mechanisms, the immunogenetics of infectious diseases including parasitic diseases and the mechanisms of escape from immunity, studies of immunopathological processes, and the possibilities for therapeutic manipulation. The final session of the conference was unstructured. The chairmen, Dr. Möller and Dr. Kirkpatrick, led the discussion back into many of the areas that had aroused the most intense discussion during the meeting and developed some new themes such as the role of immunologic surveillance in neoplasia and the use of transfer factor in clinical immunology.

LIST OF ABBREVIATIONS

ALS	antilymphocyte serum
ATS	antithymocyte serum
B cell	bone marrow or bursal equivalent-derived lymphocyte
BCG	bacille Calmette Guerin
CFA	complete Freund's adjuvant
CMI	cell-mediated immunity
CNS-BP	central nervous system myelin basic protein
CSF	cerebrospinal fluid
EAE	experimental allergic encephalomyelitis
EAN	experimental allergic neuritis
EBV	Epstein–Barr virus
FCS	fetal calf serum
HAI	hemagglutination inhibition
H Bs AG	hepatitis B antigen
HV	herpesvirus
HVT	herpesvirus tumor
MATSA	Marek's associated tumor-specific surface antigen
MD	Marek's disease
MDV	Marek's disease virus
MEM	minimal essential medium
MIF	macrophage migration-inhibiting factor
MIFIF	MIF-inhibiting factor
PFU	plaque-forming unit
PHA	phytohemagglutinin
PNS	peripheral nervous system
PNS-BP	peripheral nervous system myelin basic protein
T cell	thymus-derived or thymus-dependent lymphocyte
XC plaque	a giant cell assay for transformation
3T3	embryo fibroblast transferred every three days at 3×10^5 cells

Session I
Immunologic Mechanisms

OVERVIEW : IMMUNOREGULATION

Erwin Diener

Department of Immunology
and MRC Group on Immunoregulation
Faculty of Medicine
University of Alberta
Edmonton, Alberta, Canada

Some years ago, many of the authorities of immunology reacted with skepticism to the prophesies of some of their more
visionary colleagues who suggested the possibility that immune
surveillance embodies an intricate network of cellular and
humoral antagonists in the form of helper and suppressor cells,
antibodies, and autoantiantibodies. While the cellular antagonists have become an established reality of contemporary
knowledge, the immunological significance of autoantiantibodies
as regulatory devices is still awaiting clarification, although
their existence, under certain experimental conditions, has
been documented beyond doubt. While the above-mentioned cellular and humoral antagonists operate via specific recognition
sites, either for the antigen or for certain sites on the antibody molecule, other less specific cell-borne products known
as lymphokines constitute a further, though poorly understood,
immunoregulatory mechanism. In this introduction, I shall
briefly sketch an outline of the current understanding of the
regulatory mechanisms that keep the immune system in tune.

I. CELLULAR ANTAGONISTS: HELPER CELLS, SUPPRESSOR CELLS

A. *Helper Cells*

   1. Helper T Cells. The requirement for thymus-derived
helper (T) cells in the humoral response has been known for
more than a decade (1,2,3,4,5). The specificity of reactivity
of thymus cells was conclusively demonstrated by experiments
in which the helper activity of these cells could be specifically enhanced by exposing thymocytes to antigen in an irradiated animal prior to mixing them with bone marrow-derived
(B) cells in a second irradiated recipient (4). The discovery
that antihapten responses could be enhanced by previous priming
of T cells with the carrier (6,7) when the animal is challenged
with the hapten physically linked to the same carrier (8) led
to the definition of T-B cell cooperation by linked associative recognition (9). The postulate that the recognition by
the T cell of antigenic determinants on the carrier portion
of an antigen is mediated by Ig-like receptor molecules (10)
has found experimental support on the basis of immunochemical
and serological analysis (11) and by the recent discovery of
functional homology between T cell receptors and B cell-derived immunoglobulin idiotypes (12,13). The possibility that
T cells interact with B cells by means of a soluble carrier-
specific product derives support from both *in vitro* and *in
vivo* experiments (14,15).
   The molecular mechanism of T cell cooperation is far from
being understood. Controversy exists as to the role of the
Ig receptor on the B cell as a triggering device. One minimal
model for T-B cell interaction postulates that the binding
of antigen to the B cell receptor induces a tolerogenic signal unless T cell-derived helper factor (associative antibody) is also present, as part of the antigen receptor complex,
to elicit a B cell stimulation (16,17). This second signal
is postulated to be absent for self-antigens; hence the obvious attractiveness of this theory for offering a solution to
the problem of autotolerance. A prediction made by this hypothesis is that the number of positive signals critically depends on the capacity of the antigen (its carrier portion) to
focus helper factor molecules to the respective B cell. Optimally efficient B cell triggering, therefore, asks for a
high number of foreign antigenic sites per molecule of immunogen. Indeed, recent work in our laboratory has shown that
the molecular conditions that favor B cell triggering are optimal when the carrier molecule offers a high density of antigenic determinants that can be specifically recognized by
helper factor (18). Another popular theory on immune trigger-

ing (19) suggests that the Ig receptor merely acts as a focusing device for antigen and that B cells can receive only stimulatory signals by helper T cells or their helper products.
A formidable puzzle concerning the mechanism of T-B cell interaction is the observation that helper T cells cooperate
optimally with B cells provided the latter carry the same I-
region cell surface markers as the animal in which the T cells
have been primed (20). This phenomenon is analogous to the
phenomenon of allogeneic restriction as seen in T cell effector function against virus-infected target cells. Thus,
killer cells are only effective when the virus-infected (21)
or chemically modified (22) target cells carry the same MHC
haplotype as the stimulator cells. T cell-mediated cytotoxicity
against minor histocompatibility antigens and tumor-specific
antigens is also restricted by major histocompatibility haplotypes (23). It would seem logical that the allogeneic restriction that operates at the level of helper T and B cells
might also apply to the collaboration event between antigen-
specific T cell-derived helper factor and B cells. Such a
restriction has been found in our laboratory (18) but not in
that of other investigators (15). Helper T cells have been
analyzed most extensively as far as the humoral immune response is concerned. Extending earlier studies by others (24,
25,26), work in our department has conclusively established
the necessity for antigen-specific helper T cells in the generation of cytotoxic T cells as well (27).

    2. Helper Macrophagelike Cells. A fundamental theory of
immune triggering must identify the minimal set of cooperating
cells, which is believed to consist of immunocompetent T and
B cells and macrophagelike adherent (A) cells. While the regulatory role of A cells in the immune response has long been
recognized in studies on tolerance induction (28), their absolute requirement for antigen-mediated triggering of both T
and B cells to both T-dependent as well as T-independent antigens has only recently been established (29,30). Perhaps
the most convincing evidence that antigen-presenting cells
play a key role in immune triggering comes from the observation that allogeneic restriction is determined by the MHC haplotype of the accessory cells presenting the antigen (31,32,
33,34). For example, a population of $(A \times B)F_1$ immunocompetent B cells will give a response of comparable magnitude
when antigen is presented by either parental A/A or B/B macrophages. However, when the same population of $(A \times B)F_1$ cells
is primed with antigen-pulsed macrophages of parental origin,
secondary restimulation will only occur in response to the
same antigen in the presence of macrophages of the same parental
strain used for primary sensitization. This genetic restric-

tion appears to be controlled by the I-region of the major histocompatibility gene complex. Currently, two basic concepts
are advanced to explain the phenomenon. One concept maintains
that an immunocompetent lymphocyte has two types of receptors:
one that recognizes the extrinsic, that is, the foreign antigen, presented by the A cell, and a second with the property
of recognizing a self-antigen expressed on the A cell surface.
In the case of the mouse, the second antigen is believed to
correspond to the I-region products of the H-2 gene complex.
An alternative model suggests that the foreign antigen is
recognized in association with the self-antigen (altered self)
in a dual-recognition event mediated by only one type of receptor molecule or molecular complex. The second recognition
concept agrees with the experimental evidence that T lymphocytes are clonally compartmentalized, each clone with a capacity to recognize one type of altered self, be it via presentation of antigen by A cells in association with membrane-
bound self-antigens or via a secretory product derived from
A cells (35) and consisting in part of self-components com-
plexed with foreign antigen. To account for the experimental
evidence in favor of compartmentalization into subclones of
T cells, each recognizing the antigen in association with only
one parental MHC-haplotype, the two-receptor hypothesis must
postulate allelic exclusion for the receptor recognizing the
H-2 product.

In addition to the essential role in immune triggering
(36), A cells are also known for both their stimulatory and
inhibitory influence on the immune response (37,38,39). Recent evidence by Dr. K.-C. Lee of our department suggests
that the two functions are due to two subpopulations of A cells
with antagonistic stimulatory and inhibitory functions (40).
Depending on the type of antigenic stimulus, one or the other
of these A cell subpopulations may increase in size and thereby alter the overall functional properties of the entire A
cell population. The discovery of two types of A cell-derived
factors, one with immunostimulatory, the other with cytostatic
properties, further supports this notion (41). Our recent
work has shown that the activity of A cells, as far as the
immune response is concerned, is controlled by cortisone.
Observations concerning the dependency on the antigen concentration of the humoral response *in vitro* have revealed that
high doses of the steroid cause a dramatic decrease in the
antigen dose required to induce either immunity or tolerance
(42). There is evidence suggesting that this dose response
shift is due to an effect of cortisone on A cells (43). Further work has established that the immunosuppressive effect
of cortisone on cell-mediated immunity is also due to the functional alteration of cooperating A cells (44). These findings

may bear on the significance of stress in relationship to
immunoregulation *in vivo*. Besides these hormonal influences,
lymphokines, such as macrophage-activating and inhibitory factors, are also likely to exert immunoregulatory functions via
A cells.

B. Suppressor T Cells

The existence of suppressor T lymphocytes has been established for humoral immunity, including IgM (45), IgG, and IgE
antibody responses (46), as well as for cell-mediated immunity
(47,48), for responses to T-dependent and, to a less certain
degree, to T-independent antigens (49,50,51). Although antigen-
specific as well as nonspecific T-cell mediated suppression has
been described, the physiological significance of the latter
phenomenon is uncertain. As has been demonstrated for antigen-
specific helper T cells, antigen-specific suppressor cells also follow the rule of linked associative recognition. Thus
specific suppression by, for example, KLH-primed suppressor
cells has been shown to occur only when the hapten DNP is presented on the homologous carrier that is in the form of DNP-
KLH. Suppression fails to occur, however, when KLH-primed
T cells are tested in the presence of nonrelated carriers such
as DNP-HGG (52,53). The requirement for linked associative
recognition has recently been shown in our department also to
apply to the activity of suppressor cells that inhibit the induction of cytotoxic precursor T cells (54). In view of con-
tradictory evidence, the question whether suppressor T cells
act directly on helper T cells, the precursors of effector T
cells, or B cells, must remain unanswered at the present time.
Of interest has been the finding that genetically determined
nonresponsiveness to certain random copolymers of L-amino acids
such as GAT appears to be due to GAT-specific suppressor T
cells (55). Because in such animals an immune response to
the peptide may be provoked provided it is administered in
conjugation with an appropriate carrier (56), the role of
suppressor cells in certain types of tolerance could be established. Thus the administration of GAT to a nonresponder was
found to induce a state of suppressor cell-mediated unresponsiveness to a subsequent challenge with GAT as a hapten in
association with an immunogeneic carrier. This, together with
work by others who have demonstrated the role of suppressor
cells in low dose tolerance to bacteriophage antigens (57),
has called for reinterpretation of various models of tolerance,
including tolerance to self. This brings us to a particularly
interesting class of suppressor cells, those which are specific for allotypic or idiotypic determinants on immunoglobulin.

Extensive work on the phenomenon of allotype-specific suppressor suggests the existence of a class of suppressor T
lymphocytes capable of interfering with the ability of helper
T cells to cooperate in the induction of an immune response by
B cells expressing a particular immunoglobulin allotype (58,
59). Similarly, suppressor T lymphocytes have been described
that limit the production by B cells of antibody bearing a
particular idiotype marker (60). The fact that both these
phenomena document the existence of suppressor cells carrying
specific receptors for self-markers on receptors expressed by
T helper cells or B cells suggests a compartmentalization of
suppressor, helper, and effector cells into a number of subclasses. If so, each subclass could contain matched pairs of
antagonistically functioning lymphocytes (i.e., idiotype:
anti-idiotype).

II. CONCLUSION

The kinetic and qualitative characteristics of an immune
response reflect the development in time and space of effector cells whose specialized function we measure either in the
form of various classes of antibody or as reactions characteristic of cell-mediated immunity. Some time ago, the quantitative aspect of immunity had been worked out quite thor-
oughly: first, at the level of antigen-antibody interaction
kinetics and, with the availability of appropriate techniques,
at the level of cell population dynamics. Early concepts
trying to explain the quantitative and qualitative changes in
time of an immune response have ascribed such changes to alterations in antigen concentrations and hence alterations in
the degree to which immunocompetent cells are stimulated by
immunogens. Such interpretations have mainly been derived
from experimental work on antibody-mediated feedback inhibition. Their validity has in part been restricted, however,
when it was discovered that antibody-antigen complexes could,
under certain conditions, render immunocompetent cells unresponsive, and that therefore a decline in antibody titer may
not be due exclusively to antigen neutralization (61). Perhaps the most important expansion in our understanding of immunoregulatory processes has been the discovery of T lymphocytes with specific immunoregulatory functions affecting not
only the antibody response but cell-mediated immunity as well.
The most common immunoregulatory unit consists of two antagonists, a helper and a suppressor cell. However, there is
evidence, at least under experimental conditions, that one
and the same cell class may exert help as well as suppression,

depending on its population size. Thus, too many helper cells
appear to suppress an ongoing response (62). The more recent
discovery of suppressor T cells capable of specifically suppressing an immune response by virtue of autoanti-idiotype
antibody calls to mind the network theory on immunoregulation
(63,64), whose physiological significance has yet to be assessed. Besides T cells as immunoregulators, macrophagelike
A cells have received increasing attention in view of their
role in T cell priming and T-B cell cooperation. In addition
to their critical involvement in the actual immune triggering
event, their regulatory function in response to lymphokines
and glucocorticosteroids may prove of critical importance,
particularly from the clinical point of view.

As impressive as the current phenomonology on immunoregulatory aspects is, there is a surprising lack of interest in
trying to accommodate a formidable collection of data within
a comprehensive theoretical framework, which could help us
understand the dynamic aspects of such regulatory processes.
There has been strong emphasis on the possible significance
of suppressor cells in tolerance, notably self-tolerance, in
spite of the increasing evidence to the contrary. In view of
recent work, however, it appears more likely that the various
antagonistic functions of help and suppression by various distinct cell types and factors do in fact serve the need to
switch from one type of immune function to another.

This viewpoint has been expressed by Bretscher in a theory
on immune class regulation (65). This theory is based on the
reasonable assumption that the triggering of immunocompetent
cells, including specifically antigen-reactive helper and
suppressor cells, must be governed by parameters inherent in
the mode of antigenic stimulation. These parameters include
the quality of the antigen, such as its density of foreign antigenic determinants, as well as its concentration. According
to Bretscher, differing classes of precursor cells require
different threshold levels of stimulation by antigen and
helper cells to be triggered. For example, an immunogen that
contains only few antigenic determinants and hence is capable
of interacting with a small number of helper cells is thought
to induce cell-mediated immunity rather than humoral immunity
and vice versa. In the case of B cell stimulation, the number of triggering signals delivered to an immunocompetent cell
is believed to depend on the number of foreign sites on an
antigen and hence its capacity to focus a sufficient number
of antigen-specific helper factor molecules to the B cell in
order to reach the amount of help required for triggering.
The theory suggests that a similar mechanism will apply in
the induction of T precursor cells to become effector cells
in cell-mediated immunity. The class hierarchy of responses,

reflecting the amount of triggering signal required, is meant to extend from cell-mediated immunity with the lowest triggering threshold to IgM, and finally to IgG with the highest triggering threshold. The hypothesis most elegantly accommodates the role of regulatory cells such as helper and suppressor cells; they are thought to expand or restrict the number of available inductive signals so as to effect the expression of a particular class of immunity.

This brief review has attempted to highlight some of the prominent points of junction in the intricate network of the immune system. I am confident that this session will help set the stage on which the immunopathological phenomena to be presented during this meeting will be discussed.

References

1. Miller, J. F. A. P. *Lancet ii*, 748, 1961.
2. Martinez, C., Kersey, J., Papermaster, B. W., and Good, R. A. *Proc. Soc. Exp. Biol. Med. 109*, 193, 1962.
3. Claman, H. N., Chaperon, E. A., and Triplett, R. F. *Proc. Soc. Exp. Biol. Med. 122*, 1167, 1966.
4. Mitchell, G. F., and Miller, J. F. A. P. *J. Exp. Med. 128*, 821, 1968.
5. Nossal, G. J. V., Cunningham, A., Mitchell, G. F., and Miller, J. F. A. P. *J. Exp. Med. 128*, 839, 1968.
6. Mitchison, N. A. *J. Immunol. 1*, 68, 1971.
7. Rajewsky, K., Schirrmacher, U., Nase, S., and Jerne, N. K. *J. Exp. Med. 129*, 1131, 1969.
8. Mitchison, N. A., Rajewsky, K., and Taylor, R. B. "Developmental Aspects of Antibody Formation and Structure," Vol. 2. Czech. Academy of Science, Prague, 1971.
9. Bretscher, P. A. *Transplant. Rev. 11*, 217, 1972.
10. Mitchison, N. A. "Differentiation and Immunology," *Symp. Int. Soc. Cell Biol.*, Vol. 7, p. 29. Academic Press, New York, 1968.
11. Marchalonis, J. J., Atwell, J. L., and Cone, R. E. *Nature New Biol. 235*, 240, 1972.
12. Eichmann, K., and Rajewsky, K. *Eur. J. Immunol. 5*, 661, 1975.
13. Binz, H., and Wigzell, H. *J. Exp. Med. 142*, 197, 1975.
14. Feldmann, M., and Basten, A. *J. Exp. Med. 136*, 49, 1972.
15. Taussig, M. J., Munro, A. J., Campbell, R., David, D. S., and Staines, A. *J. Exp. Med. 142*, 694, 1975.
16. Bretscher, P., and Cohn, M. *Science 169*, 1042, 1970.
17. Bretscher, P. *Transplant Rev. 11*, 217, 1972.
18. Shiozawa, C., Singh, B., Rubinstein, S., and Diener, E. *J. Immunol. 118*, 2199, 1977.

19. Coutinho, A., and Möller, G. *Scand. J. Immunol. 3*, 133, 1974.
20. Katz, D. H., and Benacerraf, B. *Transplant. Rev. 22*, 195, 1975.
21. Zinkernagel, R. M., and Doherty, P. C. *In* "The Role of Products of the Histocompatibility Gene Complex in Immune Responses" (D. H. Katz and B. Benacerraf, eds.), p. 203. Academic Press, New York, 1976.
22. Shearer, B. M., Schmitt-Verhulst, A. M., and Rehn, T. G. *In* "The Role of Products of the Histocompatibility Gene Complex in Immune Responses" (D. H. Katz and B. Benacerraf, eds.), p. 133. Academic Press, New York, 1976.
23. Bevan, M. J. *Cold Spring Harbor Symp. Quant. Biol. XLI*, 519, 1976.
24. Cohen, L., and Howe, M. *Proc. Nat. Acad. Sci. 70*, 2707, 1973.
25. Wagner, H. *J. Exp. Med. 138*, 1379, 1973.
26. Cantor, H., and Boyse, E. A. *J. Exp. Med. 141*, 1390, 1975.
27. Pilarski, L. M. *J. Exp. Med. 145*, 709, 1977.
28. Dresser, D. W., and Mitchison, N. A. *Adv. Immunol. 8*, 129, 1968.
29. Lee, K. C., Shiozawa, C., Shaw, A., and Diener, E. *Eur. J. Immunol. 6*, 63, 1976.
30. Diener, E., Shiozawa, C., Singh, B., and Lee, K.-C. *Cold Spring Harbor Symp. Quant. Biol. XLI*, 251, 1977.
31. Rosenthal, A. S., and Shevach, E. M. *J. Exp. Med. 138*, 1194, 1973.
32. Pierce, C. W., Kapp, T. A., and Benacerraf, B. *J. Exp. Med. 144*, 371, 1976.
33. Thomas, D. W., and Shevach, E. M. *J. Exp. Med. 144*, 1263, 1976.
34. Paul, W. E., Shevach, E. M., Thomas, D. W., Pickeral, S. F., and Rosenthal, A. S. *Cold Spring Harbor Symp. Quant. Biol. XLI*, 571, 1976.
35. Erb, P., and Feldmann, M. *J. Exp. Med. 142*, 460, 1975.
36. Mosier, D. E. *J. Exp. Med. 129* 351, 1969.
37. Diener, E., and Lee, K. *Proc. 3rd Int. Congr. Immunol.*, Sydney, Australia, 1977.
38. Diener, E., Shortman, K., and Russell, P. *Nature 225*, 731, 1970.
39. Shortman, K., Diener, E., Russell, P., and Armstrong, W. D. *J. Exp. Med. 131*, 461, 1970.
40. Lee, K.-C., and Berry, D. *J. Immunol. 118*, 1530, 1977.
41. Unanue, E. R., Calderon, J., and Kiely, M. J. *In* "Immune Recognition," p. 555. Academic Press, New York, 1975.
42. Diener, E., and Lee, K.-C. *In* "Immunological Tolerance," (D. H. Katz and B. Benacerraf, eds.), p. 33. Academic Press, New York, 1974.

43. Lee, K.-C., Langman, R. E., Paetkau, V. H., and Diener, E. *Cell. Immunol. 17*, 405, 1975.
44. Lee, K.-C. *J. Immunol. 119*, 1836, 1977.
45. Gershon, R. K., and Kondo, K. *Immunology 18*, 723, 1970.
46. Tada, T., Okumura, K., and Taniguchi, M. *J. Immunol. 108*, 1535, 1972.
47. Gershon, R. K., Cohen, P., Hencin, R., and Liebhaber, S. A. *J. Immunol. 108*, 586, 1972.
48. Peavy, D. L., and Pierce, C. W. *J. Exp. Med. 140*, 356, 1974.
49. Baker, P. J., Barth, R. F., Stashak, P. W., and Amsbaugh, D. F. *J. Immunol. 104*, 1313, 1970.
50. Baker, P. J., Stashak, P. W., Amsbaugh, D. F., Prescott, B., and Barth, R. F. *J. Immunol. 105*, 1581, 1970.
51. Warr, C. W., Ghaffar, A., and James, K. *Cell. Immunol. 17*, 366, 1975.
52. Tada, T. *In* "Immunological Tolerance" (D. H. Katz and B. Benacerraf, eds.), p. 471. Academic Press, New York, 1974.
53. Basten, A. *In* "Immunological Tolerance" (D. H. Katz and B. Benacerraf, eds.), p. 107. Academic Press, New York, 1974.
54. Al-Adra, A. R., and Pilarski, L. M. (submitted).
55. Pierce, C. W., and Kapp, J. A. *Contemp. Top. Immunobiol. 5*, 91, 1976.
56. Kapp, J. A., Pierce, C. W., and Benacerraf, B. *J. Exp. Med. 140*, 172, 1974.
57. Kölsch, E., Stumpf, R., and Weber, G. *Transplant. Rev. 26*, 56, 1975.
58. Herzenberg, L. A., and Herzenberg, L. A. *Contemp. Top. Immunobiol. 3*, 41, 1974.
59. Herzenberg, L. A., Okumura, K., and Metzler, C. M. *Transplant. Rev. 27*, 57, 1975.
60. Eichmann, K. *Eur. J. Immunol. 5*, 511, 1975.
61. Diener, E., and Feldman, M. *Transplant. Rev. 8*, 76, 1972.
62. Ramshaw, I. A., McKenzie, I. F. C., Bretscher, P. A., and Parish, C. R. *Cell. Immunol. 31*, 364, 1977.
63. Jerne, N. K. *Ann. Immunol. Inst. Pasteur 125c*, 7, 1974.
64. Lindenmann, J. *Ann. Immunol. Inst. Pasteur 124c*, 171, 1974.
65. Bretscher, P. A. *In* "B and T Cells in Immune Recognition" (F. Loor and G. E. Roelands, eds.), p. 457. Wiley, London, 1977.

INDUCTION AND INHIBITION OF LYMPHOCYTE FUNCTIONS:
A NOTE ON COMPLEXITY AND CONSEQUENCES

Hans Wigzell
Robert Murgita
Ammon B. Peck

Department of Immunology
Uppsala University Medical School
Uppsala, Sweden

Hans Binz
Hannes Frischknecht

Department of Medical Microbiology
Zürich University
Zürich, Switzerland

Per Peterson
Karin Sege

Department of Medical Chemistry
Uppsala University Medical School
Uppsala, Sweden

INTRODUCTION

Triggering as well as inhibition of specific, immunocompetent lymphocytes constitute central activities within the
immune response. Through these mechanisms the immune system
may evolve with select immunity against a given set of "foreign"
substances or, alternatively, develop specific unresponsiveness
to the same group of molecules. Choices of alternative pathways of reaction take place due to an intricate set of reactions between different subgroups of lymphocytes with inter-

acting forces of positive or negative significance for the
target cells concerned. Using genetically defined systems it
has been possible to describe the existence of several functionally as well as morphologically distinct subgroups of lymphocytes as presented in Diener's overview. The development
of knowledge as to the factual existence of these subgroups
has been of great importance for our understanding of how the
immune processes may occur. However, facts obtained from complicated systems frequently are overinterpreted as to simpli-
city. It is likely that very significant yet undiscovered
complexity still lies ahead of us as to the composition of
the immune system.

The molecular events underlying the signals leading to
activation or inhibition (elimination) of the relevant immunocompetent lymphocytes when confronted with antigen are obscure.
In the B lymphocyte group it is clear that so-called thymus-
independent antigens carry an inherent property to be mitogenic for maybe all B cells, irrespective of their antigen-
binding specificity (Coutinho, 1975). The antigen-binding
specific receptors on those B cells, which do carry significant avidity for the antigenic determinants on such a T-independent antigen would here merely seem to function as focusing
devices for the mitogen. Thus, the "true" antigen-specific B
cells will be triggered by much lower concentrations of T-
independent antigens compared to the polyclonal activation of
any B cell occurring at a much higher concentration of the
same antigen. The underlying events at the cellular level
leading to division and initiation of high-rate immunoglobulin
synthesis are, however, unknown. When studying B cell activation by so-called T-dependent antigen, it would seem likely
that such antigens in order to trigger the B cells must acquire
mitogenic properties for the B cells. This may occur via a
combination between the antigen and antigen-specific "helper"
factors from T cells (Mozes *et al.*, 1975). Again, the actual
events at the level of cell triggering are unknown.

When discussing triggering of T lymphocytes by antigen the
situation would seem even more complicated and unclear as to
molecular events. T lymphocytes will seemingly always react
against antigen in conjunction with histocompatibility molecules on the surface of the "triggering" cells. The superior
triggering cells using conventional, soluble antigens in this
regard are the macrophages, whereas it is possible that histoincompatible cells of other types may function as triggers
for antihistocompatibility reactions.

Helper T cells do seem to recognize antigen together with
the Ia antigens of the macrophages (Rosenthal and Shevach,
1973) whereas suppressor and killer T cells normally "see"
the antigen in conjunction with the SD-determinants (the K or
D region molecules of the H-2 in the mouse) (Bach *et al.*, 1976).

The striking thing is that there is a clonal expression of T
cell reactivity not only with regard to conventional antigens
but also with regard to the major histocompatibility complex
antigens even in the self-MHC context (Zinkernagel and Doherty,
1976). This means among other things that *in vivo* generated
immune T cells will normally only respond to the same antigen
if presented in the context of a given, self-MHC antigen, a
fact of significant importance not only for theoretical reasons
but also of practical consequence, for instance, in studies
of tumor-specific immune reactions. The receptor structure
used by T cells in the cognition and recognition of antigen
would thus carry as a major requirement the ability to react
with specificity not only to any conventional antigen but to
simultaneously also carry reactivity toward a certain MHC
structure. A number of models as to how such a receptor may
be created exist (Janeway *et al.*, 1976). As the present knowledge of the T cell receptor for antigen is still by no means
complete, it would follow that our understanding of the specific triggering of T cells by antigen is even less complete
than that of B cell triggering.

Despite this ignorance, our understanding of the build-up
of the immune system is rapidly expanding. The interested
reader is referred to the summaries from a recent symposium to
gather the present stage of knowledge as to the present consensus of the immune system (*Cold Spring Harbor Symp. Quant.
Biol. 46*, 1976). We shall consider the reader acquainted with
the "normal" behavior of lymphocytes during triggering with
antigen. Assuming this to be the case, we shall describe how
changes in the surroundings may affect the normal reactions
to make them quite abnormal, discuss what may be the "real"
driving force during immune induction and present some data
as to how autoimmune reactions against the antigen-specific
receptors themselves may result in drastic triggering of reactions both within and outside the normal frameworks of immune
reactions.

TRIGGERING OF IMMUNOCOMPETENT T CELLS BY HISTOINCOMPATIBLE
STIMULATOR CELLS: MODIFICATION OF THE "NORMAL" RESPONSE AS
TO QUANTITY AND QUALITY BY EXTERNAL FACTORS

It is commonly conceived that induction of immunocompetent
T cells by histoincompatible stimulator cells will proceed
according to a certain, fixed pathway according to the nature
of the stimulator antigens. Thus, stimulation with Ia associated antigens does under normal conditions lead to the proliferation of T cells, which by and large are characterized

as "helper" T cells with only minor contributions of proliferating killer T cells. Likewise, triggering with SD-differences (K and D differences in the murine system) is considered to cause the proliferation and induction of specific killer T cells (Alter *et al.*, 1973), although this proliferation of anti-SD T cells is frequently found to require a simultaneous induction of proliferation of anti-Ia helper T cells functioning as triggering cells for the potential killer T cells (Cantor and Boyse, 1975). The reader should understand that this is very likely the most common pathway of induction occurring under normal conditions. However, this normal route of triggering may well succumb to distraction by changes in the environment in ways telling us not only of our ignorance of activating conditions for lymphocytes but also to the flexibility of the immune system. Here, we would like to discuss changes in the immune reaction patterns achieved *in vitro* by the addition of a protein, alfa-feto-protein (AFP) to the tissue culture media. AFP is a controversial agent in this regard, found to inhibit a variety of immune reactions *in vitro* with a dominating target being the helper T cells for antibody formation against T dependent antigens. One mechanism is known whereby AFP will induce inhibitory T cells *in vitro* capable of highly efficient inhibition of helper T cells (Murgita *et al.*, 1977). These AFP-induced inhibitory T cells display a different setup of differentiation antigens compared to the "normal" suppressor T cells of the mouse being of the Ly 1^+2^- phenotype in contrast to the conventional phenotype Ly 1^-2^+. Likewise, newborn mouse T cells are found to be efficient suppressor T cells (Murgita *et al.*, 1978). These newborn suppressor T cells also have the Ly 1^+2^- phenotype. It is tempting to suggest that *in vivo* contact with AFP may at least in part be responsible for this.

Be that as it may, AFP can be shown to have profound but highly variable consequences when present during primary or secondary MLC:s. In the murine system there exist at least four different genetic systems that allow the stimulation of primary MLC:s with significant vigor (Peck *et al.*, 1978). These four are Ia and SD differences encoded by the major histocompatibility compolex genes, the M locus, and a fourth "group" of differences here merely called the non-MHC loci. Presence of AFP during cultures *in vitro* can be shown to practically wipe out the proliferation against Ia and/or M locus structures, whereas normal numbers of T blasts will develop when stimulation is carried out against SD or non-MHC loci determinants. However, although normal numbers of T cells respond via cellular division when confronted with SD antigens, in the presence of AFP there will be no generation of cytolytic T cells (Peck *et al.*, 1978). Products of the non-MHC

TABLE I. *Summary of Effects of AFP on Primary or Secondary MLC or CML in Murine Systems*

Antigenic barrier	AFP	Proliferation	Generation of CTL
Ia only	−	++++	+
	+	+ or −	−
SD only	−	++	++
	+	++	−
M locus only	−	+++	−
	+	−	−
Non-MHC only	−	++++	−
	+	++++	−
SD or non-MHC	−	++++	++++
	+	++++	++++

loci, on the other hand, cannot stimulate efficient killer cells against their own specificities but as stated above do stimulate normal T cell proliferation even in the presence of AFP. The results are summarized in Table I.

What can be concluded from these findings? Here, a fetal substance is found with selective ability to interfere with immune cell triggering against histocompatibility antigens. The inhibitory actions may seem appropriate for a substance with hypothetical, beneficial immunosuppressive ability during embryonic life, but surely this does not prove that AFP does function in this manner *in vivo*. However, it is very clear from the present investigations that a "normal" pathway of stimulation by antigen may be significantly changed in direction by external agents. The consequences of this may be selective dramatic changes of the immune response exemplified here by the abolition of proliferation by AFP of the anti-Ia response or the elimination of cytolytic T cell generation against the isolated SD differences. It would seem likely that several agents of this type may be endowed with ability to cause a similar perturbation of an immune reaction. Changes in immune responses under various conditions of disease may thus at least in part be caused by abnormal presence of such modifying substances.

SUPPRESSOR CELLS: A NOTE AS TO THE REQUIREMENT FOR STRINGENT
DEFINITIONS OF SPECIFICITY AND CELL TYPES INVOLVED

Suppressor cells of specific or "nonspecific" nature can
be found within several subgroups of cells. In this regard,
specific suppressor T cells have attracted particular interest
during the last few years. It would now seem clear that such
suppressor lymphocytes, at least in the mouse, can be characterized not only by functional criteria but also via unique
serotypic markers (Gershon, 1976). Complications have already
arisen in this regard, as other subsets of T cells may serve
as amplifiers for the suppressor T cells (i.e., they function
as helper cells for the actual suppressor cells) (Feldmann *et
al.*, 1976). Also, suppressor T cells of a nonspecific nature
have also been reported to exist with an antigenic phenotype
distinct from that of the conventional suppressor T cells
(Watanabe *et al.*, 1977). It should be noted, however, that
the term nonspecific may only conceal our ignorance as to
the actual specificity of the so-called nonspecific suppressor
T cells and it may well be that within such a subset there
exist still additional subgroups with varying selectivity as
to function. Whereas it should be realized that some specific
suppressor T cells have helper T lymphocytes as their major
target (Gershon, 1976) it may be wise to consider how specific suppression may occur via other routes. In this regard
we would like to describe a system that we have analyzed in
some detail (Binz and Wigzell, 1977).
    Here idiotypes and anti-idiotypes can be shown to coexist
in a system measuring antigen-specific reactions against major
histocompatibility antigens are equipped with idiotypic,
antigen-specific receptors on their surface signifying their
specific immune capacity. The host is, however, not tolerant
toward its own idiotypic receptors and can be "cheated" to
make autoanti-idiotypic immune reactions against a particular
group of idiotype-positive molecules. Such reactions can be
shown to lead to the actual elimination of the relevant idiotypic lymphocytes and this may be paralleled by a simultaneous
elimination of the relevant immune capacity (Binz and Wigzell,
1975, 1977). As the present antigens studied are histocompatibility antigens, this elimination may cause selective transplantation tolerance. This approach is obviously of interest
as a possible means of obtaining specific immune tolerance in
adult immunocompetent individuals (Binz and Wigzell, 1975).
In this regard we noted that such spleen cells from autoanti-
idiotype immunized animals were able to transfer the specific
suppression to other, normal syngeneic recipients (Binz and
Wigzell, 1978). Our way of inducing specific suppression of

immune reactivity against a given set of major histocompatibility antigens was to use autologous blasts with specific idiotype-positive receptors as autoimmunogen (Andersson *et al.*, 1976). Such blasts were generated from normal autologous T cells via contact with the allogeneic antigens using mixed leukocyte cultures. The results with such autoblast immunization procedures indicate that it is comparatively easy to induce specific reduction in MLC reactivity against the relevant alloantigens (Andersson *et al.*, 1976). Production of autoanti-idiotypic antibodies in these autoblast-immunized individuals is infrequently detected but can be shown to occur in several of the animals. The specific reduction in immune reactivity can be caused by two major pathways: through autoanti-idiotypic immune reactions or through the induction of antigen-specific suppressor T cells. The latter cells could arise via the transfer of alloantigens derived from the stimulator cells present on the outer surface of responding, idiotype-positive T cells. That such stimulator cell alloantigens indeed can exist on the surface of responding T blasts is well established (Nagy *et al.*, 1976).

We have investigated the cell type responsible for inducing specific unresponsiveness using the transfer system described above (Binz and Wigzell, 1978). Spleen cells from autoblast-immunized animals could transfer the suppression. Purified B cells could also transfer suppression, albeit significantly less efficiently than normal spleen cells. T cells were more efficient than unfractionated spleen cells. When subfractionated according to Ly-antigen phenotypes, Ly 1^+2^- cells were less capable than Ly 1^-2^+ of causing the suppressed response. The results are summarized in Table II. From this we deduce that in this system suppressing ability resides in several subgroups of lymphocytes although with varying efficiency. From our point of view we would deem it likely that these B and T lymphocyte subgroups may all exert their immunosuppressive ability via an autoanti-idiotypic immune reaction. If so, immune B cells could do this via the release of autoanti-idiotypic antibodies, which in concert with complement may lead to irreversible inactivation of the relevant idiotype-positive cells (Binz and Wigzell, 1975, 1977). The Ly 1^+2^- T cells having the phenotype of "classical" helper T cells could exert their immunosuppressive function by acting as true helper T cells for the autoanti-idiotypic B cells, thus facilitating the production of suppressive antibody molecules. The Ly 1^-2^+ cells, finally, may function either directly as killer T cells for the relevant idiotype-positive target cells (Andersson *et al.*, 1976) or as classical T suppressor cells using the pharmacological batteries of reactions ascribed to such cells.

TABLE II.   *Characteristics of Spleen Cells from Autoblast-Immunized, Suppressed Animals*

(a)   *Functional properties: May express specific ability to kill idiotype-positive target cells in vitro; may produce autoanti-idiotypic antibodies; may transfer specific suppression*

(b)   *Groups of cells equipped with suppressor cell ability in ranking order: Ly 1^-2^+ T cells < whole T cells > whole spleen cells < Ly 1^+2^- T cells > B cells*

(c)   *Specificity: Suppressor cells will not bind to alloantigen-positive cells but will react with idiotype-positive, alloantibodies*

The availability of the transfer system coupled with affinity fractionation procedures allowed us to analyze whether the most efficient suppressor cells have specificity for the idiotype receptors or if they were functioning as alloantigen-specific suppressor T cells.

First, attempts were made to remove the suppressor T cells by incubation on fibroblast monolayers *in vitro*, a method known to remove antigen-specific T cells reactive against histocompatibility antigens in other systems. The cells remaining in the supernatant of such monolayer incubated cells were, however, still able to transfer suppression (Binz and Wigzell, 1978). Thus, no evidence was obtained of alloantigen-specific suppressor T cells as measured by this assay. Such negative results could be easily explained on the basis of technical failures or because of faulty expression of relevant, i.e., Ia antigens, on the allogeneic monolayers. Another approach was to see whether the suppressor cells displayed significant binding to idiotype-positive alloantibody molecules. This was done by first producing T cells from spleen cells from suppressed, autoblast-immunized mice by filtration through anti-Ig coated-beat columns. The cells were then incubated with normal serum or relevant alloantiserum. In our experiments the cells were from C57BL/6 mice autoimmunized with anti-CBA/H blasts. We then incubated the C57BL/6 spleen T cells with C57BL/6 normal serum or with C57BL/6-anti-CBA/H antiserum, washed the cells once, and then filtered them through a second anti-Ig bead column (Binz and Wigzell, 1978). Cells retained on the second bead column were recovered by mechanical means using procedures known to allow the recovery of functionally intact T cells (Binz and Wigzell, 1977). The passed or eluted cells were then analyzed for their ability to transfer suppression into normal C57BL/6 mice. The results

were very clear-cut. The passed cells showed no suppressive
ability, while the retained cells were excellent in conveying
suppression upon transfer. Thus, the overwhelming majority
of the suppressor cells in the present system have anti-idiotype specificity rather than specificity for the relevant
alloantigens. From these results we would like to draw certain conclusions. In the system analyzed there was selective
suppression of immune reactivity against a given set of antigens. The suppressive action was directed against the relevant idiotype-positive lymphocytes and could be exerted by
several sets of immune cells. Our data thus show in the
present system that immune B lymphocytes, helper, as well as
suppressor and killer T cells may all express significant suppressing ability. This by no means excludes or argues against
the factual existence of a special kind of T cell with pharma-
cologically unique features of a "suppressor" cell, as this
is well proven (Gershon, 1976). However, the present results
have been mentioned as they may be found in other autoanti-
idiotypic immune systems. They have to be distinguished from
the antigen-specific, "conventional" T suppressor cells.

ANTI-IDIOTYPIC ANTIBODIES: A NOTE ON THEIR POSSIBLE FUNCTIONS
AS INDUCERS OR INHIBITORS OF IMMUNE OR HORMONAL FUNCTIONS

Autoanti-idiotypic immunity may occur as a natural consequence of immunization with antigen. This has been shown
true for several immunogens involving both T and B lymphocytes
(Wigzell, 1978). It is still quite open, however, as to whether the production of autoanti-idiotypic immune reactions
against multivalent antigens have any practical importance in
significantly changing the immune process. It is obvious that
in cases of unusual clonal dominance of the immune response
against a given antigen determinant, the existence of such
autoanti-idiotypic immunity may cause a significant change in
the immune reaction against that antigenic determinant
(Cosenza *et al.*, 1976). The possible consequence of autoanti-
idiotypic immune reactions and their possible role in the immune system have been well discussed in the form of the "network theory" of the immune system (Jerne, 1974).
      Anti-idiotypic antibodies may in the presence of comple-
ment eliminate relevant idiotype-positive T and B lymphocytes,
thus eradicating the corresponding immune potential of the
treated-cell population (Binz and Wigzell, 1975). It is also
true that anti-idiotypic antibodies of different immunoglobulin classes when administered *in vivo* may cause either the
priming of idiotype-positive lymphocytes or elimination of the

very same cells (Eichmann and Rajewsky, 1975). The underlying
reasons for this paradoxical effect depending on immunoglobulin class are unclear. *In vivo* induction conditions do not,
however, lend themselves easily to the ananlysis of the actual
ongoing events.

We have worked with anti-idiotypic immune reactions against
antigen-specific receptors for histocompatibility antigens
(Binz and Wigzell, 1975, 1977). It is here clear that autoanti-
idiotypic antibodies can become induced, as previously stated.
Such anti-idiotypic antibodies will in the presence of complement wipe out T and B cells having specific reactivity toward
the relevant histocompatibility antigens (Binz and Wigzell,
1975). However, when adding such autoanti-idiotypic antisera
to normal spleen cells of the same strain as the antiserum
donors *in vitro* in the absence of complement we did sometimes
observe significant induction of DNA synthesis. It was subsequently found that autoanti-idiotypic antiserum added to
primed T cells specific for the same antigens as the idiotypic,
alloantibody molecules may cause a second set stimulation *in
vitro* as measured by DNA synthesis (Frischknecht *et al.*, 1978).
In a detailed analysis of the undergoing events using relevant
autoanti-idiotypic antibodies added to syngeneic normal or immune T cells *in vitro*, autoanti-idiotypic antibodies could be
shown able to completely replace alloantigen in the specific
proliferative stimulation of the relevant idiotypic, antigen-
specific T cells (Frischknecht *et al.*, 1978). The kinetics
of induction of DNA proliferation by the autoanti-idiotypic
antibodies using normal spleen cells was significantly slower
than when using allogeneic cells as stimulating agent, reaching a DNA peak 1-2 days after the peak caused by allogeneic
stimulation. The specific immune ability of normal T cells
triggered *in vitro* by mere contact with relevant autoanti-
idiotypic antibodies was analyzed in cytolytic assays. Here
it could be shown that autoanti-idiotypic primed T cells could
function as excellent killer cells against syngeneic T blasts
carrying the proper idiotypic receptors. Results are presented in a summary form in Table III.

The above results strengthen our beliefs that immune processes are of extreme complexity. Here, an agent such as an
anti-idiotype antibody could be shown in the presence of adequate amounts of complement to kill the relevant idiotype-
positive lymphocyte (Binz and Wigzell, 1975, 1977). In the
absence of such concentrations of complement the opposite results, namely, priming of the idiotypic cells, may ensue. It
is easily perceived that during immunization, antigen can induce idiotype-positive, antigen-specific lymphocytes, where-
upon anti-idiotype immune reactions may occur. Some of the
latter reactions may lead to elimination of the idiotype-
positive cells, whereas other reactions may cause the opposite,

TABLE III. *Consequences of Allowing Anti-Idiotypic Antibodies to Make Contact with Idiotype-Positive T Cells in vitro. A System Using Anti-Idiotypic Antibodies against Receptors with Specificity for Histocompatibility Antigens*

Cells	Treatment	Consequences
Normal spleen cells	Anti-idiotypic antibodies in presence of complement	Elimination of MLC and CTL activity against the relevant transplantation antigens
	Anti-idiotypic antibodies in absence of complement	Triggering of MLC and CTL activity against the relevant transplantation antigens
Immune T cells	Anti-idiotypic antibodies in presence of complement	Elimination of immune reactivity measured both by functional and direct lytic measurement
	Anti-idiotypic antibodies in absence of complement	Second set triggering of proliferation of idiotype-positive T cells

namely, acceleration of the immune reaction against the inoculated antigen. The mere fact, however, that anti-idiotypic antibodies in the absence of antigen may lead to nearly identical consequences with regard to immunization as introduction of the antigen itself, may have both theoretical as well as practical implications. Immunization without ever having to introduce the actual antigen should thus be possible under certain conditions. This may cause the reader to reconsider which is the "real" immunogen during the immunization: the actual immunogen administered or the idiotypic receptors in combination with antigen serving as a possible autoantigen for anti-idiotype specific helper or suppressor cells.

It is thus possible to consider an anti-idiotypic antibody to be functionally (and maybe also in some steric ways) similar to the actual antigen for which the idiotype-positive

TABLE IV. *Characteristics of Certain Antianti-Insulin*
Antibodies as to Specificity and Function

(a)   *Bind to fat cells with known insulin receptors on the*
      outer surface

(b)   *Compete with radiolabeled insulin for such receptors*

(c)   *Induce uptake of aminobutyric acid in thymocytes in ana-*
      logous manner to insulin

(d)   *Reduce the blood glucose levels in diabetic mice*

antibody has an antigen-combining site. This may lead to interesting possibilities insofar as certain anti-idiotypic antibodies may, besides displaying specific binding to the idiotypic antibody molecules, also express some functional properties of the initial antigen. In an attempt to analyze
such a possible action of anti-idiotypic antibodies, anti-insulin antibodies were induced followed by the production of
anti-idiotypic antibodies against the purified anti-insulin
antibodies (Sege and Peterson, 1978). The assumption was
then made that some anti-anti-insulin antibodies may in part
"look like" insulin as far as the insulin-binding receptors
on the target cells were concerned. Experiments summarized in
Table IV show that this was indeed the case. It was thus
possible using such specific anti-anti-insulin antibodies to
block the binding of radiolabeled insulin to the insulin receptors on fat cells to show direct binding to the insulin receptors of the radiolabeled antianti-insulin antibodies, and
actually in analogous manner to insulin to induce a significant uptake of alpha-aminobutyric acid in young rat thymocytes
in vitro. The most drastic evidence for an insulinlike activity of the anti-anti-insulin antibodies was obtained, however,
using diabetic mice, which when receiving such antibodies would
display a highly significant reduction in their blood glucose
levels.
     Replacement of hormone activity may thus be achieved using
anti-idiotypic antibodies of select quality. It is tempting
to speculate that this may sometimes occur as a secondary consequence to the induction of antihormone antibodies. Whether
such anti-idiotypic antibodies would have an inducing or
blocking function when reacting with the specific hormone receptor would most likely vary between systems. That such antireceptor antibodies can be found in certain clinical situations is known in the system of the long-acting thyroid stimulating factor (Manley *et al.*, 1974; Smith and Hall, 1974)
found in certain hyperthyreotic patients. It would be inter-

esting to know if the antireceptor antibodies were initially
induced directly against the receptor itself or via the induction of autoanti-idiotypic antibodies.

CONCLUSION

Lymphocytes can express their specific immune function via
genetically predetermined receptors. The triggering conditions
for the respective subgroups of lymphocytes are only in part
known as to phenomenology with virtually nothing known as to
the actual molecular events. The actual antigen-binding receptors on lymphocytes may primarily function as concentrating
devices for various triggering substances, with the actual
differentiation pathways in part determined by the cell itself,
in part by the environment and the triggering substance. We
have concentrated here on complicating new findings as to the
induction or inhibition of lymphocyte functions using either
antigen-nonspecific substances like alfa-fetoprotein as a
selective agent in *in vitro* modulation of the responding cell
types; the possible consequences of autoanti-idiotypic immunity have been discussed in relation to inhibition or induction of humoral or endocrine functions. If the reader considers his appreciation of the complexity of the immune response to be enlightened by this contribution, then its aim has
been fulfilled.

Acknowledgments

The present work was supported by the Swedish Cancer Society, the Swedish Medical Research Council, the Swiss National Science Foundation grant 3.688-0.76, NIH grant AI.CA.13485-
01, and the Nordiska Insulinfonden.

References

Alter, B., Schendel, D. J., Bach, M. L., Bach, F. H., Klein,
    J., and Stimpfling, J. (1973). *J. Exp. Med. 137*: 1303.
Andersson, L., Binz, H., and Wigzell, H. (1976). *Nature 264*:
    778.
Bach, F. H., Bach, M. L., Kuperman, O. J., Sollinger, H. W.,
    and Sondel, P. M. (1976). *Cold Spring Harbor Symp. Quant.
    Biol. 41*: 429.
Binz, H., and Wigzell, H. (1975). *J. Exp. Med. 142*: 197.

Binz, H., and Wigzell, H. (1977). *Contemp. Top. Immunobiol.* 7: 113.

Binz, H., and Wigzell, H. (1978). *J. Exp. Med.*, in press.

Cantor, H., and Boyse, E. A. (1975). *J. Exp. Med. 141*: 1390.

Cosenza, H., Augustin, A. A., and Julius, M. H. (1976). *Cold Spring Harbor Symp. Quant. Biol. 41*: 709.

Coutinho, A. (1975). *Transplant. Rev. 23*: 49.

Eichmann, K., and Rajewsky, K. (1975). *Eur. J. Immunol. 5*: 661.

Feldmann, M., Beverly, P., Erb, P., Howie, S., Kontiainen, S., Maoz, A., Methies, M., McKenzie, I., and Woody, J. (1976). *Cold Spring Harbor Symp. Quant. Biol. 41*: 113.

Frischknecht, H., Binz, H., and Wigzell, H. (1978). *J. Exp. Med.*, in press.

Gershon, R. K. (1976). *Transplant. Rev. 26*: 170.

Janeway, C., Wigzell, H., and Binz, H. (1976). *Scand. J. Immunol. 5*: 993.

Jerne, N. K. (1974). *Ann. Immunol. (Inst. Pasteur) 125c*: 373.

Manley, S. W., Bourke, J. R., and Hawker, R. W. (1974). *J. Endocrinol. 61*: 437.

Mozes, E., Isac, R., and Taussig, M. J. (1975). *J. Exp. Med. 141*: 703.

Murgita, R. A., Goidl, E. A., Kontiainen, S., and Wigzell, H. (1977). *Nature 267*: 257.

Murgita, R. A., Goidl, E. A., Kontiainen, S., Beverly, P. C. L., and Wigzell, H. (1978). *Proc. Nat. Acad. Sci.*, submitted.

Nagy, Z., Elliott, B. E., Nabholz, M., Krammer, P. H., and Pernis, B. (1976). *J. Exp. Med. 143*: 648.

Peck, A. B., Murgita, R. A., and Wigzell, H. (1978). *J. Exp. Med.*, in press.

Rosenthal, A., and Shevach, E. (1973). *J. Exp. Med. 138*: 1194.

Sege, K., and Peterson, P. (1978). *Proc. Nat. Acad. Sci.*, in press.

Smith, B. R., and Hall, R. (1974). *Lancet ii*: 427.

Watanabe, N., Kojima, S., Shen, F., and Ovary, Z. (1977). *J. Immunol. 118*: 485.

Wigzell, H. (1978). *In* "Autoimmunity" (N. Talal, ed.). Academic Press, New York, in press.

Zinkernagel, R., and Doherty, P. (1976). *Cold Spring Harbor Symp. Quant. Biol. 41*: 505.

DISCUSSION

DR. BLOOM: Why do only a small fraction of autoanti-insulin antibodies react with insulin receptors?

DR. WIGZELL: Insulin has many antigenic determinants, only a few of which are relevant for binding to the receptors. Thus, only a fraction of the autoidiotypic antibodies would be expected to have "antireceptor" specificity.

DR. WALDMANN: If one were to immunize an animal with a purified hormone receptor (e.g., an insulin receptor), do you feel that this would function as an anti-idiotype molecule to the antigenic determinants of the insulin molecule that normally interacts with the hormone receptor but not the determinant at other regions of the insulin molecule? Would this be an easier way to generate anti-idiotype antibodies to a specific region of the molecule than the procedures Peterson is using?

DR. WIGZELL: I do not think so. Such antireceptor antibodies would to a certain degree be autoanti-idiotypic for anti-insulin antibodies. However, I would assume that the majority would fail to react with such anti-insulin antibodies.

DR. SCHWARTZ: I have a comment. Antibodies against receptors for hormones may block the receptor as well as stimulate it. For example, in the disease partial lipodystrophy, there is extreme insulin resistance and autoantibodies to insulin receptors. Also, in myasthenia gravis, an auto-antibody against the receptor for acetylcholine blocks its function. Moreover, some anti-idiotypic antibodies may trigger B cells, whereas others may block B cell responses. It seems that the effect of antireceptor antibodies may be heterogeneous and perhaps dependent on antibody class or other intrinsic properties of the immunoglobulin molecule.

DR. WIGZELL: I fully agree.

DR. DOHERTY: If anti-idiotype antibodies will bind to hormone receptor, this could have disastrous consequence. Binding of antibody and complement might lead to deletion of the relevant cells.

DR. WIGZELL: It sure would.

DR. VAN ROOD: How reproducible is the production of auto-anti-idiotype antibodies?

DR. WIGZELL: Detectable "useful" titers of autoanti-idiotype antibodies in the transplantation antigen system are rare. I believe this is in part due to the need of multiple auto-idiotypic specificities in the serum to allow a significant deleting or reacting power.

DR. SELL: I would like to comment on our experience with chimps. It was interesting that it took as many as five or

six immunizations before the antibody appeared and before
there was decreased MLC or PLT reactivity. In fact, during
the early phases of immunization, there was increasing reactivity. If we continued to immunize, during the first two
or three shots we got better and better Plts from the chimp
along the way and then, after the antibody appeared, inhibition of the MLC. The chimp cells' reactivity dropped very
sharply but not to levels that were any lower than the original reactivity in the chimps that gave the original MLC.
So that in our hands, if you keep immunizing you eventually
get to the point where autoantibodies appear. They appear to
be quite specific; we now have two chimps to that stage and
we have another group being immunized that are about at their
third or fourth immunization dose. It is clear that, if you
persist, antibody may appear more regularly, like Dr. Wigzell
described. In other words, if you have a limited immunization
schedule, you might not get to the point where the autoantibodies actually appear. I have no evidence regarding persistence.

DR. WIGZELL: There's another problem in the autoblast
immunization procedure and that's what I was alluding to as
to the problem of stimulator alloantigens being transferred.
In the experiments that Dr. Sell was mentioning, they transferred enormous amount of blasts, the purity of which is significantly less than ours, something like 65%. We normally
have a much higher cut-off level. But the antisera that are
made in the chimps do behave exactly similarly like our auto-
anti-idiotypes in the mouse relative to stimulation of the T
cells *in vitro*.

DR. AMOS: I have a comment and a related question. One
of our experimental subjects, RC, produced two antibodies to
HLA, one against Aw29, one against Bw16. After a time his
titer fell off and we decided to reimmunize to produce only
anti-Aw29. To do this we took RC serum, absorbed out the
Aw29 activity, and coated lymphocytes from the immunizing
donor (ToH) with the anti-Bw16 antibody. These were injected
into RC. He failed to make an appreciable response to either
Aw29 or Bw16. We rested him for 2 months and restimulated
with untreated ToH cells. Again RC did not produce detectable
antibody. Restimulated after 9 months he responded briefly.
Do you have any knowledge of comparable animal experiments
and of what the mechanism of turnoff is? Do you think it is
possible to inhibit a preformed immunity by antibody-antigen
complexes?

DR. WIGZELL: At least in part, yes. We tried to wipe out
existing immunity using autoanti-idiotype therapy. Here, inbred mice immune across an H-2 barrier were treated with autologous anti-H-2 blasts of the same specificity. A reduction

in a specific manner amounting to approximately 75% was thus achieved. It is possible that we could have reached complete elimination of immunity if further treatments had been carried out.

DR. DIENER: In the case when you were talking about alpha-fetoprotein, which suppresses Ly 1 suppressors...

DR. WIGZELL: No, it doesn't suppress, it induces them.

DR. DIENER: It induces Ly 1 suppressors?

DR. WIGZELL: I want to make this clear. Murgita has found that alpha-fetoprotein, in the presence of adult mouse spleen cells for about 4 days, would lead to the appearance of very efficient suppressor T cells. One thousand such cells per 10^6 normal spleen cells would lead to significant suppression of T-dependent antibody responses *in vitro* without touching T-independent antibody formation.

DR. DIENER: This is Ly 1?

DR. WIGZELL: Yes. They're Ly 1^+, 2^-. Normal mouse serum under these conditions does not generate efficient suppressor cells. The newborn suppressor T cells that you find in the mouse in our hands are also Ly 1^+, 2^-, contradicting what Moshier had published. We have found this in the CBA series of mice, which have, of course, a different kind of series of Ly like the C57 blacks, and we find it in both.

DR. DIENER: You're sure they've never helped? I mean you don't think that you could actually observe too much help, which is known to suppress?

DR. WIGZELL: Well, when doing a dilution curve, you will find that this is not the case.

DR. KANTOR: Do nude mice make autoanti-idiotypic antibodies? In other words, are they thymus dependent?

DR. WIGZELL: I really do not know. I believe nude mice should be able to make autoanti-idiotypic antibodies in systems using thymus-independent antigens.

DR. DIENER: How do complement-deficient mice behave? Have you tried them?

DR. WIGZELL: I don't know.

DR. DIENER: With reference to your data, which indicate that anti-idiotype antibody may in some cases initiate C'= dependent killing, did you test what this antibody does in C'-deficient mice?

DR. WIGZELL: No.

DR. DOHERTY: Immunization with some killed viral antigens results in rather long-term production of antibody. Can we visualize this as operating through a dynamic, self-perpetuating idiotype-anti-idiotype network?

DR. WIGZELL: I believe this to be unlikely. I would rather favor persistence of antigen or the stimulation of immune cells by cross-reacting viral antigens.

DR. DOHERTY: Can interaction depend in a directly quantitative sense on cell numbers? For instance, a cell-to-cell interaction mechanism might be expected to operate much less effectively *in vivo*, when the number of cells available falls off.

DR. WIGZELL: I think it's probably a qualitative matter; from a single cell standpoint, it really doesn't matter if it meets one cell every hour or one cell every week.

DR. DIENER: Can you tell us something about the physiologic meaning of your observations? Would you comment on the vicious circle of anti-idiotypic antibody in physiological terms.

DR. WIGZELL: If you ask whether anti-idiotypic immunity plays a biologically relevant role in regulating the immune response, there are several immune systems where individual animals have been followed for prolonged periods of time and clonal analysis of the immunoglobulin product has been done for the same period. The rabbit, for example, immunized for a period of 1 to 2 years, might express, when boosted, the very same clonotypes as it did quite early during immunization. This kind of information leads me to believe that autoantiidiotype regulatory forces are by no means a general factor of relevance. However, if you ask if anti-idiotype antibodies function in either a positive or negative way in any kind of system, it would be interesting to examine the clonal dominance systems such as those of Dr. Eichmann and Dr. Cantor. It is now clear, for example, from Dr. Eichmann's studies, that anti-idiotypes can prime helper T cells, which predominantly have activity for B cells of the same idiotype. In other words, helper T cells and B cells do not have the same idiotypes; one is the anti-idiotype of the other. Also, if you look at the anti-alpha-1,3-dextran response or the antiphosphorylcholine response, you frequently see antibody of one idiotype appearing after antigen injection, then autoantiidiotype antibody appears, after which both disappear. If you give antigen again, the same pattern appears without any obvious limiting capacity. To summarize, under normal conditions, the regulatory function of anti-idiotype antibody is probably not of major consequence; however, in selected systems, it could be important.

DR. DIENER: In cell-mediated allotype suppression, there appears to be a specific set of suppressor T cells that recognize a specific allotype marker. Since there are markers on idiotypes, is it now necessary to envisage subclasses of anti-idiotype active cells in a similar manner? Is there any evidence for this?

DR. WIGZELL: You're really asking about the specificity of B cells; there's really no answer to your question now.

I'm reminded of experiments by Dr. Cebra, who was able to completely pervert the immunoglobulin class by varying the form and timing of antigen administration. It's obvious that, in his system, this effect results from T cells regulating expression of antibody by B cells.

DR. DIENER: Rather than think of suppressor cells in terms of suppressors of a given immune response, we must consider the concept stated by Bretscher in which these cells are regarded as the mediators of immune class regulation. Thus, suppressor cells may suppress, for example, a humoral response and allow a cell-mediated response to take place.

DR. BRITTON: Did you say that the helper cell idiotypes may not have "antigen" specificity, but rather anti-B idiotype specificity?

DR. WIGZELL: With regard to dominant B cell idiotype expression, the data from Dr. Eichmann and from Dr. Cantor would support such a concept. I do not believe, however, that this is the dominant way of expressing T cell helper specificity. They are rather antigen specific.

REGULATORY ROLES OF ANTIBODY*

Gregory W. Siskind

Division of Allergy and Immunology
Department of Medicine
Cornell University Medical College
New York

I would like to deal primarily with the regulation of antibody synthesis and especially with possible regulatory roles
that antibody may play in controlling the immune response.

The immunologic system has been classically viewed as
operating in accordance with a clonal selection theory such
as originally proposed by Burnet (1). The fundamental postulates of such theories are: (a) that individual lymphoid cells
(both antigen-binding cells and antibody-secreting cells) are
restricted in regard to their capacity to produce different
antibodies; (b) that individual precursors of antibody-secreting cells have on their surface antigen receptors with binding
properties identical to those of the antibody produced by the
antibody-secreting cells derived from them; (c) that the interaction of antigen with antigen receptors on the surface of
precursors of antibody-secreting cells is of critical importance in imparting specificity to the immune response.

It should be emphasized that the clonal selection theory
deals with the selection of antibody secreting cells from a
preexisting array of antigen-binding cells. It does not deal
with questions relating to the mechanism of generation of diversity or the mechanism of the restriction of information expressed by individual cells. Furthermore, the theory does not
deal with additional signals, or cell cooperation events, which
may be important in lymphocyte triggering. It deals only with
the putative process involved in the selection of specific

*Supported in part by research grants from the National In-
stitutes of Health, USPHS Numbers AI 11694, CA 20075, and AG
00541.*

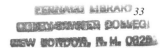

cells and thereby the introduction of specificity into the response. Finally, it should be emphasized that according to such a theory the entire repertoire of potential antibody producing cells is present prior to antigen exposure and that antigen merely serves to select, from the preexisting array, those cells which, by chance, have antigen receptors complementary to epitopes (antigenic determinants) on the antigen molecule.

A variety of evidence has been consistent with the basic tenets of a clonal selection theory. The most direct support has been derived from studies that have specifically deleted antigen-binding cells, by procedures that depend upon their ability to bind antigen, and thereby specifically eliminated the capacity of the population of lymphoid cells to produce the corresponding antibody. A variety of procedures have been employed in such specific deletion experiments, in particular: (a) adsorption of cells onto antigen-coated immunoadsorbant columns; (b) "suicide" of those cells which bind a highly radioactive or toxic antigen; (c) elimination of antigen-binding cells by use of the fluorescence-activated cell sorter. In each case the capacity to produce the corresponding antibody is specifically deleted (2-4). Recently, similar results have been obtained through the use of anti-idiotype antibodies.* Thus, the injection of anti-idiotype antibodies, of appropriate class, can lead to a deletion of the capacity of the animal to produce the particular idiotype following immunization with an antigen to which the idiotype is complementary (5-7). It has also been shown that anti-idiotype antibodies, of certain classes, can specifically activate B and T lymphocytes bearing that idiotype in a manner that appears to be comparable to that by which antigen, interacting with cell surface antigen receptors, activates the cell (8). All of these studies strongly support the hypotheses: (a) that the precursors of antibody-secreting cells are antigen-binding cells having antigen receptors identical in binding properties to that of the antibody produced by antibody-secreting cells derived from them following appropriate triggering; (b) that the antigen-binding precursors of antibody-secreting cells are restricted with respect to the number of different antibodies they can produce.

*The term idiotype refers to antigenic determinants in the variable region of an antibody molecule, that is, the variable region (antigen binding site) of the antibody molecule viewed as an antigenic determinant. Anti-idiotype antibody would be an antibody specific for such determinants in the variable region of an antibody molecule.

It can be predicted, from the basic clonal selection theory, that the antibody produced by an individual animal will be heterogeneous for any given antigenic determinant. Since antigen-binding cells are present prior to antigen exposure there is every reason to believe that there should be a number of different antibody molecules (that is, differing in the amino acid sequence of their hypervariable regions) that will bind to any given epitope. For example, on the basis of cloning experiments Williamson and Askonas (9) concluded that there were approximately 7000 different antibody species (clones) that could respond to the 2,4-dinitrophenyl haptenic determinant. These antibodies will, of course, differ in regard to the strength of the bond they form with the antigenic determinant or epitope. Thus, some antibodies interact with the corresponding epitope to form a highly stable bond that has relatively little tendency to dissociate (high affinity). Other antibody molecules interact with the epitope to form a weak bond (low affinity) that readily dissociates. One would expect that the antibodies produced in response to any given epitope represent a highly heterogeneous population with respect to their affinity for the epitope. It has been established that most antigens do indeed elicit a heterogeneous response to each of the individual epitopes that they bear and to which the animal is stimulated to produce antibody (10-11).

Consideration of the heterogeneity of the immune response led to a modification of the clonal selection theory to include the existence of an affinity-dependent selection process (10). That is, it was suggested that precursors of high-affinity antibody-secreting cells have high-affinity antigen receptors and therefore preferentially capture antigen and preferentially proliferate. It is expected that at the time of initial antigen exposure most of the antigen-binding cells would have receptors of low affinity for the antigenic determinant in question. With time after immunization, antigen dependent, preferential proliferation of high-affinity antigen-binding cells will occur. In this manner, a type of microevolutionary process will take place in which there is a gradual shift of the population of antigen-binding cells. Cells bearing high-affinity receptors gradually come to predominate in the population. In agreement with this hypothesis it has been shown that there is a progressive increase in antibody affinity with time after immunization and that the rate of increase in affinity is inversely related to antigen dose (10-12). Furthermore, it has been shown that B-cell tolerance induction preferentially effects high-affinity antibody production (13).

It should be noted that very late after immunization there is a preferential loss of high-affinity antibody-secreting cells; there is a decrease in the average affinity of serum antibody; and there is a shift toward a broadly heterogeneous population of serum antibody molecules and plaque-forming cells (PFC) ranging from very low to very high in affinity. The explanation for this late decrease in high affinity PFC and serum antibodies is not known. It does not appear to be predictable from the simple clonal selection theory described above. It should be emphasized that high-affinity memory cells persist, since boosting promptly (5 days) elicits very high-affinity PFC and serum antibodies (14). If it is assumed that the cessation of high-affinity antibody production is a consequence of "running out" of antigen, then one would have to ask why low-affinity antibody production continues. One possible explanation is that the production of low-affinity antibody is stimulated by cross-reacting environmental antigens. However, evidence in support of this hypothesis is not available.

    In the context of a clonal selection theory, such as described above, at least one possible regulatory role for serum antibody is predictable. It is expected that serum antibody will bind antigen, will thereby reduce the effective free-antigen concentration, and will thus decrease the stimulation of specific B and T lymphocytes. That is, serum antibody can be viewed as competing with specific lymphocytes for available antigen. This effective reduction in antigen concentration will result in a more efficient selection for high-affinity antibody synthesis. One would expect that the injection of specific antibody at the time of immunization will cause a specific reduction in the magnitude of the immune response and an increased rate of increase in antibody affinity. This prediction has been confirmed in several system (12, 15). One would therefore expect that the serum antibody produced during the immune response will operate to limit the magnitude of the immune response and to facilitate the selection for high-affinity antibody-secreting cells. In addition, it has been shown that antigen-antibody complexes (in appropriate ratios) can induce specific immunologic tolerance *in vitro* (16). Whether this effect can also operate *in vivo* is not known. It is also possible that antigen-antibody complexes can stimulate specific suppressor T-lymphocyte activity and in this manner indirectly contribute to the regulation of the immune response.

    A number of additional factors have been identified that probably influence the basic process of cell selection by antigen, which was summarized above.

    (A) If one views the immune response as a microevolutionary system in which positive selection by antigen operates as the principal driving force, then it is apparent that the extent of proliferation is critical in determining the efficiency of selection for high-affinity antibody synthesis. Since the entire catalog of antigen-binding cells is present prior to antigen exposure it is to be expected that initially most of the cells specific for a given epitope would be of low or intermediate affinity, while precursors of high-affinity antibody-secreting cells would be rare. It is only as a consequence of selective proliferation that the initially rare high-affinity antigen-binding cells come to predominate in the population of specific cells.

In this regard it should be mentioned that if high-affinity cells are rare and low-affinity cells are relatively common, then one should expect, on a chance basis, that the initial antibody produced would be of low affinity. Furthermore, if limiting amounts of antigen are administered so that only a few cells are stimulated one should expect them to be of low affinity. Results consistent with these predictions have been obtained (12).

(B) The epitope density on the antigen should influence cell selection. In addition to the possible role of cross-linking receptors in providing activation or deactivation signals, a high epitope density favors multiple bond formation between an individual antigen molecule and antigen receptors on the surface of an individual B lymphocyte. This would stabilize binding and result in a marked increase in effective affinity. High epitope density would thus be expected to permit the triggering of cells having receptors of lower intrinsic affinity for the antigenic determinant than could be triggered by an antigen of low epitope density.

(C) In a similar manner, increasing the antigen receptor density on the cell surface will favor multiple-bond formation to polyvalent antigens and will probably thereby favor triggering. Some evidence has been offered to suggest that the receptor density on B memory cells is greater than on naive B cells (17).

(D) Specific (and perhaps in some cases nonspecific) suppressor and helper T cell activity can clearly influence B cell selection. It has been reported that in the absence of helper T cells efficient selection for high-affinity antibody synthesis does not take place (18). To what extent this is secondary to reduced cell proliferation and to what extent this may be due to more specific selective effects of helper T cells is not known. Specific suppressor cell activity has been shown to preferentially effect high-affinity antibody synthesis in several systems (19-24). This is possibly the result of a preferential localization of antigen-bound specific suppressor substance to high-affinity B cells as a consequence of

their preferential capture of antigen. Reduced proliferation
during the response, as a consequence of suppressor activity,
would, of course, also tend to reduce the efficiency of selection for high-affinity antibody production.

(E) Recently a variety of studies have defined a phenomenon referred to as clonal dominance. In certain experimental
systems, where immune responses of restricted heterogeneity
are elicited, it appears that one or a small number of dominant clones produce all or most of the antibody. As long as
these clones function, other potential antibody-secreting
clones are not expressed and, in fact, appear to be actively
suppressed (25, 26). The mechanism of clonal dominance is
not known. While clonal dominance has thus far been identified in responses of restricted heterogeneity, it seems likely that a similar process operates in the usual heterogeneous
immune response. It appears that only a small fraction of
the total clones capable of producing antibody complementary
to a given epitope normally respond. What factors (other
than chance) determine and maintin this restriction of the
antibody response is not known. It appears that as long as
these initially stimulated dominant clones produce antibody
other clones will not be triggered. It may well be that the
microevolutionary process, by which high-affinity antibody-
producing clones come to predominate in the responding population, operates only upon the subset of dominant clones
that was initially triggered.

(F) Recent studies have emphasized a possible role for
autoanti-idiotype antibodies (and T cells) in the regulation
of the immune response (27). It is clear that anti-idiotype
antibody and idiotype-specific T cells can specifically depress the synthesis of the corresponding idiotype. The concept has developed that the immune system behaves like a network (28) of interacting elements that normally exist in an
equilibrium condition. Antigen entering the system stimulates
a set of idiotypes to proliferate. This perturbs the system
from equilibrium. The expanded idiotypes act as "foreign"
epitopes and stimulate an anti-idiotype response and a new
equilibrium state is achieved. In this context the immune response can be viewed as the perturbation of the system from a
preexisting equilibrium state by antigen and the subsequent
alterations in the network, which are required to reestablish
equilibrium. On the cellular level an immune response would
result in a change in the distribution of specificities among
the array of T and B lymphocytes.

Thus, it would appear that an affinity-dependent clonal
selection process, which operates in a microevolutionary manner, is probably primarily responsible for controlling the
immune response. A number of additional factors have been

discussed above, which are undoubtedly involved in regulation
of immune reactivity, although the relative importance of
these factors cannot be fully evaluated on the basis of available information. The view of the immune system as a network
of interacting cells emphasizes the highly regulated quality
of the immune response and probably provides a more sophisticated framework for speculation about control of immune reactivity.

In a general overview of regulatory roles of antibody in
the immune response, it is probably useful to briefly consider one additional characteristic of antibody. From the
discussion above it is clear that the antibody response to
any given epitope is, in general, highly redundant. That is,
an extensive array of different antibody species are produced
that are complementary to the epitope. Theoretically, the
existence of this redundancy is a logical consequence of the
clonal selection theory, which posits that the information required to produce all antibody species is present prior to
antigen exposure (that is, the generation of diversity is regarded as operating independently of antigen). In addition
to this redundancy in the immune system, it should be emphasized that individual antibody species are, in all probability,
degenerate with regard to their ability to interact with different epitopes. That is, it can logically be proposed that
individual antibody molecules can bind to a number of different chemically related and chemically unrelated epitopes.
It has been formally established by Richards and co-workers
(29,30) that an individual antibody species can bind two
different epitopes. The two epitopes were shown to be bound
at different positions within the antigen-combining region of
the antibody molecule. Extending these findings, one might
suggest that an individual antibody molecule can bind a large
number of different epitopes to different subsites within the
overall antigen-binding region. The extent of this degener-
acy is, of course, unknown but might be considerable. Thus,
with regard to serum antibody, the immune system is both redundant and degenerate.

Since individual antibody molecules are at least somewhat
degenerate and might be highly degenerate with respect to
the number of different epitopes that they bind, the question
may be raised as to why antisera generally exhibit a marked
degree of specificity in their interactions. In this regard
it is reasonable to assume that the epitopes that different
antibody molecules can bind are randomly assorted. If one
considers the set of antibody molecules that bind epitope A
then the individual molecules will bind different sets of
antigenic determinants. That is, the capacity to bind epitope A will be associated with the ability to bind a different

group of epitopes in different antibody molecules. Thus, the
ability to bind any given second determinant will be a property of only a small subset of the set of molecules that bind
epitope A. In this manner, individual antibody molecules may
be highly degenerate, while the heterogeneous population of
antibody molecules normally produced in response to any given
epitope will behave in a highly specific manner.

In conclusion, it appears that individual antigen-binding
cells are restricted with respect to the number of different
types of antigen-binding sites present on their surface.
Antibody-secreting cells are derived from antigen-binding
cells following interaction with antigen (and possibly other
signals). Antibody-secreting cells produce a homogeneous
antibody that has binding properties identical to those of the
antigen receptors on the surface of the antigen-binding cells
from which they were derived. Affinity-dependent cell selection by antigen operates, in a microevolutionary manner, to
bring about the production of high-affinity antibodies. Antibody acts, by binding antigen and thereby blocking further
activation of immunocompetent cells, to regulate the immune
response. The increased concentration of a set of idiotypes
stimulates an autoanti-idiotype response that may have an important regulatory role. Activity of helper and suppressor
T lymphocytes is probably also involved in the normal control
of the immune response. This complex array of cells very
likely exists in a type of network at equilibrium. Introduction of antigen stimulates proliferation of a set of cells
within this network, perturbing the preexisting equilibrium
state. Stimulation of idiotype-specific cells (and probably
other factors) leads to a reestablishment of equilibrium with
a new distribution of specificities in the population of immunocompetent lymphocytes. The immune response in this sense can
be viewed as an antigen-induced, affinity-controlled perturbation of the lymphoid system followed by "compensatory" changes
resulting in the reestablishment of equilibrium. The antibody
produced by individual cells and individual clones is homogeneous. In most immune responses a large number of different
clones is activated and the antibody produced is consequently
heterogeneous. Thus, the antibody response to a given epitope
is generally highly redundant and consists of a large number
of different antibody species, which can be shown to differ
in their affinity for the epitope. In addition, individual
antibody molecules are probably degenerate in that they can
bind a number of different epitopes. The typical, marked
specificity of serological reactions probably is, in part, due
to a random assortment of the capacity to bind different epitopes in the set of antibody species (clonotypes) produced.

References

1. Burnet, Sir M. "The Clonal Selection Theory of Acquired Immunity," The Abraham Flexner Lectures. Vanderbilt University Press, Nashville, 1959.
2. Wigzell, H., and Andersson, B. *J. Exp. Med.* *129*, 23, 1969.
3. Ada, G. L., and Byrt, P. *Nature (London) 222*, 1291, 1969.
4. Julius, M. H., Masuda, T., and Herzenberg, L. A. *Proc. Nat. Acad. Sci. 69*, 1934, 1972.
5. Cosenza, H., and Köhler, H. *Proc. Nat. Acad. Sci. 69*, 2701, 1972.
6. Eichmann, K. *Eur. J. Immunol. 4*, 296, 1974.
7. Hart, D. A., Wang, A.-L., Pawlak, L. L., and Nisonoff, A. *J. Exp. Med. 135*, 1293, 1976.
8. Eichmann, K., and Rajewsky, K. *Eur. J. Immunol. 5*, 661, 1975.
9. Williamson, A. R., and Askonas, B. A. *Nature 238*, 337, 1972.
10. Siskind, G. W., and Benacerraf, B. *Adv. Immunol. 10*, 1, 1969.
11. Eisen, H. N., and Siskind, G. W. *Biochemistry 3*, 996, 1964.
12. Siskind, G. W., Dunn, P., and Walker, J. G. *J. Exp. Med. 127*, 55, 1968.
13. Theis, G. A., and Siskind, G. W. *J. Immunol. 100*, 138, 1968.
14. Goidl, E. A., Barondess, J. J., and Siskind, G. W. *Immunology 29*, 629, 1968.
15. Heller, K. S., and Siskind, G. W. *Cell. Immunol. 6*, 59, 1973.
16. Diener, E., and Feldmann, M. *Transplant. Rev. 8*, 76, 1972.
17. Klinman, N. R. *J. Exp. Med. 136*, 241, 1972.
18. Gershon, R. K., and Paul, W. E. *J. Immunol. 106*, 872, 1971.
19. Tada, T., and Takemori, T. *J. Exp. Med. 140*, 239, 1974.
20. Takemori, T., and Tada, T. *J. Exp. Med. 140*, 253, 1974.
21. Taniguchi, M., and Tada, T. *J. Exp. Med. 139*, 108, 1974.
22. Bell, E. B., and Shand, F. L. *Eur. J. Immunol. 5*, 481, 1975.
23. Bell, E. B., and Shand, F. L. *Eur. J. Immunol. 5*, 1, 1975.
24. Warren, R. W., Murphy, S., and Davie, J. M. *J. Immunol. 116*, 1385, 1976.
25. Willcox, H. N. A., and McMichael, A. J. *Eur. J. Immunol. 5*, 131, 1975.
26. McMichael, A. J., and Willcox, H. N. A. *Eur. J. Immunol. 5*, 58, 1975.
27. Binz, H., and Wigzell, H. *Contempt. Top. Immunobiol. 7*, 113, 1976.

28. Jerne, N. K.   *Ann. Immunol. (Inst. Pasteur) 125c*, 373,
    1974.
29. Rosenstein, R. W., Masson, R. A., Armstrong, M. Y. K.,
    Konigsberg, W. H., and Richards, F. F.   *Proc. Nat. Acad.
    Sci. 69*, 877, 1972.
30. Varga, J. M., Koningsberg, W. H., and Richards, F. F.
    Proc. Nat. Acad. Sci. 70, 3269, 1973.

DISCUSSION

DR. DIENER: Early work by Nossal indicated that IgG antibody could "switch off" the production of IgM (*Cold Spring Harbor Symp. 1*). Could you briefly comment on this aspect in view of current knowledge?

DR. SISKING: It is probably still true as a first approximation. However, I suspect that additional factors are probably involved in controlling the persistence and turn-off of IgM antibody synthesis.

DR. THEIS: What is the nature of the heterogenous antibody response late after immunization? Do IgM-producing cells reappear, or are there only IgG-producing cells?

DR. SISKIND: There are predominantly IgG-producing cells. They are highly heterogeneous with both low- and high-affinity antibodies. In fact, the low-affinity antibodies are never "turned off," but continue to be produced even in the presence of high-affinity antibody production. Initially there is a heterogenous response of mainly low affinity. With time (3 months in the rabbit; 3 weeks in the mouse) there is a shift to give a predominant population of high- and a tail of low-affinity antibodies (skewed distribution). Late in the response (1 year in the rabbit; 1 month in the mouse) there is a preferential loss of high-affinity antibody production and a broadly heterogenous population is present. What maintains the production of low-affinity antibodies is not known. One possibility is that they are stimulated by cross-reacting environmental antigens.

DR. STANLEY COHEN: Why doesn't anti-idiotype antibody induce anti-idiotype antibody to itself, and so on ad infinitum until the entire immunologic environment is preempted by the animal's first immune response to its first contact with antigen? What stops or controls the process.

DR. SISKIND: Obviously, these are processes we do not really understand. You should probably direct this question to Dr. Wigzell. One possibility is that the antibody and the anti-idiotype antibody form a murually complementary pair in which each is capable of stimulating and inhibiting the other. Thus the system does not proceed "to infinity" but rather forms a series of pairings. Obviously, reality is more complex than this since there are undoubtedly a number of anti-idiotype antibodies to any idiotype and so heterogeneity probably exists on both sides of the equation. Additional factors are probably also involved.

DR. MUSHER: I have two questions. Are low-affinity antibodies effective in protecting the host against microorganisms?

Do high-affinity antibodies put themselves out of business leaving persisting low-affinity antibodies?

DR. SISKIND: Little is known about the effectiveness of low-affinity antibodies in protective immunity.   More low-than high-affinity antibody is required to elicit PCA reactions or Arthus reactions.   One would expect that, in functions requiring the binding of antigen, high-affinity antibody would be more effective than low-affinity antibody.   The mechanism of the decrease in high-affinity antibodies late after immunization is not known.   It is certainly not an absorption of high-affinity serum antibody since high-affinity antibody-secreting cells (PFC) are also decreased late after immunization.   It should be noted that high-affinity memory cells persist, since boosting promptly (5 days) elicits high-affinity antibody-secreting cells.   Possibly the decrease in high-affinity antibody-secreting cells is merely the consequence of "running out" of antigen.   If this is true, then the key question is why low-affinity antibody synthesis persists. This might be due to stimulation by cross-reacting environmental antigens.   It is also possible that autoanti-idiotype antibodies are responsible for the late decrease in high-affinity PFC.

REGULATION OF LYMPHOKINE PRODUCTION AND ACTIVITY*

Stanley Cohen

Department of Pathology
University of Connecticut Health Center
Farmington, Connecticut

INTRODUCTION

It is now generally accepted that the majority of the reactions that comprise "cell-mediated" immunity are dependent
upon the production of non-antibody-soluble mediators by
lymphocytes called lymphokines. For the most part, the lymphokines have been defined in terms of *in vitro* activity, although much evidence is now available documenting their *in
vivo* role (1). In general, they fall into three main categories: lymphokines that damage their target cells (lympho-
toxins), lymphokines that cause cell proliferation (mitogenic
factors), and lymphokines that modulate inflammatory and possibly reparative responses. Under usual circumstances, the
cellular source of lymphokines is the T lymphocyte; in certain
cases, however, B lymphocytes and even nonlymphoid cells can
produce similar mediators (2). The latter category of mediators have been defined as "cytokines." There is good evidence
for the identity or close similarity of one cytokine with conventional lymphocyte-derived MIF (3). This suggests that the
lymphokines may represent a subset of the cytokines.

Given the wide range of lymphokine activities, the multiple possible sources of lymphokines, and the great variety
of biologic reactions in which they have been implicated, it
is clear that they are ubiquitous agents. Moreover, the conditions for their production often involve positive feedback
loops. For example, mitogenic agents can stimulate nonsensi-

*The work described here was supported by Grants AI-12477,
AI-12225, and CA-19286 from the National Institutes of Health.*

45

tized lymphocytes to produce lymphokines. Following antigenic
stimulation, one of the lymphokines made is a mitogenic factor.
Presumably, this can trigger other, uncommited cells to make
lymphokines, including mitogenic factor, which can trigger
other cells, and so forth. Obviously, there must be control
mechanisms that limit and regulate this process so that it
proceeds in an orderly manner, and terminates itself at the
appropriate time and place. Unfortunately, virtually nothing
is known about these regulatory events.

Many experimental models exist that deal with situations
in which either the production of lymphokines or the expression
of their activity is suppressed. Many of these, such as those
involving exogenous pharmacologic agents, have no obvious
relationship to possible normal internal homeostatic mechanisms. However, a few situations involve suppressive effects
that could be operative in the unmanipulated animal. These
involve (1) desensitization, especially as it involves the
activity of lymphokines present systemically, and in large
amounts; (2) inhibition of B cell-derived MIF by a T cell product, which may serve as a model for similar effects on T cell
production of lymphokines; (3) monosaccharide inhibition of
lymphokine activity; and (4) inhibition of *in vivo* lymphokine
activity by antilymphokines, a mechanism that could be operative in certain immunopathologic states.

In this presentation, I shall focus in detail on these
experimental models, and discuss their possible relevance to
an understanding of how lymphokine-dependent regulatory mechanisms might operate in the intact animal.

DESENSITIZATION IN RELATION TO MEDIATOR PRODUCTION

Various manifestations of delayed hypersensitivity in
guinea pigs injected previously with antigen in complete
Freund's adjuvant (CFA)* can be suppressed by the systemic
injection of the same antigen. This effect is best seen when
the antigen is presented intravenously or intramuscularly, in
large doses and without adjuvant. The process leading to the
loss of reactivity is known as desensitization.

Uhr and Pappenheimer (4) presented evidence that suggested
that desensitization was an antigen-specific phenomenon although they reported that early stages of desensitization included a transient anergic state that is nonspecific. Re-

*CFA includes a form of mycobacterium, which is often M.
butyricum, but was originally dead M. tuberculosis, together
with lipids.

cently, however, it was shown by Asherson and Stone (5) that
desensitization of doubly immunized animals could be accom-
plished by unrelated antigens. For example, when animals are
immunized with bovine γ-globulin (BGG) in CFA, they show positive delayed skin reactions to purified protein derivative
(PPD) as well as to BGG. This proved to be a useful model
for study. Injection of 20 to 30 mg of BGG into such animals
reduced the skin reactivity to both PPD and BGG. Similar observations have been reported in *in vitro* systems. Lipsmeyer
and Kantor (6), using animals sensitized with multiple antigens, showed that lymphocytes from these animals exposed to
one of the immunizing antigens had decreased ability to produce migration inhibitory factor (MIF) when subsequently stimulated by the other antigen .

In contrast to these observations, passive transfer of
desensitization appears to be antigen specific. Lymphocytes,
from donors immunized with BGG in CFA and desensitized with
BGG, were shown to have a normal ability to transfer skin reactivity to PPD, whereas they lacked the ability to transfer
skin reactivity to BGG (5).

These observations are difficult to reconcile with a single
mechanism for the desensitization of delayed hypersensitivity.
It is more likely that the effects of desensitization may be
expressed differently in various experimental systems. We investigated the phenomenon using the macrophage disappearance
reaction (7,8) as well as cutaneous delayed hypersensitivity
as the test responses. Guinea pigs exhibiting delayed hypersensitivity were desensitized by a single large dose of antigen
administered intramuscularly. In our studies, we found that
desensitization with a soluble protein such as egg albumin
(EA) or bovine γ-globulin (BGG) was nonspecific in that they
suppressed both cutaneous reactivity and the macrophage disappearance reaction (MDR) to unrelated antigen in doubly
immunized animals. The MDR, in brief, is a manifestation of
cell-mediated immunity in which intraperitoneal antigen causes
a reduction in macrophage content of a peritoneal exudate induced in delayed hypersensitive animals. In contrast, mycobac-
terial antigen, at the dose studied, showed limited specificity
in that it could suppress the MDR but not a skin test to an unrelated antigen (9).

Induction of an MDR was shown to be associated with the
appearance of macrophage migration inhibitory factor (MIF) and
macrophage chemotactic factor (MCF) activity in the peritoneal
exudate fluid. Pretreatment with desensitizing doses of mycobacteria prevented the EA-induced appearance of MIF in the
peritoneal fluids. In contrast, chemotactic activity could
still be recovered, even though the MDR was suppressed. Mycobacteria functioned as a specific desensitizer not only with

respect to cutaneous reactivity, as stated above, but also
with respect to the production of chemotactic factor by peritoneal exudate cells. In contrast, mycobacteria functioned as
a nonspecific desensitizer with respect to both the MDR and
MIF production (9).

These observations, taken in conjunction with previous
studies, suggest that desensitization is a complex phenomenon
that may be the result of several different mechanisms acting
separately or in concert. The apparent discrepancies in the
literature as to whether or not desensitization is a specific
process would appear to arise from differences in the experimental model and the particular antigen used.

In any case, the fact that nonspecific desensitization can
be achieved by appropriate experimental manipulation suggests
the presence of an inhibitory environment in the desensitized,
anergic animal. In support of this contention is the observation of Kantor that immune lymphocytes could not transfer reactivity to animals made anergic to an unrelated antigen (10).

There are obviously many possible mechanisms that could
lead to the "inhibitory environment," since an enormous number
of endogenous suppressive factors have been described. However, a number of observations led us to consider the effects
of lymphokines themselves in this regard. We had reported
previously that guinea pigs immunized so as to produce delayed
hypersensitivity, when injected with specific antigen intravenously, developed detectable MIF activity in their serum (11).
The appearance of serum MIF paralleled a transient reduction
in peripheral blood monocyte levels. The regimen for inducing
serum MIF was similar to that used for desensitization. To
ascertain whether there might be a causal relation between the
anergy and the serum lymphokine, we studied the effect of ad-
ministering exogenous lymphokines to actively immunized animals. We found that intravenous injection of MIF-containing
lymphocyte culture supernatants (but not control supernatants)
resulted in a marked reduction in the number of monocytes in
the peripheral blood of recipient guinea pigs. This treatment resulted also in the suppression of delayed-type skin reactions to unrelated antigens in such recipients (11).

We had previously reported that MIF-containing supernatants
injected intraperitoneally could mimic a MDR in nonsensitized
animals (12). Thus, supernatant fluids from antigen-stimu-
lated lymphocyte cultures may modify intact animals in three
ways: these fluids can decrease the number of macrophages
in preexisting peritoneal exudates, they can diminish the
level of circulating monocytes, and they can partially inhibit the expression of skin reactivity. The peritoneal effect
is due to increased adhesiveness of macrophages, which causes
them to clump and adhere to peritoneal surfaces. It is con-

sidered to represent an *in vivo* analog of the migration inhibition reaction and, as such, may be mediated specifically by MIF. One could similarly explain the reduction of monocytes in the circulation. The mechanism of suppression of skin reactivity is probably more complicated, since reactions are diminished at 24 hours, at a time when effects of lymphokine-containing supernatants on either circulating monocytes or peritoneal macrophages are no longer detectable. It is, of course, possible that the specific immunologic events that set the skin reaction in motion occur early, and that the subsequent slow evolution is based upon nonspecific factors that influence the behavior of the infiltrating macrophages. In any case, even if the suppression of skin reactivity is due to a MIF-induced sequestration of the monocytes that are the precursors of the infiltrating macrophages, this does not implicate MIF in the pathogenesis of the skin reaction itself. Indeed, although it has been possible to recovery both a skin-reactive factor and various chemotactic factors from skin delayed hypersensitivity reaction sites (13), it has not been possible to recover MIF from these sites. The point here is that the suppressive lymphokine need not be the same as the lymphokine responsible for the reaction itself, provided that they affect the same target cell.

The ability of exogenous lymphokine to reduce the level of circulating monocytes suggests that the similar reduction that follows challenge of immune animals with specific antigen may reflect the activity of endogenous lymphokine, such as MIF. The possibility was strengthened by the observation of Salvin *et al.* (14) that mice infected with BCG develop detectable migration inhibitory activity in their serum. Sephadex chromatography revealed this activity to be mainly present in pools corresponding to molecular weights of 45,000 and 80,000, which suggests that the results were not due to immune complexes. Similar results were obtained in the guinea pig by Yamamoto and Takahasi (15) as well as ourselves (11).

The experiments described above all suggest that densensitization is a state that should be capable of passive transfer with serum. Our observations on the appearance of serum lymphokine, and on the effects of administration of exogenous lymphokines, all suggested that timing would be crucial. We immunized prospective donors with DNP-BSA or DNP-EA in CFA. These were desensitized on the eighth day after immunization with 0.5 to 2 mg doses of the immunizing antigen intravenously and/or subcutaneously. These animals were bled by cardiac puncture 12 to 16 hours after the desensitizing treatment. These sera were used in the transfer experiments. Serum taken immediately 1-3 hours after antigen injection, or later than 24 hours after injection were shown to be ineffective in preliminary studies.

    Recipient animals in these transfer of experiments were
initially immunized with 100 Lf of diptheria toxoid-antitoxin
complex in IFA. For skin test studies, 13 days after immunization, they were given 6 ml of serum from desensitized
animals (1 ml intravenously, 5 ml intraperitoneally). When
suppression of the MDR via desensitized serum was under study,
recipient animals received 2.5 ml of serum intravenously and
2.5 ml subcutaneously; the treatment was given on the thirteenth
day after immunization, one day before evaluation of the MDR.
Some of the control animals received "immune serum" obtained
from animals immunized with the same antigen 7-8 days previously, but which had not received the desensitization treatment.

    We found in these experiments that a humoral factor was in
fact capable of inducing desensitization with respect to both
cutaneous delayed hypersensitivity and the macrophage disappearance reaction (16). Using various antigenic combinations,
we were able to show that transfer of desensitization is nonspecific and is not due to residual antigen in the donor sera.
Sephadex G-100 chromatography located the inhibitory activity
in the size range of 10,000-45,000 daltons; since larger molecular weight fractions were devoid of inhibitory activity, this
provides evidence that antibodies and immune complexes are not
responsible for the effect observed, and the inhibitory serum
component is not associated with macroglobulins.

    We have consistently found strongest desensitization ac-
tivity in sera obtained from animals at times when circulating
MIF was present (maximally 12 hours after antigen-induced desensitization). This plus the physicochemical data obtained
suggests that one possible mechanism for the desensitization
involves the presence of MIF or other lymphokines that participate in *in vivo* manifestations of cell-mediated immunity.
The ability of exogenous lymphokines to induce anergy (11)
supports this contention. However, definitive proof of this
point would require a degree of characterization of the putative mediator beyond what is presently available for any of
the known lymphokines. Studies on monosaccharide inhibition
profiles, and reactivity with antilymphokine antibodies, currently in progress, should shed further light on this important
point.

    It should be noted that if systemic lymphokine activity
should prove to be involved in the mechanism of desensitization,
this would not be inconsistent with our studies, which failed
to detect lymphokine production by lymphocytes exposed to
desensitizing doses of antigen *in vitro* (9). This finding
merely provides evidence against mediator exhaustion as a mechanism for desensitization. *In vivo*, small degrees of mediator
production by each reactive cell, triggered by appropriate
amounts of specific antigen in the microenvironment, would

likely be adequate for the serum levels of mediator observed. The large bolus of antigen is required to ensure the delivery of adequate antigen doses to the bulk of the available lymphocytes specifically responsive to that antigen.

In this regard, it should be noted that desensitization could be obtained even after the skin test had been initiated. Thus, if the mechanism of desensitization in this system is lymphokine-dependent, it would seem to affect the reaction at some stage or stages beyond the initial triggering event.

INHIBITION OF B CELL-DERIVED MIF

Since lymphokines are the putative mediators of cellular immunity, and since cellular immunity is a manifestation of T cell function, it was initially assumed that lymphokines were exclusively T cell products. We have demonstrated that under appropriate conditions guinea pig B lymphocytes, as well as T lymphocytes, can make migration inhibition factor (MIF). We found that both purified protein derivative (PPD) and endotoxin lipopolysaccharide (LPS), which are B cell mitogens, can induce B cells from nonsensitized animals to make MIF (17). Similarly, the capability of human B cells to make MIF (18), human (19), and guinea pig (20) B cells to make macrophage chemotactic factor as well as MIF (21) as well as human B cells to make (mitogen-induced) interferon (22) have all been recently described. In most of these studies, a requirement for B cell activation by mitogenic factors has been demonstrated, although in one report (18) specific antigen was found capable of serving as inducing agent as well.

Since it now appears unequivocal that B cells have the capacity to produce MIF and several other lymphokine mediators, it becomes necessary to understand the requirement for T cells, rather than B cells, in the various *in vivo* reactions whose mechanism seems to involve lymphokines. One clue comes from the observation that all of the studies demonstrating mediator production by B cells, of necessity, involve purified B cell-rich subpopulation of lymphocytes. In our experimental design, which involves the effect of PPD or LPS on nonsensitized lymphocytes, incubation of whole, unfractionated lymph node or spleen cell suspensions with these agents does not lead to MIF production, although as stated above, relatively pure B cell preparations can be stimulated under these conditions to produce MIF. Although it is possible that the separation procedure modifies the B cells in some manner that enables or enhances this activity, a more likely explanation is that T cells present in the original suspensions exert a suppressive effect on the B cells.

We explored this simple hypothesis in a series of experiments involving mixing of lymphocyte cell subpopulations and of cell products (23).

We found that the presence of T cells inhibits the production of detectable MIF by B cells, both in unseparated lymphocyte syspensions and in 1:1 reconstituted mixtures of T and B cells. This effect is clearly proportional to the ratio of T to B cells, since even our purified B cell populations are contaminated with up to 10% of T cells. Of course, it is possible that more pure B cell preparations would give even higher MIF activity.

In other experiments, we incubated B cells with supernatants of T cell cultures. We found that the suppressive effect described above was at least in part mediated through the production of a heat labile, nondialyzable factor by the T cells on exposure to PPD or LPS. This substance, which inhibits the expression of MIF activity, represents an inhibitory factor for MIF, and we therefore defined it as MIFIF. The mechanism of this effect remains to be elucidated. MIFIF could either act directly on the B cells to prevent synthesis or release of MIF, or it might even be cytotoxic for those cells. An alternative possibility is that it could interact with the MIF as it is formed. However, preliminary evidence obtained by incubating MIFIF-containing supernatants directly with MIF-rich supernatants has shown that MIFIF does not appear to act directly on MIF or to compete with it for a receptor site on its target cell. Another, but less likely possibility, is that the T cell is modifying the PPD or LPS and that this modified material is then suppressive. This would be an unusual mechanism for B cell control.

In any case, the results presented demonstrate that the presence of T cells in sufficient numbers can suppress the production or expression of MIF activity by B cells and that this effect is mediated by a soluble factor, which itself by definition is a lymphokine. In addition to defining a new kind of suppressor activity by a T cell on a B cell, these results point to the ability of PPD and LPS, two substances whose mitogenic and lymphokine-inducing activities are directed at B cells, to activate T cells as well. This finding also raises the possibility that, in analogy with the situation for antibody production, the production of other B cell-derived lymphokines might be under similar T suppressor cell control. This would explain why reactions of cell-mediated immunity *in vivo* appear to be T-dependent. If this is so, it would suggest that in certain immunodeficient states characterized by pure

T cell deficiency, B cells might be potentially capable of sub-
serving T cell functions. This possibility awaits further
study.

As a final point, it should be noted that although a number
of studies have provided evidence for the regulation of various manifestations of cell-mediated immunity by suppressor
cells (23-25), no data are currently available as to suppressor activity with respect to the lymphokines themselves. It
may well be that mechanisms similar to those described here
will be found operative with respect to conventional T cell-
derived MIF as well.

MONOSACCHARIDE INHIBITION OF LYMPHOKINES

Evidence has accumulated to show that carbohydrates in
plasma membranes play an essential role in many biological
activities of cells that are dependent upon recognition of
molecules of other cells. Although the mechanisms involved
in cellular recognition of various substances are still unclear, a variety of terminal monosaccharides have been shown
to be important for various cellular functions such as the
binding of viruses to infectable cells (26), cellular receptors for endotoxins (26), proper homing of lymphocytes (26-
28), blocking of lectin binding sites (29), contact inhibition (30), cytotoxic responses (31), T cell rosette formation
(32), and intercellular adhesion (33).

Based upon such considerations, Remold (34) has presented
data suggesting that α-L-fucose may be part of a guinea pig
macrophage cellular receptor site for migration inhibitory
factor (MIF). This conclusion was based upon the ability of
L-fucose to inhibit the macrophage migration inhibition reaction, and the ability of fucosidase to cause macrophages to
become transiently refractory to the action of MIF. Similar
results were also reported by Fox *et al.* (35) utilizing MIF
obtained from PPD-stimulated lymphocyte cultures and MIF-like
substances obtained from fetal calf serum.

More recently, Rocklin (36) has investigated the role of
monosaccharides in the interaction of human MIF and human leukocyte inhibitory factor (LIF) with macrophages and neutrophils, respectively. He found that the 5- methylpentose
sugars L-fucose, L-rhamnose, and 6-deoxy-D-glucose could inhibit MIF but not LIF. Conversely, N-acetyl-D-galatosamine,
which had no effect on MIF, could inhibit LIF activity. The
limited specificity of the inhibition of the MIF-macrophage
interaction by L-fucose, and the necessity for using large
concentrations of sugar (0.1 *M*), raise questions as to whether

the active monosaccharides are intrinsic components of a receptor site or whether they interfere with the activity of
MIF by indirect means, especially since it is known that the
presence of various sugars in the incubation medium can lead
to alterations of cell morphology including changes in shape
and loss of microvilli (37).

We explored the ability of monosaccharides to inhibit
lymphokine activity in order to focus on the specificity of
the effect in terms of class of inflammatory mediators affected (lymphokines vs. other factors), kind of lymphokine affected, and kinds of sugars capable of inhibition.

In contrast to the previous reports cited above, we found
that L-rhamnose as well as L-fucose was capable of inhibiting
guinea pig MIF activity. These sugars also inhibited the activity of macrophage chemotactic and neutrophil chemotactic
factors (38). Thus, fucose is not a specific inhibitor of
MIF, nor its activity confined to that lymphokine.

Preincubation of these sugars with the lymphokines was
required for inhibition of chemotactic activity. This finding,
as well as the results of dose-response experiments, suggested
that the mechanism of chemotactic inhibition is similar to the
mechanism of inhibition of MIF by monosaccharides, i.e., it is
possible that the lymphokines possess receptor sites that
recognize cell sites bearing a structural or conformational
similarity to these sugars. In contrast, L-xylose, the only
other sugar out of 12 found inhibitory in our study, appeared
to exert its activity by a direct effect on the target cells
themselves rather than by interaction with the mediator.
These preincubation studies suggested that the putative receptor is of low affinity, that binding occurred slowly, and
that the interaction was a reversible one. Curiously, when
we performed dose-response studies, we found that the effect
of L-fucose on inhibition of either lymphokine activity is
inversely proportional to the amount of lymphokine activity
initially present.

A major finding that emerged from our study is that the
monosaccharide inhibition of inflammatory mediator activity
appears to be confined to either lymphokines themselves or
cytokines (lymphokine-like factors derived from nonlymphoid
cells). Three other biologic mediators with chemotactic
activity, fragments from trypsin-treated C3 and C5, and bacterial factor could not be inhibited by either L-fucose or
L-rhamnose. This suggests that there may be multiple and distinguishable cell sites for interaction with factors possessing
similar biologic activity, and thus, for example, different
chemotactic factors need not have similar active regions or
molecular homology. This finding may be also of considerable

practical importance since it could provide a simple way to distinguish different sources of chemotactic activity in complex biologic mixtures such as serum or tissue extracts.

ANTILYMPHOKINE ANTIBODIES

We initially began studies on the possibility of producing antilymphokine antibodies in order to obtain potentially useful probes of lymphokine structure and function. The ultimate goal would be the accumulation of monospecific antisera for each of the known lymphokines. This goal has proven elusive in many laboratories because of the multiplicity of such substances in biologic preparations, their presence in minute quantities, and the presence of a large number on contaminating materials in these preparations. We have attempted the first step toward this goal, namely the preparation of an antiserum directed against a supernatant with multiple lymphokine activities. We have partially circumvented the difficulties mentioned by a two-stage immunization procedure in which the lymphokine-containing supernatant is first treated with an antibody directed against the control supernatant. By this means, one might hope to reduce the level of contaminants common to each supernatant. The partially purified lymphokine preparation is then used as immunogen to obtain the final antiserum. The reaction between lymphokine and anticontrol antiserum is allowed to occur in the solid phase, using conjugated Sepharose bead immunoadsorption so as to obviate the necessity for precipitating antibody in the system. Indeed, with the relatively crude reagents available, it is difficult to detect antibody activity using precipitation techniques. For similar reasons, we treat lymphokine-containing fluids with antilymphokine serum on immunoadsorbents, rather than simply mixing the two preparations together.

We found it possible to prepare an antiserum with significant biologic activity. We were able to almost completely remove MIF, SRF, and macrophage chemotactic factor activities from culture supernatants (39). This justifies the use of the term "antilymphokine antiserum."

This antilymphokine antibody had no effect on lymphotoxin, mitogenic factor, or neutrophil chemotactic activity (40).

In these studies, we found that it is possible to suppress the delayed hypersensitivity skin reactions in actively immunized guinea pigs by local administration of antilymphokine antibody. In this regard, it should be noted that the presence of any contaminating antilymphocyte activity would have no effect on the results discussed above, where mediator substances

rather than lymphocytes were involved. On the other hand,
antilymphocyte antibody, if present, could inhibit the evolution of the skin reaction in actively immunized animals, since
the triggering event here is the reaction between antigen and
sensitized lymphocyte. It is unlikely, however, that the experimental and control antisera, both prepared against lymphocyte culture supernatants, would differ with respect to any
antilymphocyte activity. In support of this contention, we
observed no diminution in viability (by trypan blue exclusion)
after as much as 24 hour incubation of lymphocytes at 37°C in
20% serum (antilymphokine or control). Incubation in 50% serum
led to a reduction of approximately 30% in viability, but
there were no differences regardless of whether antilymphokine
or control antiserum was used. The addition of fresh guinea
pig serum as an additional complement source has no effect on
these results.

These results demonstrate the efficacy of antilymphokine
antibody in an *in vivo* setting, and provide evidence that cutaneous delayed hypersensitivity reactions are at least in
part lymphokine-mediated.

SUMMARY AND CONCLUSION

In this brief presentation, we have focused on various experimental procedures by which one can modify lymphokine production or the expression of lymphokine activity. Of these,
desensitization provides the clearest model for a process that
could have general biologic significance. Many disease processes exist in which a large antigen load is present systemically; this is most common in infectious and in neoplastic disease. Other, less well-defined diseases such as sar-
coidosis may also involve "overload" mechanisms. It is of
interest that in many of such cases, so-called clinical anergy
is seen.

It is also possible that under normal, nonpathologic circumstances, local fluctuations in antigen distribution and
antigen levels lead to imbalances of mediator production, with
local activation of target cells in one area preempting their
availability elsewhere.

MIFIF, an inhibitor of MIF, may also represent a good model
for immunoregulation. First, it provides a means for preventing
the expression of a B cell potentiality (lymphokine production)
that is not needed, in a teleological sense, when T cells are
available. Under pathologic conditions where T cells are absent, then B cells might express this function. In this sense,
in addition to its role in antibody production, the B cell
provides a fail-safe mechanism for lymphokine production.

Second, factors similar to or identical with MIFIF could control lymphokine production by T cells themselves.

A possible biologic role for simple sugars is less easy to visualize. However, such sugars are found in various cell membranes, including those of invading pathogens, and in blood group substances. It is not inconceivable that monosaccharides derived from these sources at sites of inflammation or tissue destruction could limit the expression of mediator activity.

Finally, since experimentally produced antilymphokine antibodies are capable of inhibiting delayed hypersensitivity reactions *in vivo*, it is possible that similar kinds of activity could arise spontaneously in the course of disease. Thus, one could envision an autoimmune mechanism for the suppression of lymphokine-dependent reactions.

These examples most likely represent a mere fraction of the available mechanisms for containing or limiting reactions of cell-mediated immunity. They are probably not even the most important, in a biologic sense. For the moment, however, they serve as convenient, readily manipulable systems for exploration of the factors that are operative in the control of this form of immunologic reactivity.

References

1. Yoshida, T., and Cohen, S. *In* "Mechanisms of Cell-Mediated Immunity" (R. T. McCluskey and S. Cohen, eds.), p. 43, Wiley, New York, 1974.
2. Cohen, S. *Am. J. Pathol. 88*, 502, 1977.
3. Yoshida, T., Bigazzi, P. E., and Cohen, S. *Proc. Nat. Acad. Sci. 72*, 1641, 1975.
4. Uhr, J. W., and Pappenheimer, A. M., Jr. *J. Exp. Med. 108*, 891, 1958.
5. Asherson, G. L., and Stone, S. H. *Immunology 13*, 469, 1967.
6. Lipsmeyer, E. A., and Kantor, F. S. *J. Immunol. 102*, 1074, 1969.
7. Nelson, D. A., and Boyden, S. V. *Immunology 6*, 264, 1963.
8. Sonozaki, H., and Cohen, S. *J. Immunol. 106*, 1404, 1971.
9. Sonozaki, H., Papermaster, V., Yoshida, T., and Cohen, S. *J. Immunol. 115*, 1657, 1975.
10. Kantor, F. S. *N. Engl. J. Med. 292*, 629, 1975.
11. Yoshida, T., and Cohen, S. *J. Immunol. 112*, 1540, 1974.
12. Sonozaki, H., and Cohen, S. *Cell. Immunol. 2*, 341, 1971.
13. Cohen, S., Ward, P. A., Yoshida, T., and Burek, C. L. *Cell. Immunol. 9*, 363, 1973.
14. Salvin, S. B., Youngner, J. S., and Lederer, W. H. *Infect. Immun. 7*, 68, 1973.

15. Yamamoto, K., and Takahashi, Y. *Nature (New Biol.) 233*, 261, 1971.
16. Papermaster, V., Yoshida, T., and Cohen, S. *Cell. Immunol.*, in press.
17. Yoshida, T., Sonozaki, H., and Cohen, S. *J. Exp. Med. 138*, 784, 1973.
18. Rocklin, R. E., MacDermott, R. P., Chess, L., Schlossman, S. F., and David, J. R. *J. Exp. Med. 140*, 1303, 1974.
19. Mackler, B. F., Altman, L. C., Rosenstreich, D. L., and Oppenheim, J. J. *Nature 249*, 834, 1974.
20. Wahl, S. M., Iverson, G. M., and Oppenheim, J. J. *J. Exp. Med. 140*, 1631, 1974.
21. Bloom, B. R., Stoner, G., Gaffney, J., Shevach, E., and Green, I. *Eur. J. Immunol. 5*, 218, 1975.
22. Epstein, L. B., Kreth, H. W., and Herzenberg, L. A. *Cell. Immunol. 12*, 407, 1974.
23. Asherson, G. L., and Zembola, M. *Br. Med. Bull. 32*, 158, 1976.
24. Turk, J. L., Polak, L., and Parker, D. *Br. Med. Bull. 32*, 165, 1976.
25. Neta, R., and Salvin, S. B. *J. Immunol. 117*, 2014, 1976.
26. Winzler, R. J. *Int. Rev. Cytol. 29*, 77, 1970.
27. Gesner, B. M., and Woodruff, J. J. *In* "Cellular Recognition" (R. T. Smith and R. A. Good, eds.), p. 79. Appleton-Century-Crofts, New York, 1969.
28. Spiro, R. J. *Ann. Rev. Biochem. 39*, 599, 1970.
29. Powell, A. E., and Leon, M. A. *Exp. Cell. Res. 62*, 315, 1970.
30. Nicolson, G., and Lacorbiere, M. *Proc. Nat. Acad. Sci. 70*, 1672, 1973.
31. Brondz, B. D., Sneiginova, A. E., Rassulin, Y. A., and Shamborant, O. G. *Immunochemistry 10*, 175, 1973.
32. Bentwich, A., Douglas, S. D., Sketelsky, E., and Kunkel, H. G. *J. Exp. Med. 137*, 1532, 1973.
33. Roth, S., McGuire, E. J., and Roseman, S. *J. Cell. Biol. 51*, 536, 1971.
34. Remold, H. G. *J. Exp. Med. 138*, 1065, 1973.
35. Fox, R. A., Gregory, D. S., and Feldman, J. D. *J. Immunol. 112*, 1867, 1974.
36. Rocklin, R. E. *J. Immunol. 116*, 816, 1976.
37. Amos, H., Leventhal, M., Chu, L., and Karnovsky, M. J. *Cell 7*, 97, 1976.
38. Amsden, A., Ewan, V., Yoshida, T., and Cohen, S. *J. Immunol.*, in press.
39. Yoshida, T., Bigazzi, P. E., and Cohen, S. *J. Immunol. 114*, 688, 1976.
40. Kuratsuji, T., Yoshida, T., and Cohen, S. *J. Immunol. 117*, 1985, 1976.

DISCUSSION

     DR. KANTOR: What is the relationship between lymphokine-
producing cells (Ly 1 or Ly 2,3) and helper cells (Ly 1)?
     DR. COHEN: This is a complicated system since, in the
mouse, mediators with antagonist activity and precursor lymphokines with blocking activity can be produced.   Thus, it is
hard to assay the production of specific mediators by subpopulations of cells.   Our own unpublished data suggest that MIF
can be made by both types of cells.
     DR. BLOOM: We have evidence on this point (Newman, W.,
Hammerling, U., and Bloom, B. R., *J. Immunol.*, in press).
Using a secondary mouse MLC system in which we could be certain that both Ly 1 and Ly 2,3 T cells could be engaged by
antigen, we found that MIF was produced by both Ly 1 and Ly 2,3
cells.   These *in vitro* data are consistent with the results of
cell transfers *in vivo* by Vadas and Miller, who found that,
while passive transfer of DTH to protein antigens in the mouse
was mediated by Ly 1 cells, contact hypersensitivity could be
transferred by both Ly 1 and Ly 2,3 cells.   It is our view
that the nature of the T cell subpopulation activated by lymphokines *in vivo* is likely to be determined by the mode of antigen presentation rather than the intrinsic capabilities of
the subpopulations.
     DR. BRITTON: Is it true that, in one of your desensiti-
zation models, there is nothing wrong with the T cells; rather
to the contrary, they make too many lymphokines, which block
receptors of the target cells (monocytes-macrophages) so that
they cannot orientate themselves toward a site of intravenous
injection of specific antigen even if plenty of T cells are
there signaling for them?
     DR. COHEN: There are at least four possible mechanisms
of desensitization: defective or absent sensitized cells,
mediator exhaustion, suppressor cells or factors, and target
cell preemption.   I know of no firm data for the first two.
In the models I've discussed, I gave evidence for target cell
preemption by systemic lymphokines as well as the production
of suppressive factors that inhibit lymphokine production.
Although, at first glance, these appear paradoxical, they are
temporally separated.   Indeed the high lymphokine level seen
shortly after challenge with desensitizing doses of antigen
may be the signal for the subsequent production of the
suppressor factor.   The various puzzling findings reported
in the literature are probably due to a failure to take into
account this dual mechanism of desensitization.   In any case,
the main point here is that desensitization is probably a good

model for other kinds of physiologic homeostatic mechanisms for the fine-tuning and the expression of lymphokine activity.

DR. DOHERTY: Does an allogeneic interaction result in production of mediator? For instance, is mediator produced when T cells specific for Ia are generated?

DR. COHEN: I don't know.

DR. BLOOM: If you take ATH and ATL and run them in an MLC, you see mediator production, as measured by migration inhibition, but you don't see it clearly. That is, it's not there until the fourth day and the cells die on the sixth day. However, in a secondary MLC, which was the system I mentioned earlier, we found it within the first 24 hours.

DR. DOHERTY: Is it yet known whether there is any MHC-related restriction in mediator production?

DR. COHEN: Allogeneic interaction can give rise to lymphokine production, although it is not usually observed in the guinea pig system. There is no apparent histocompatibility restriction in the production of MIF or expression of MIF activity.

DR. DOHERTY: Is it known whether any of the mediators contain Ia antigenic specificities?

DR. COHEN: Such specificities have not been detected in the mouse system by us or, as far as I am aware, in other laboratories. The guinea pig mediators are harder to study in this regard, but they also appear to lack histocompatibility-type specificities.

DR. BLOOM: Ethan Shevach explored both guinea pig and mouse systems and could not find any Ia component.

DR. BRITTON: I wanted to ask about antibody to cytotoxic lymphocytes.

DR. COHEN: We don't have antibody to lymphotoxin--we can't make it. Zoltan Lucas can make an antilymphotoxin antibody that, interestingly, does not cross react with these factors and I believe his will inhibit, at least in the *in vitro* model. Whether it has *in vivo* activity, I don't think has been looked at. You would think from Chris Henney's work that this should not be. This would be a very good use for his reagent, but as far as I know, he has not done those experiments. These restrictions and the kind of antibody you can make are interesting when you consider that all of the starting preparations are relatively crude. It's very hard to have situations in which you have production of any one of the mediators in isolation. What it will tell us ultimately is that there are distinguishable parts of these molecules. From the lymphotoxin work, it begins to look as if they behave as if functionally they contain two subunits, one of which codes for the target that the mediator is going to affect, and another which tells it what to do to that target. Of those, it looks like the most immunogenic part is the part that finds its proper cell.

DR. PLATE: Is any allospecificity or species specificity detected in the antilymphokine sera?

DR. COHEN: The anti-guinea pig lymphokine does not react with lymphokines from man or mouse, but does react with some monkey-derived cytokine MIF preparations; thus there is limited specificity.

DR. YUNIS: What is the role of Australian antigen in your observation of alteration of MIF production in patients?

DR. COHEN: I don't know. The correlations we observed were between SGOT elevation and serum MIF levels. As only half of these patients had detectable Australian antigen, its role in the generation of the MIF is unclear.

DR. DIENER: What is the physiologic significance of MIF in terms of immune induction and immune regulation? If it is true that any Ly 1 helper cell can make these factors, what does this mean in terms of B cell triggering if the same thing happens in cell-mediated immunity?

DR. COHEN: What it really tells you is just that there is heterogeneity, not only with respect to different properties of T cell function but even with respect to mediator production, because there are Ly 1,2,3, restrictions in terms of helper kinds of activities but not with respect to the effector molecules such as MIF. It's a semantic problem; when we say lymphokines, we tend to think of nonantibody substances made by lymphocytes. But there really are two kinds, those involved in the affector side of the thing, to kick over B cells, for example, and those involved at the other end, where they do things to inflammatory cells, so that it's not hard to understand a design where these things are functioning differently.

Session II
Immunogenetics and Escape Mechanisms

OVERVIEW: IMMUNOGENETICS AND ESCAPE MECHANISMS

Frank Lilly

Department of Genetics
Albert Einstein College of Medicine of Yeshiva University
Bronx, New York

The study of genetically controlled susceptibility or resistance to induced disease has often been a rewarding means
of approaching the factors involved in the genesis of the disease. It is an approach that depends, of course, on the existence of polymorphism within a species in response to the inducing agent. Analysis of the polymorphism may allow identification of a gene responsible for susceptibility or resistance, and analysis of the mechanism of the gene may then elucidate an important step in the disease process.

A major impediment to realization of this strategy is the
fact that, in many cases, the genetic control of disease susceptibility turns out to be multifactorial, and traits governed
by several genes rather than a single gene can be exceedingly
difficult to analyze. At this point, two further substrategies
are generally brought into play to aid in pulling individual
genes out of the black box, which contains a diversity of them.
First, it may be possible, often by luck, to find a family or
a cross of strains in which only one of the several genes is
segregating. Thereafter one may be able to map this gene and
thus differentiate its effects from those of the remaining
genes. Second, one may take advantage of existing knowledge
or hypotheses concerning discrete events in the disease process and then be able to distinguish susceptibility genes affecting this step from those affecting other steps in the
generation of the disease.

The first two papers in this session concern a particular
system: viral leukemogenesis in the mouse. This is a good
example of a multiple-gene system, since a dozen or so genes
have been identified as capable of playing a role in susceptibility to mouse leukemia (1). Only a few of these genes

have been ananlyzed sufficiently to give a clear indication
of the level at which they act, but it is already clear that
some of them govern immunologic processes, whereas others do
not. Those which do not operate immunologically appear to
act at one or another stage of the virus penetration or replication cycle (e.g., *Fv-1*). Those which do operate by way of
an effect on the immune system share the perhaps surprising
property of being within or closely linked to the major histocompatibility locus, *H-2*. (Although immune response genes in
other mouse systems have sometimes proved to be independent of
H-2, this has not yet been true of mouse leukemia.)
     That even the subclass of *H-2* linked susceptibility genes
is heterogeneous is indicated by the fact that, among the
different viral isolates studied in this manner, some have
proved to be strongly influenced by the hosts' genotype in
the *K* end of the *H-2* complex (2,3), whereas others are more
strongly influenced by genes mapping in the *D* end of the complex (4,5). Very closely associated with the *K* end of the
complex is the *I* region, itself complex, identified as govern-
ing immune responsiveness to certain specific antigenic determinants (6). Thus a major hypothesis to explain the mechanism of *K* end-associated susceptibility genes in mouse leukemia
has long been that the animals are either good or poor res-
ponders to virus-induced, tumor-specific antigens of their
leukemic cells and thus either strongly or weakly capable of
rejecting them by immunologic means, according to their *I* region genotype. Strong evidence pointing in this direction
has emerged from certain studies, but further definition of
the exact mechanisms involved remains as an urgent need. For
example, some sets of data imply that the control mechanism
involved is a positive one, in the sense that the immune response studied is dominant in heterozygotes involving a responder and a nonresponder strain (7); other studies, by contrast, have suggested that a negative control or a suppressor
factor is involved (8).
     The *D* end of the *H-2* complex is not known to be closely
associated with immune response genes in any previously defined sense, and it has been necessary to seek novel approaches
to the mechanism of genes mapping within this chromosomal segment. Recently, studies of the cytotoxic T-cell response to
virus-induced cellular antigens have provided a promising lead
that may help to solve this problem. These cytotoxic T cells
exhibit the phenomenon of *H-2* restriction, or linked associative recognition; i.e., the cytotoxic activity of the T cells
appears to be effective only on targets bearing both the same
viral antigen(s) and the same *H-2* antigen(s) as the cells used
for immunization of the T cell donors. Studies in one leukemia
virus system have suggested that the antigen recognized by the

T cells results from the formation of an *H-2*/viral antigen
molecular complex on the cell surface (9). A most interesting
feature of this finding is that formation of the molecular
complex appears to occur with certain *H-2* molecules and not
with others. Thus resistance to leukemia might represent the
capacity of the *H-2* molecules on the leukemia cell to generate
an antigen that T cells can recognize and to which they can
respond, and it is possible that this sort of phenomenon is
the basis of the *D* end effect on leukemogenesis.

Clearly these observations and ideas represent a bare beginning in the analysis of immunologic factors in disease resistance, even in the one system considered. Most other systems are even less well understood, and the final paper of
this session will summarize the status of immunologic factors
in parasitic diseases, an area where our understanding is especially rudimentary. We immunologists do not lack interesting
and urgent problems to tackle.

References

1. Steeves, R. A., and Lilly, F. *Ann. Rev. Genet. 11*, 277-
   296, 1977.
2. Lilly, F. *In* "Comparative Leukemic Research 1969" (R. M.
   Dutcher, ed.), pp. 213-220. Karger, Basel, 1970.
3. Lonai, P., and Haran-Ghera, N. *J. Exp. Med. 146*, 1164-
   1168, 1977.
4. Chesebro, B., Wehrly, K., and Stimpfling, J. *J. Exp. Med.
   149*, 1457-1467, 1974.
5. Meruelo, D., Lieberman, M., Ginzton, N., Deak, B., and
   McDevitt, H. O. *J. Exp. Med. 146*, 1079-1087, 1977.
6. Benacerraf, B., and McDevitt, H. O. *Science 175*, 273-279,
   1972.
7. Sato, H., Boyse, E. A., Aoki, T., Iritani, C., and Old, L.
   J. *J. Exp. Med. 138*, 593-606, 1973.
8. Meruelo, D., Deak, B., and McDevitt, H. O. *J. Exp. Med.
   146*, 1367-1379, 1977.
9. Blank, K. J., and Lilly, F. 1977.

GAMES PARASITES PLAY

Barry R. Bloom
Herbert Tanowitz
Murray Wittner

Albert Einstein College of Medicine
Bronx, New York

I. INTRODUCTION

The games parasites play are, in fact, a serious matter.
It is estimated that between 500 million and a billion people,
primarily in the developing countries, suffer from tropical
diseases and parasitic infections. The figures shown in Table
I indicate current estimates on the prevalence of some parasitic
diseases. Exact figures are difficult to obtain (9); for
some diseases, few if any epidemiologic surveys have been
carried out. In addition to the diseases of man, only some
of which can be touched on in this article, it should be mentioned that unknown millions of cattle, vitally needed for the
world's food supply particularly in the developing countries,
die of parasitic diseases each year, and at least 700 million
are estimated to be at risk (10). In Africa alone, 7 million
square kilometers of grazable land capable of supporting 120
million head of cattle remain largely unproductive chiefly because of two parasitic diseases, trypanosomiasis and East
Coast fever. Some of the parasitic diseases of animals important for the human food chain are listed in Table II.
    The basic challenge in parasitic diseases is the obvious
fact that the survival of parasites and the extent of their
ability to live in the host species reflect the fact that
they have evolved mechanisms for surviving in the face of the
best the body has to offer in the way of natural and acquired
immunity. The challenge to the immunologist, in trying to en-

Portions reproduced from
Nature, Vol. 279, No. 5708, pp. 21–26, May 3 1979

TABLE I. Some Parasitic Diseases of Man

	Morbidity
Hookworm	700,000,000
Trachoma	400,000,000
Schistosomiasis	200,000,000
Malaria	150,000,000
Filariasis	200,000,000
Chagas disease	12,000,000(?)
Sleeping sickness	unknown
Leishmaniasis	unknown

gender resistance or immunity to these parasites, is to do
something better and beyond what the body's immune system is
ordinarily capable of.

The level of understanding of the immunology of parasitic
infections is embarrassingly rudimentary, attributable as much
to lack of interest by the immunologists as to lack of funding
for this area. The organisms are complex, with varied life
cycles and mechanisms of pathogenesis, and until reasonable
understanding of some of the basic immunological mechanisms
became available, it would indeed have been difficult to probe
deeply the mechanisms underlying immunity or pathogenesis of
various parasitic infections. There is currently a resurgence
of interest in tropical diseases and in the possibility of providing immunological protection for many of them. It is to be
expected that as these approaches are applied, they will be
recognized by the parasites as selective pressures to be over-

TABLE II. Some Parasitic Diseases in Cattle

	Estimated mortality
African trypanosomiasis	3,000,000
Anaplasmosis	1,000,000
East Coast fever	500,000
Babesiosis	250,000

come, and they will devise even more sophisticated mechanisms for eluding the host's immune response. But the time frame of evolution is a great deal longer than the time frame required to bring under some control most infectious diseases.

In the simplest of terms, the ground rules of the game may be sketched as follows: if parasites totally eluded the immune response and were sufficiently virulent, they would kill their hosts upon whom their survival depends and preclude their own survival. Conversely, if they were too easily destroyed by an immune response, their survival would be similarly jeopardized. Consequently, immunity and escape from surveillance are relative phenomena, which are ordinarily in a constant balance and tension.

The examples that follow are fragmentary bits of information on known mechanisms that *could* explain escape from surveillance, but what is currently known may be only the top of the iceberg in view of the wealth of our ignorance of the immunology of these organisms. The findings are here suggested as possibilities, in some cases very strong, in some cases likely to be artifacts, but in all cases, we believe, interesting and worthy of pursuit.

OLD-TIME GENETIC ENGINEERING

In order to ensure the survival of both their mammalian hosts and the parasites themselves in a wide variety of geographical and climatic environments, it is hardly surprising that an almost infinite variety of genera, species, classes, and families of parasites have evolved, only a fraction of which produce disease in man. There are some parasites within a simple classification that have enormous host ranges and are capable of infecting and growing in virtually all domestic mammals, such as *Trypanosoma brucei* and *Trypanosoma cruzi*; there are others such as *T. simiae* that produce fulminating infection in only a few, apparently unrelated species such as monkeys and pigs; and there may be others that produce infections with more limited host range, such as the exclusive infection of cattle by *Theileria parva* or of certain species of monkeys by the monkey malaria agent *Plasmodium knowlesi*. In the vast majority of instances the mechanisms underlying these host restrictions remain unknown; yet were such mechanisms understood, it might be possible to learn much about the parameters that govern host-parasite interactions. Obviously the genetic factors in escape from surveillance that should be considered include not only the nature of the parasite and

host, but also the species of vectors, available and susceptible, the parasites' tissue tropisms, immunogenicity, and
susceptibility to immune mechanisms.

In West Africa, there is a great variability in susceptibility among various breeds of cattle to infections produced by *Trypanosoma congolense*. Cattle introduced to Africa
from Europe during the time of the Roman empire as well as
native Zebu cattle are highly susceptible to this parasite.
Indigenous West African short-horned cattle such as the n'dama
and muturu appear to be naturally much more resistant (11,12).
This is an example of what is generally termed "natural immunity." The principal approach to the mechanisms of natural
immunity, in general, appears to involve the study of the
toxicity of fresh serum from many species of animals for various parasites. It is well known that human serum is quite
toxic for *Trypanosoma brucei*, an African trypanosome not pathogenic for man, whereas *Trypanosoma b. rhodensiense* and *gambiense*, the causative agents of sleeping sickness, are relatively resistant, although *T. rhodensiense* is not primarily
a human parasite. But as Fairbairn (13) has commented, "it
is extraordinary that *T. gambiense* which is completely resistant to human serum should produce a chronic infection in man
while *T. rhodensiense*, which is conparatively susceptible to
human serum (even on first isolation) should produce an acute
rapidly fatal disease." Another example of the problem in
this approach to the mechanisms of natural resistance is reflected in recent observations of *Trypanosoma cruzi*, the pathogenic protozoan responsible for Chagas disease in man. Here
the culture form of the organism, which is *not* found *in vivo*
in man, is almost totally susceptible to normal human serum
(14), probably because it activates the third component of complement by the alternative pathway and initiates its own destruction (15). Of interest, however, is the fact that the
trypomastigote form, that form found in the blood of infected
animals and man, and which is the most pathogenic form of the
organism, is essentially totally resistant to lysis by human
serum. Thus in man serum apparently offers no protection
against the disease-causing form and probably contributes
little to natural immunity. In fairness, it should be noted
that, in avian species, sera are lytic for the blood form,
and this may partially explain why these species have such
high natural resistance to this parasite. Thus, while
there may be factors in serum and tissues in resistant animals
capable of inactivating parasites *in vitro* and possibly *in
vivo*, it is clear that many well-studied organisms can elude
this simple type of natural resistance, and in some cases, this
kind of natural resistance may actually select for the survival of more virulent forms *in vivo*.

Another example of the mysterious ways in which the outcome of infection is modified by the genetics of both host and
parasite is provided by three extraordinarily different clinical entities in three different parts of the world caused by
Leishmania, a species of protozoan parasites that grows exclusively in macrophages in man. *Leishmania donovani* is the
cause of a systemic, progressive nonhealing disease called
visceral leishmaniasis (known in South Asia as *kala azar*);
Leishmania tropica is the cause of Oriental Sore found mostly
in the Middle East and which is a local, cutaneous, self-
healing lesion; and *Leishmania brasiliensis* is the cause of
mucocutaneous leishmaniasis in Central and South America with
its most fulminating form known as espundia, a disease in
which the parasite destroys the soft tissue and literally
makes its victims faceless. How can three so different diseases be produced by related organisms that grow in the same
cell type? The subtlety of the genetic factors is emphasized
by the fact that the same organisms inhabiting different host
species can produce different effects. Pursuing the above
examples, *L. donovani* produces only a localized disease in
dogs, while *L. tropica* can produce a visceral disease in rodents. The point is that the evolved adaptations and genetic
changes are extraordinarily complex and not usually susceptible
of simple interpretation.

In spite of the current enthusiasm about immune response
genes, in a wide variety of experimental bacterial, viral
(with the debatable exception of lymphocytic choriomeningitis,
LCM), and parasitic infections studied in inbred mouse strains,
it has not yet been demonstrated that host resistance is primarily dependent on genes associated with the major histocompatibility complex. However, within a host species, there may
be striking genetic differences in susceptibility to parasitic
infection. This is perhaps best illustrated by studies on two
protozoa that cause quite different diseases in man--*Leishmania donovani*, discussed above, and *T. cruzi*, which produces
Chagas disease in Latin America. When various inbred mouse
strains were studied for susceptibility to *L. donovani* by Bradley (17), C3H/He mice appeared to be most resistant and C57Bl
most susceptible. By appropriate crosses it was possible
to show that there was a single major autosomal dominant gene
that controlled resistance, and that this gene was not H2
linked. In parallel studies by Dr. T. Trischmann in our laboratory on resistance to *T. cruzi* in the same strains of mice,
an almost reciprocal pattern of susceptibility was found (16)
(Table III). Here the C3H is the most susceptible strain and
the C57Bl relatively resistant. Again we have found resistance
to be unlinked to H2. It is obviously of great interest to
pursue the mechanism by which these major autosomal genes con-

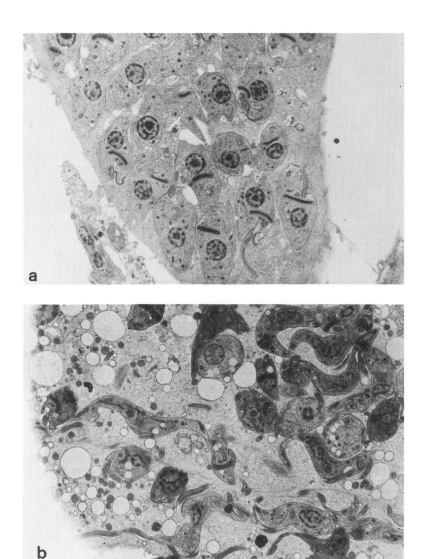

FIGURE 1. (a) *Heterogenous cells of primary culture of the heart of C57B10 mice infected 8 days previously with tryp-omastigotes of* T. cruzi *(2100×).* (b) *Same as* (a) *except that cells are derived from the heart of C3H/He mice (2100×).*

TABLE III. Mouse Strain Differences in Resistance to Two Protozoal Parasites

Mouse strain	L. donovani	T. cruzi
C57Bl	Susceptible	Resistant
Balb/c	Susceptible	Intermediate
C3H/He	Resistant	Susceptible
DBA/2	Resistant	Susceptible
A/J	Resistant	Susceptible

trol resistance. We have ruled out the obvious possibility that the major gene controlling resistance in mice to *T. cruzi* might control receptors required by the parasite for entry into host cells. As can be seen from Fig. 1, heart cells from both resistant and susceptible strains are equally susceptible to infection by the organism *in vitro*.

It is important to note that most such studies are carried out in mice, which are not the natural hosts for these parasites, and it may not be too surprising to learn that mice have not evolved Ir genes to deal with parasites they are unlikely to have encountered in evolution. Nevertheless, even in the case of the murine leukemia viruses, the principal genetic determinants of susceptibility are the Fv-1 and Fv-2 genes, which are not H2 linked (18), and the Rgv-1 gene, which is H2 linked, plays a secondary role. In both Bradley's studies and our own, there is some evidence that an H2-linked gene does exert a secondary influence on resistance following infection. In this regard studies of HLA patterns in Sardinia by Piazza *et al.* (19) showed significant differences in the HLA-B locus antigens between inhabitants of the highlands, an area in which malaria was essentially nonexistent, and the lowlands, an area in which malaria flourished until recently. This is suggestive that there may have been a selection for certain HLA-B-linked, possible Ir gene functions by the malarial parasite.

Although the focus of the essay is on means by which parasites adapt to the immunologic pressures of the host, one cannot fail to comment on the probability that parasites may in fact have selected for mutations in the human species, which enables them to resist the parasite. A case in point is malaria. It was Allison (21) who first pointed out the fact that the sickle cell hemoglobin gene, which codes for the substitution of a valine for a glutamic acid in the protein, confers partial resistance to *Plasmodium falciparum* and limits its

intraerythrocytic multiplication. Subsequently, it has been
observed that thalassemia and glucose-6-phosphate dehydrogenase
deficiency reduce susceptibility to malaria. In the case of
the sickle cell trait, people with the normal hemoglobin A/A
genotype are highly susceptible to falciparum malaria; those
with homozygous sickle cell genotype (Hb S/S) suffer serious
and usually lethal sickling disease, and those with heterozygous
Hb A/S are selected for on the basis of their resistance to
falciparum malaria. It may be a rare instance in which hybrid
vigor or balanced polymorphism of a single genetic locus in
man is selected for by a known agent. While the epidemiological evidence is very strong, it is only very recently that
this conclusion has been experimentally verified. In studies
in vitro on the growth of *P. falciparum* in heterozygous Hb A/S
erythrocytes, it has been found that those cells which are
sickled, but curiously not the unsickled cells, are unsuitable
for permitting growth of the malaria parasite (78). Reflecting
on this, it is possible to speculate that the high incidence
of sickle cell anemia in American Blacks (the frequency of
the heterozygote Hb A/S is 10%) is the legacy of an earlier
genetic adaptation to resist the pressure of malaria in Africa.

Malaria may have selected another human gene, as well.
Miller *et al*. (28) have recently demonstrated that the receptor of erythrocytes recognized by *P. vivax*, which produces a
malaria in man, and by *P. knowlesi*, a monkey malaria, is the
Duffy blood group determinant. The Duffy negative genotype
(FyFy), while rare in most of the world's populations, is present with a frequency of over 90% among West Africans. Again,
it is suggestive that the malaria parasite selected against the
Duffy blood group antigens in Africa, and consequently Blacks
are almost totally resistant to vivax malaria.

HOW PARASITES CHANGE THEIR SPOTS: ANTIGENIC VARIATION

There is no more striking example of successful adaptation
of a parasite to the host's immune response than that exhibited
by African trypanosomes, which live entirely extracellularly
in the blood stream of ungulates or man, where they cause
sleeping sickness. As long ago as 1907 Massaglia (cf. 21)
observed that following infection through the bite of the
tsetse fly, the numbers of parasites in the blood fluctuated
periodically, and suggested that this succession of parasitemia,
remission, and recrudescence was due to the destruction of
trypanosomes by host antibody and the emergence of parasites
of different antigenic constitution. The course of these
waves of parasitemia in a single patient described in 1910 is

illustrated in Fig. 2. Human sleeping sickness is caused primarily by two subspecies of *T. brucei* known as *gambiense* and *rhodesiense*. Following each wave of parasitemia, antibodies, generally agglutinins or lysins are produced, which are exclusively individual variant-specific.

What are the possible genetic and regulatory mechanisms that could explain antigenic variation? The simplest hypothesis would be that most infections contain a mixed population of parasites comprising several strains, and as the predominant strain grows and is killed, there is simply outgrowth of another variant type present in the original inoculum. This hypothesis was essentially disconfirmed by experiments in which single trypanosomes were cloned and maintained in immunologically compromised animals and antigenic variation was not seen. When transferred to conventional animals, even though all of the population derived clonally from a single organism, antigenic variation was seen (22).

A second hypothesis would be mutation, possibly involving small determinants in the molecule, which are immunodominant and which could vary randomly to elude the immune response. In fact, a mutation frequency of 1.2×10^{-5} has even been calculated as being adequate to explain the appearance of variants in a clone at 3-4 day intervals (23). Opposed to this hypothesis are the findings of Grey that antigens of a clone tend to appear in an apparently programmed sequence (24).

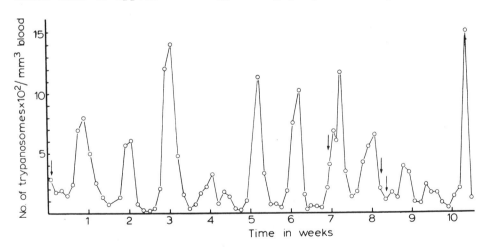

FIGURE 2. Parasitemia occurring in a patient with African trypanosomiasis (from Vickerman, reference 21).

Thus, display of variant antigens A-B-C-D-? appears to be non-random, and passage of variants at any stage back through the tsetse fly results in reversion to the basic antigenic variant type A of the strain. It is difficult to explain this programmed sequence on the basis of simple random mutation.

A third possible mechanism is an adaptive phenotypic variation, in which the parasite has a finite number of genes that can code for its surface antigens and that it can switch on and off in a regular sequence. There are several precedents relevant to this process in classical genetic studies on antigenic variation in other microorganisms. Studies on antigenic variants of paramecia revealed a cytoplasmic regulatory factor (plasmid) that controls the differential expression of surface antigens in the presence of antibody. In phase variation of H or flagellar antigens of *salmonella*, there are only two phases and two gene loci with many alleles at each locus that can vary. This gene-switching model is the one currently held out to be most likely and relevant to antigenic variation in African trypanosomes.

Does antibody select or induce variants? As early as 1909 Ehrlich found that trypanosomes incubated with homolygous antiserum and then injected into mice produced a parasitemia of a different variant type. As mentioned before, passage of clones of trypanosomes or variants in immunologically incompetant animals results in clonal fidelity without antigenic variation. Grey (25) was able to perturb the programmed antigenic succession in the rabbit by passively protecting animals against four variants of a strain and then challenging with that strain. The rabbits thereupon produced antibody to a fifth variant when challenged with the original strain, which is suggestive that antibody has both an inductive as well as a selective role in antigenic variation.

What is the nature of the antigens that vary? Cross (26, 27) has demonstrated that the outer coat of *T. brucei* contains a surface coat or glycocalyx that is comprised principally, if not exclusively of the variant specific glycoprotein antigen. This antigen has a molecular weight of 67,000 and constitutes 10% of the entire cell protein and 30% of the soluble proteins. The variant glycoprotein molecules contain between 7 and 17% carbohydrate, and have widely varying isoelectric points from pH 5 to 10. Enzymic digestion studies indicate that the carbohydrate-containing portion is that closest in apposition to the plasma membrane. Approximately 7×10^6 molecules are found per trypanosome, a number sufficient to cover the entire surface of parasite, and Cross has suggested that this coat, which projects 12-15 nm from the plasma membrane, may serve as a spacer or barrier sufficient to prevent antibody and complement from ever reaching the plasma membrane.

When the amino acid sequence ananlysis was carried out on isolated purified variant glycoproteins, Cross found in the N-
terminal 20-30 residues essentially no structural homologies.
Each had a unique sequence, and there was no obvious evidence
for deletions or frame-shifts, thereby virtually eliminating
the mutational hypothesis for antigenic variation.

It has become possible for the first time to cultivate
African trypanosomes *in vitro* (75) using a bovine cell feeder
layer, and it may now be possible to study the inductive or
selective effects on antibodies on antigenic variation *in
vitro* with cloned parasite populations, to provide insights
on the molecular mechanisms of genetic and regulatory control
underlying antigenic variation.

Antigenic variation has also been well documented in the
genus Plasmodium, which causes malaria, and in *babesia*, a tick-
borne parasite of cattle rather similar to malaria (28,31).
However, the importance of antigenic variation in the survival
of these parasites is much less well documented than in the
case of trypanosomes. Something often referred to as "antigenic variation" has been found in a nematode, *Nippostrongylus
brasiliensis*, a worm that parasitizes the small intestine of
rats and serves as a model for many worm infections of man.
Ogilvie (32) has found that larvae obtained from rats immunized by previous infection develop into adult worms that are
less immunogenic than adult worms obtained from hosts undergoing primary infection.

Lastly, it is important to mention the possibility that
parasites can "cap" their surface antigens off to elude the
immune response. Doyle *et al.* (33) have shown that within
minutes after exposure of *leishmania* to fluorescent antibodies
at 37°C, the parasites capped off their surface antigens and
became refractory to the effects of immune sera and complement.
It is not known whether capping occurs *in vivo* and represents
an important mechanism for escape of protozoa from immune
attack.

ANTIGENIC MIMICRY AND CONCOMITANT IMMUNITY

While the term "concomitant immunity" is most familiar to
immunologists in the context of a tumor-bearing animal in which
an autochthonous transplant of the primary tumor is rejected
while the primary tumor grows progressively to kill the animal,
there is a precisely analogous phenomenon that occurs during
infection with a number of parasites. The terms "concomitant
immunity" (34) or "premunition" (30) are used to describe a
form of acquired immunity in which the established parasitic

infection persists long after resistance has developed against
a challenge infection, perhaps the best example being that of
schistosomiasis. This disease, which afflicts an estimated
200 million people worldwide, is a chronic disease caused by
the trematode, *schistosoma*. *S. mansoni* and *S. japonicum* invade in the portal and mesenteric systems and produce a hepa-
tosplenic disease and *S. haematobium* causes a disease of the
urinary tract.

Adult schistosome worms reside in the mesenteric venules
often for many years. This persistence is characteristic of
infection by some types of worms, and for many there is little
evidence to indicate that they stimulate any immune response
at all. However, in the case of schistosomes, adult worms do
induce an immune response that can prevent reinfection of the
same animal with immature schistosome forms (34). Adult worms
were transferred to portal veins of monkeys that had never ex-
perienced the immature migrating forms. When challenged with
the immature form called cerceria, the monkeys resisted infection, but they could not reject the transferred adults.
Thus the immunologic paradox is how it is possible for adult
worms to engender an immune response that can prevent infection by immature forms while remaining unaffected by the immune response that they engender.

Two explanations have been proposed for parasitic concomitant immunity. One would hold that the parasite, by natural
selection, evolved some antigenic determinants similar or identical to those of the host. One difficulty with this hypothesis, at least with respect to schistosomes, is that the organism can grow in a variety of mammalian hosts, and it is unlikely that an organism would have evolved major antigens
common to a wide variety of hosts. An alternative hypothesis,
originally suggested by Smithers and Terry (34), is the possibility that schistosomes adapt to the range of hosts in which
they grow by appropriating some host molecules onto their surface layer or tegument. This has been amply demonstrated for
S. mansoni (35). In initial experiments, worms were grown in
both mice and gerbils, and transferred either to normal rhesus
monkeys, or to monkeys immunized against erythrocytes of mice
or gerbils. The results indicated that adult worms transferred to normal monkeys resumed their egg laying and were
viable after about 5-6 weeks. Adult worms transferred from
mice to monkeys immunized against mouse erythrocytes were
killed, and failed to establish themselves. Monkeys immunized
against mouse erythrocytes failed to inhibit the growth of
adult worms grown in gerbils. These experiments demonstrated
the acquisition of mouse antigens onto adult worms.

In order to explain concomitant immunity, it is necessary
to argue that these host antigens may be acquired by the adult

worms but would not be found on the immature forms, since the
immune response of the chronically infected host can kill the
immature forms. In point of fact Clegg (36) demonstrated that
the most immature form, the cercaria, is not killed by the
monkeys immunized against mouse erythrocytes, and hence does
not appear to have host antigens, but that by 7 days, the
intermediate stage of the parasite, the schistosomula, has
already acquired host antigens. This finding has been confirmed in a reciprocal experiment in which the ability of an
antibody and complement to kill was tested on schistosomulas
cultured *in vitro* in medium containing the red cells and/or
serum of the host species (37,38). If acquisition of host
antigens indeed contributes to escape of the parasite from
immune recognition, then immune serum should be less effective
on schistosomula maintained in the presence of host erythrocytes and serum, and that was found to be the case.

What are the host antigens found to be acquired by these
organisms? When schistosomula are cultured with human type A,
type B, or type O erythrocytes, the schistosomula have been
shown to have group A, group B, and the H blood group antigens,
respectively, on their outer layer (39). Blood group Rh or
MN determinants are not found but several other host serum
proteins have been found. One wonders whether other host antigens, such as histocompatibility antigens, are adsorbed to
parasites as well (*c.f.* paper by Sher, this volume). As intriguing as the present data are, there unfortunately is as yet no
compelling evidence to establish that "mimicry" is responsible
for the failure of adult worms to be rejected by the host.

LEARNING TO LIVE IN YOUR MACROPHAGES

From the time of Metchnikoff, macrophages have been described as highly phagocytic cells capable of killing and degrading a wide variety of microbes. Nevertheless, a number of
microorganisms including *M. tuberculosis*, *M. leprae*, and protozoa such as *toxoplasma*, *besnoitia*, *leishmania*, and *T. cruzi*
survive and grow for part or all of their stay in the mammalian host inside macrophages. At least three different mechanisms can be defined to account for the ability of these parasites to evade killing by the macrophage, although the molecular basis for these phenomena remains largely unknown. It
is similarly unclear how important these mechanisms studied
in vitro are to the survival of the parasites *in vitro*.

Extracellular particles that are phagocytized by macrop-
phages enter by invagination of the plasma membrane and appear
in phagocytic vesicles (43). There follows a fusion between

TABLE IV. *Lysosomal Fusion and Killing by Mouse Macrophages Infected with Some Parasites*

	Fusion	Killing
T. gondii	−	−
L. donovani	+	−
T. cruzi	+	−/+*
M. lepramurium	+	−
M. tuberculosis	−	−
M. tuberculosis + antibody	+	−

^{a}*Some escape killing in normal macrophages and penetrate into cytoplasm; most can be killed by BCG macrophages.*

the phagocytic vesicle and primary lysosomes, known to contain degradative enzymes, and probably peroxisomes to form secondary lysosomes. In addition, fusion between secondary lysosomes and phagocytic vesicles is known also to occur (see Table IV).

A. *Failure to Fuse*

A number of parasites have evolved mechanisms to prevent fusion of primary and secondary lysosomes with the phagocytic vesicle containing the invader. Human virulent *M. tuberculosis* grows intracellularly in vesicles within macrophages, but these fail to fuse with lysosomes (44). When secondary lysosomes were labeled with electron-dense ferritin, it was shown that the ferritin was not found in the vesicles containing the mycobacteria, and the organisms were not killed. However, when the mycobacteria were killed or damaged by irradiation, fusion readily occurred. Ironically, fusion could be induced by coating viable mycobacteria with antibody (45), but the organism, even after lysosomal fusion, remained viable. A very similar pattern has been recorded for *T. gondii* (46). Once again, viable organisms are readily ingested by macrophages *in vitro*, but there is a failure of lysosomes, e.g., secondary lysosomes labeled with thorotrast, to fuse with the phagocytic vesicle. Opsonization of the parasite with antibody permits fusion of secondary lysosomes with the phagocytic vesicle. In this case, the effect of antibody is to facilitate killing of the *toxoplasma*. A third case is that of *Chlamydia psittaci*, a model for the chlamydia that causes trachoma,

which is phagocytized by L-cells and seems to block lysosomal
fusion. The mechanism by which the living parasites are able
to block lysosomal fusion in host cells remain largely unknown.

B. *Resistance to Killing*

As mentioned above, when *M. tuberculosis* is opsonized,
lysosomal fusion occurs, but the mycobacteria are perfectly
capable of surviving within the lysosome. An even more dramatic instance of this phenomenon of resistance to the killing
mechanisms of macrophages is provided by *M. lepramurium*, which,
even in the absence of antibody, is found in vesicles that fuse
avidly with primary and secondary lysosomes. In spite of
this, the organism grows unimpeded (44). Similarly, *leishmania*
grow exclusively in macrophages, and survives and multiplies
in lysosomes even after fusion has occurred (40).

A subtle example of survival in macrophage lysosomes is
provided by two species of *leishmania*. *L. enrietti* produces
a disease similar to human cuteneous Leishmaniasis or Oriental
sore in the guinea pig; *L. tropica* produces a similar disease
in mice. When mouse macrophages were activated by sensitization for delayed hypersensitivity either to *L. enrietti* or its
soluble protein antigens and then challenged *in vitro*, Mauel
and Behin (47) found them to be resistant. However, when similar procedures were used for activating guinea pig macrophages,
L. enrietti was not killed. Conversely, activated guinea pig
macrophages were highly resistant to *L. tropica*, but failed
to resist challenge with *L. enrietti*. Thus, these leishmania
have developed quite specific, but unknown, mechanisms for
eluding the destructive capability of macrophages from the
species they normally infect, while being susceptible to the
killing mechanisms of activated macrophages from animal species
that are resistant to infection by them. An elegant control
in these experiments was the simultaneous infection of activated guinea pig macrophages with *L. enrietti* and *Listeria
monocytogenes*, to ascertain whether the Leishmania survived
by nonspecifically blocking the macrophage cytocidal mechanisms (48). The results obtained were striking in that, under
these conditions, *listeria* in the same phagosomes were in fact
killed, but the Leishmania survived. Thus, there is an extraordinary selectivity in the evolution of resistance to macrophage killing by *leishmania*.

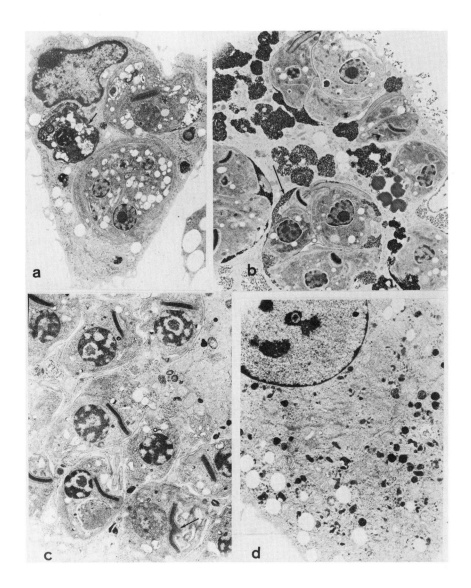

FIGURE 3.   (a)   Normal mouse peritoneal macrophages infected with epimastigotes of T. cruzi at a ratio of 1:1 after
2 hours. Note that parasites are in the process of being digested (→) (3000×). (b) BCG-activated macrophages infected
with T. cruzi at a ratio of 10:1 after 2 hours. Thorium dioxide is seen in secondary lysosomes and fusion with parasite
containing vacuole (→) (3000×). (c) Normal mouse peritoneal
macrophage at a 1:1 infection ratio after 96 hours. Trypanosomes are present in cytoplasm where division has begun to

C. *Escape from the Lysosomes*

In studies on the interaction of *T. cruzi* with normal and activated murine macrophages, we and others (49-51) have observed that virtually all phagocytized trypanosomes were found, after 2 hours, intracellularly in phagocytic vesicles, and that lysosomal fusion almost invariably occurred (Fig. 3b). Resident, unstimulated peritoneal macrophages within the first 24 hours were as effective as BCG-activated macrophages in killing and degrading a high proportion of the infection organisms. However, when infected cultures were examined at 72-96 hours, a remarkable picture was seen. Resident macrophages were found to have large numbers of trypanosomes growing within the cytoplasm, and when the thorotrast labeling technique was used, virtually none of these parasites could be found in a vesicle containing the lysosomal marker (Fig. 3c). They appeared to be able to escape from their precarious predicament within the lysosome, and take up residence in the cytoplasm, where the macrophage has no specialized mechanism for killing foreign invaders. In contrast, by 3-4 days following infection, macrophages nonspecifically activated by BCG had essentially killed and degraded virtually all of the parasites, and only debris was seen (Fig. 3d).

While escape from lysosomes is in general not seen in bacteria, there is evidence that *M. leprae* may be an exception (44), and that during the period of logarithmic growth in the mouse footpad, the organism appears to reside in the cytoplasm. Interestingly, when infected mice ultimately develop cell-mediated immunity to the human lepra bacillus, the growth of the organism plateaus and mycobacteria are found in vesicles surrounded by double membranes, suggesting they indeed are being contained and killed within the lysosomes (76).

A word of caution, however, is in order regarding interpretation of the *in vitro* interaction of parasites and macrophages. For example, while BCG-activated macrophages effectively destroy carefully chosen numbers of infecting *T. cruzi* *in vitro*, BCG immunized mice of highly susceptible strains show little or no resistance to challenge with *T. cruzi in vivo*. Interestingly, however, the most susceptible strain of mouse is the C3H, which, in fact, appears not to be responsive to the adjuvant effect of the BCG (42). Similarly, it has been shown that chronic infection of mice with *toxoplasma* or *besnoitia* establishes a state of chronically activated macrophages (79). Macrophages from such chronically infected ani-

---

occur (→). There is no evidence of lysosomal fusion (4800×). (d) BCG-activated mouse peritoneal macrophage after 192 hours of infection with T. cruzi. *There is no evidence of trypanosomes and some evidence of secondary lysosomes (2400×).*

mals are resistant not only to the infecting organism, e.g., *toxoplasma*, but are also resistant nonspecifically to infection with listeria and kill tumor cells (52). However, the animals themselves appear to be quite specifically resistant to the immunizing organisms. Thus, Toxoplasma-infected animals resist challenge with Toxoplasma but are susceptible to *besnoitia,* and vice versa (53,77).

Another potential hazard is interpreting the *in vitro* macrophage studies is the failure to discriminate between growth inhibition and killing. While activated macrophages have well demonstrated ability to *inhibit the growth* of L. *monocytogenes* and *T. gondii*, it is not clear that they have an enhanced capability to *kill* the infecting inoculum any better than unstimulated macrophages (54,55).

JAMMING THE IMMUNE RESPONSE

One of the obvious adaptive mechanisms for eluding a normal host response, which was unlikely to be passed up in evolution, is suppression of the immune response by parasites. A number of parasites have availed themselves of this possibility. For example, immunosuppression has been reported in hamsters infected with L. *donovani* (56), mice infected with *T. gondii* (57), and rats infected with the roundworm *Nippostrongylus brasiliensis* (58). However, by far the most impressive and clinically important instances of the immune suppression of the host response occur in African trypanosiasis (58,80), malaria (60), and kala azar. In the case of human sleeping sickness malaria and visceral leishmaniasis (kala azar), elevated levels of IgM are characteristic, on occasion rising to 5 gm/100 ml (61). In spite of the high levels of IgM, 5% or less of these immunoglobulins have been found to react specifically with antigens of *P. falciparum* or *T. gambiense*, the parasites responsible for malaria and sleeping sickness, respectively, in West Africa (61, 80). At the same time, in the case of malaria and African trypanosomiasis it is well documented that responses of patients to salmonella antigens and tetanus toxoid, and animals to SRBC, is markedly reduced. In this paradoxical situation there is markedly heightened production of antibodies to the parasites with depressed humoral immunity to other antigens.

A number of animal models have been developed to probe the mechanisms of this type of immunosuppression. For example, mice infected acutely or chronically with *P. berghei* malaria show a marked depression in development of both direct and indirect Jerne PFC, the effect being more pronounced on the IgG

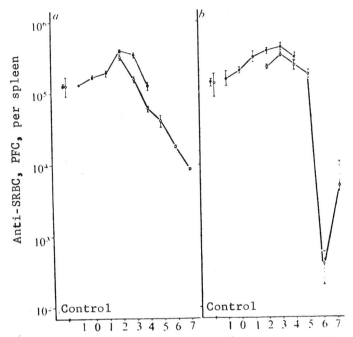

Day of SRBC administration in relation to infection day

FIGURE 4. Rise in SRBC background IgM PFC in T.b. brucei
*in infected mice in relation to blood parasitemia. Male
Balb/c mice were infected with 1000 parasites i.p. (from Hudson et al., reference 62).*

plaques (60). Even more striking suppression is seen in mice
infected with *T.b. brucei* (62). When a careful study was made
of these systems, even more impressive than the suppression of
specific antibody production was the marked increase in the
background of direct plaque-forming cells to SRBC, generally
at least a log higher in infected than in uninfected animals
(Fig. 4). Thus, infection with *plasmodia* or *trypanosomes*
caused a marked increase in the background PFC not only to SRBC
but also for spontaneous plaque-forming cells on donkey, horse,
or TNP-RBC. The high background and lack of specificity are
strongly reminiscent ob the observations made on mouse spleens
treated 1-2 days prior to immunization with a plyclonal mitogen, such as endotoxin (LPS) (63). There is an increase in
immunoglobulin, an increase in polyclonal antibodies, which
account for the background, and a diminution in specific PFC.
On the basis of these experiments, it has been proposed that
one mechanism for inducing immunosuppression is a polyclonal

mitogenic activity of the malaria and trypanosome parasites
(80). These experiments raise the concern that in conditions
of unknown etiology in which there are increased levels of immunoglobulins, as in the cerebrospinal fluid (CSF) in patients
with multiple sclerosis or in rheumatoid joint fluids, the
possibility exists that the elevated immunoglobulins may not
in fact be specific antibodies, but polyclonal immunoglobulins
induced either directly or indirectly by an infectious agent.

A further mechanism for parasite-induced immunosuppression
has recently been suggested for the African trypanosomes in
mice (64). Spleen cells from infected conventional mice showed
a diminished response to mitogens: spleens of infected nu/nu
mice did not. When spleen cells from infected conventional
were mixed with normal spleens, they had the ability to suppress the response to mitogens. It was suggested that this
immunosuppressive effect was mediated by suppressor T-cells,
and possibly suppressor macrophages, although the suppression
could not be eliminated by treatment of the infected spleens
with anti-thy 1 and complement.

The observations on the immunosuppression by parasites
have implications beyond merely the survival of the specific
parasite. It is well known that patients with sleeping sickness have an increased susceptibility to secondary bacterial
infections, a problem recognized in some of the earliest
studies on the disease. Children in the tropics with acute
falciparum malaria have similarly high rates of bacterial infection, although it must be noted that many also have other
parasitic infections, and more importantly, protein calorie
malnutrition and avitaminosis. Nevertheless, responses in
children to tetanus toxoid from villages with malaria prophylaxis are higher than those from comparable villages where
malaria infection is frequent. It may furthermore not be co-
incidental that Burkitt's lymphoma (65) occurs mainly in
geographical areas coincident with holoendemic malaria. It is
conceivable that the malaria-induced immunosuppression could
provide a favorable environment for development of lymphoma
viruses. This possibility has received experimental confirmation from the studies of Wedderburn in mice in which the incidence of lymphomas in mice infected with both malaria and
murine leukemia virus was dramatically higher (60, 66).

SUBVERSION OF THE IMMUNE SYSTEM

While the above examples illustrate the ability of parasites to evade the immune system, there are at least two fascinating examples in which the immune system may be requisite
for survival of the parasite. *Babesia rodhaini* and Theileria

species are protozoan blood parasites that can infect mammalian hosts and are transmitted in nature by ticks. They are
of considerable importance because they infect cattle, **babesia**
producing a malaria-like disease in cattle all over the world
and *Theileria parva* causing a disease known as East Coast
fever, which affects cattle primarily in East Africa. Babesia
rarely produce disease in humans, and three of the first reported cases involved individuals who had undergone splenec-
tomy, though there have recently been a number of cases reported in the northeast United States.

In the case of *babesia*, it has recently been found that
this organism appears to require complement activation, specifically C3, factor B, and possibly C5, in order to penetrate
the erythrocyte in which it grows. C3- or C5-deficient mice
or mice treated with cobra venom are protected from infection
(67).

Unquestionably the most fascinating case of subversion of
the immune system is that of *T. parva*. This parasite enters
lymphocytes where it transforms the lymphocytes into lymphoblastoid cells (68,69). The intracellular parasite, in its
large form called the macroschizont, divides by binary fision
and increases in number tenfold every 3 days until almost all
the lymphoid cells are parasitized (70). During this process
there is a marked lymphocytosis resembling the uncontrolled
growth of a leukemia or lymphoma. From about the tenth day of
infection, increasing numbers of the macroschizonts break a-
part into large numbers of microschizonts. In the process,
host lymphocytes are destroyed and small infectious particles
termed micromerozoites are released, which invade red cells.
There the parasite develops an intraerythrocytic stage, which
rapidly infects and destroy RBCs until anemia and death result. In enzootic areas in East Africa, 40% of the calf crop
may die from this disease (75).

The most extraordinary aspect is that when lymphoblasts
obtained from cattle infected with *T. parva* are put into
tissue culture, they develop into continuously growing lymphoblastoid cell lines (71). Bovine cells from uninfected animals are not known to develop into continuous cell lines.
Thus, *T. parva* appears to be the only parasite other than oncogenic viruses capable of transforming lymphocytes into continuous growth. In culture, there is an extraordinary syn-
chrony between mitosis of the macroschizont and its host lymphoid cell (70), although this is not obligatory, since the
macroschizonts continue to divide within lymphoid cells that
have been irradiated to block their division (72). In culture,
the transition of the macroschizonts to the infectious fragments does not occur unless the normal culture conditions are

TABLE V

Protozoa	Vector	Host
T. cruzi	triatomid bug	man and other mammals
T.b. gambiense T.b. rhodensiense	tsetse fly	man, cattle

P. vivax
  (benign tertian malaria)
P. falciparum
  (malignant tertian)
P. malaria
  (Quartan malaria)
P. Ovale
	anopheles
	  mosquito
		man

L. donovani	sand fly	man
L. tropica	sand fly	
L. braziliensis	sand fly	man

T. gondii	congenital; in-
	  fected meat, o-
	  ocysts in cat stool
		man, animals

Babesia	tick	cattle, occa- sionally man
T. parva	tick	cattle

Helminths
  S. mansoni
  S. japonicum
  S. hematobium
	snail
	snail
	snail
		man

Primary geographic area	Disease
Central-South America	Chagas' disease (South Am. try-panosomiasis) Acute: myocarditis, hepatospleno-megaly, menintoencephalitis; 10% mortality primarily in children Chronic: cardiomyopathy, mega-colon megaesophagus
Africa	African sleeping sickness, lymph-adenopathy, splenomegaly
South America, Africa, Asia	Intraerythrocytic parasite of man, hemolytic anemia, splenomegaly
South America, Africa, Asia	
Africa, Asia	
Africa	
Mediterranean, Asia, South America	Visceral Leishmaniasis, kala azar, fever, hepatosplenomegaly, leu-kopenia
Asia, Middle East	Cutaneous Leishmaniasis, "orien-tal sore"
South America	Espundia; mucocutaneous ulceration of naso-oral area
	Lymphadenopathy, myocarditis, pneumonitis, encephalitis, ce-rebral calcifications
Worldwide in cattle; predo-minantly Nantucket Island, Long Island	Intraerythrocytic parasite of man and animals; causes hemolytic anemia
East Africa	Causes hemolytic anemia and lym-phocytosis
Caribbean, Brazil, Africa Asia Africa	Chronic hepatosplenic disease, portal hypertension, pulmonary hypertension; hematuria, urinary tract disturbance

perturbed, e.g., by incubating infected lymphoblastoid cultures at 42°C (73). It is tempting to speculate that *in vivo* this process may be initiated by a spike of fever.

While skeptics may insist that it is unlikely for a protozoan to induce a neoplastic transformation of lymphoid cells, and that the parasite may be carrying an oncogenic virus, it is notable that the continuous persistently infected bovine lymphoblastoid cell lines, when transferred back to susceptible cattle, have been demonstrated to induce protection to tick-borne infection with *T. parva* in about 80% of the instances (74). This does not rule out a virus, however, and one would like to see an attempt to cure the lines of the parasite with antibiotics, to ascertain whether they remain transformed. On the other hand, when lymphoblastoid cell lines obtained from one of a pair of freemartins or identical twins is injected into the other, East Coast fever and death have followed, suggesting that one of the properties of the continuously infected lymphoblastoid cell lines that may enhance their efficacy as vaccines is the probability that the cells are histoincompatible with the majority of recipients, and the host-versus-graft allogeneic reaction that ensues may serve as a useful adjuvant.

COMMENT

The purpose of this essay has clearly not been to provide a comprehensive or even critical review of what is known about mechanisms for escape of immune surveillance by parasites. The hope has been to indicate that the immunology of parasites, and the sophisticated and subtle mechanisms by which they interact with the immune system is an extraordinarily challenging subject. It is also a very important one for millions of people in the world. Enough is now known about fundamental mechanisms of immunology applicable to specific problems in parasitic immunity to ensure real progress in medical intervention in some, but probably not all parasitic diseases (see Table V). Lastly, as in the other area in which the scientific method is applied to disease-related problems, e.g., the studies of Avery and his collaborators on pneumococcal pneumonia at the Rockefeller Institute in the 1940s, the study of immunity to parasites is likely to provide new and fundamental knowledge of far wider application than to the individual organism or disease initially studied.

Acknowledgments

We are grateful to Dr. Thomas Trischmann for allowing to present his unpublished results, and to Ms. Yvonne Kress for generously providing the electron micrographs. We wish also to express our appreciation to Drs. L. Miller, M. Rifkin, and M. P. Cunningham for helpful discussions.

References

It would have been impossible to prepare this article without the help of several excellent reviews of the immunology of parasites. We have "parasitized" many of these, and both gratefully acknowledge our indebtedness to these sources and recommend them to immunologists who wish to pursue problems of immunity to parasites in more detail. The principal reviews are listed as follows:

A. *Reviews*

1. Ogilvie, B. M., and Wilson, R. J. N. Evasion of the immune response by parasites. *Br. Med. Bull. 32*, 177, 1976.
2. *Ciba Foundation Symposium 25.* "Parasites in the Immunized Host: Mechanisms of Survival." Elsevier, Amsterdam, 1974.
3. Cohen, S., and Sadun, E. "Immunology of Parasite Infections." Blackwell Publ., Oxford, 1976.
4. Jackson, J., Herman, R., and Singer, I. "Immunity to Parasitic Animals." Appleton-Century-Crofts, New York, 1970.
5. Soulsby, E. J. L. The control of parasites: The role of the host. *Proc. Helminth. Soc. 44*, 28, 1977.
6. Miller, L., Pino, J., and McElvey, J. "Immunity to Blood Parasites in Animals and Man." Plenum Press, New York, 1978.
7. Warren, N., and David, J. R., eds. *Am. J. Trop. Med. Hyg. Suppl.*, 1977.
8. *Transplantation Reviews 19.* "The Immune Response to Infectious Diseases."
9. W.H.O. "World Health Statistics Report," Vol. 30. WHO, New York, 1977.

B. *Specific References*

10. Bloom, B. R. *Nature 260*, 380, 1976.
11. Desowitz, R. S. *Ann. Trop. Med. Parasitol. 53*, 293, 1959.

12. Stewart, J. L. *Vet. Rec. 63*, 453, 1951.
13. Fairbairn, H. *Ann. Trop. Med. Parasitol. 27*, 185, 1933.
14. Muniz, J., and Boriello, A. *Rev. Brasil Biol. 5*, 563, 1945.
15. Nogueira, N., Bianco, C., and Cohn, Z. *J. Exp. Med. 142*, 224, 1975.
16. Trischmann, T., Tanowitz, H., Wittner, M., and Bloom, B. R. *Exp. Parasit. 45*, 160, 1978.
17. Bradley, D. J. *Nature 250*, 353, 1974.
18. Steeves, R., and Lilly, F. *Ann. Rev. Genet. 11*, 1977.
19. Piazza, A., Belvedere, M. C., Bernoco, D., and Cepellini, R. *In* "Histocompatibility Testing 1972" (J. Dausset and J. Colombani, eds.), p. 73. Munksgaard, Copenhagen, 1975.
20. Allison, A. C. *In* "Immunity to Protozoa" (P. C. C. Garnham, A. E. Pierce, and I. Roitt, eds.), p. 109. Blackwell Publ., Oxford, 1963.
21. Vickerman, K. *Ciba Found. Symp. 25*, 53, 1974.
22. Doyle, J. *In* "Immunity to Blood Parasites in Animals and Man" (L. Miller, J. Pino, and J. McElvey, eds.). Plenum Press, New York, 1978.
23. Watkins, J. F. *J. Hyg. 62*, 1964.
24. Gray, A. R. *J. Gen. Microbiol. 41*, 195, 1965.
25. Gray, A. R. *Ann. Trop. Med. Parasitol. 59*, 27, 1962.
26. Cross, G. A. M. *Parasitology 71*, 303, 1975.
27. Cross, G. A. M. *Am. J. Trop. Med. Hyg. Suppl.*, 1977.
28. Miller, L. H., Mason, S. J., Dvorak, J. A., McGinniss, M. H., and Rothman, I. K. *Science 189*, 561, 1975.
29. Brown, K. N. *Ciba Found. Symp. 25*, 35, 1974.
30. Sergent, E. *In* "Immunity to Protozoa" (P. C. C. Garnham, A. E. Pierce, and I. Roitt, eds.), p. 39. Blackwell Publ., Oxford, 1963.
31. Brown, K. N. *Nature 230*, 163, 1971.
32. Ogilvie, B. M. *Ciba Found. Symp. 25*, 81, 1974.
33. Doyle, J. J., Behin, R., Manuel, J., and Rowe, D. S. *J. Exp. Med. 139*, 1061, 1974.
34. Smithers, S. R., and Terry, R. J. *Adv. Parasitol. 7*, 41, 1969.
35. Smithers, S. R., Terry, R. J., and Hockley, D. J. *Proc. Roy. Soc. London B. Biol. Sci. 171*, 483, 1969.
36. Clegg, J. A., Smithers, S. R., and Terry, R. J. *Int. J. Parasitol. 1*, 43, 1971.
37. Dean, D. A., and Sell, K. W. *Clin. Exp. Immunol. 12*, 525, 1972.
38. Clegg, J. A. *Ciba Found. Symp. 25*, 161, 1974.
39. Clegg, J. A., Smithers, S. R., and Terry, R. J. *Nature 232*, 653, 1971.
40. Chang, K.-P., and Dwyer, D. M. *Science 193*, 678, 1976.

41. Friis, R. R. *J. Bacteriol. 110*, 706, 1972.
42. Lagrange, P. Cited in *WHO Rep. 34d IMMLEP Sci. Working Group*, TDR/SWG/IMMLEP (3)/77.
43. Van Furth, R., ed. "Mononuclear Phagocytes." Blackwell Publ., Oxford, 1975.
44. Draper, P., and Hart, P. D. *In* "Mononuclear Phagocytes" R. Van Furth, ed.), p. 575. Blackwell Publ., Oxford, 1975.
45. Armstrong, J. A., and D'Arcy Hart, P. *J. Exp. Med. 142*, 1, 1975.
46. Jones, T. C., Yeh, S., and Hirsch, J. G. *J. Exp. Med. 136*, 1173, 1972.
47. Mauel, J., and Behin, R. *Transplant. Rev. 19*, 121, 1974.
48. Behin, R., Mauel, J., Biroum-Noerjasin, and Rowe, D. *Clin. Exp. Immunol. 20*, 351, 1975.
49. Kress, Y., Bloom, B. R., Wittner, M., Rowen, A., and Tanowitz, H. *Nature 257*, 394, 1975.
50. Hoff, R. *J. Exp. Med. 142*, 299, 1975.
51. Noguiera, N., and Cohn, Z. *J. Exp. Med. 143*, 1402, 1976.
52. Hibbs, J. B., Jr., Lambert, L. H., Jr., and Remington, J. S. *J. Infect. Dis. 124*, 587, 1971.
53. Hoff, R. L., and Frenkel, J. K. *J. Exp. Med. 139*, 560, 1974.
54. Borges, J. S., and Johnson, W. D., Jr. *J. Exp. Med. 141*, 483, 1975.
55. Fowles, R. E., Fajardo, I. M., Leibowitch, J. L., and David, J. R. *J. Exp. Med. 138*, 952, 1973.
56. Clinton, B. A., Stauber, L. A., and Pulczuk, N. C. *Exp. Parasitol. 25*, 171, 1969.
57. Strickland, G. T., Voller, A., Pettit, L. E., and Fleck, D. G. *J. Infect. Dis. 126*, 54, 1972.
58. Keller, R., Ogilvie, B. M., and Simpson, E. *Lancet 1*, 678, 1971.
59. Urquart, G. M., Murray, M., and Jennings, F. W. *Trans. Roy. Soc. Trop. Med. Hyg. 66*, 342, 1972.
60. Wedderburn, N. *Ciba Found. Symp. 25*, 123, 1974.
61. Cohen, S. *Ciba Found. Symp. 25*, 3, 1974.
62. Hudson, K. M., Byner, C., Freeman, J., and Terry, R. J. *Nature 264*, 258, 1976.
63. Coutinho, A., and Moller, G. *Adv. Immunol. 21*, 113, 1975.
64. Jayawardena, A., and Waksman, B. H. *Nature 265*, 541, 1977.
65. Burkitt, D. P. *J. Nat. Cancer Inst. 42*, 19, 1969.
66. Wedderburn, N. *Lancet 2*, 1114, 1970.

67. Chapman, W. E., and Ward, P. A. *Science 196*, 67, 1977.
68. Barnett, S. A. *In* "Immunity to Protozoa" (P. C. C. Garnham, A. E. Pierce, and I. Raitt, eds.), p. 180. Blackwell Publ., Oxford, 1963.
69. Ristic, M. *In* "Immunity to Blood Parasites in Animals and Man" (L. Miller, J. Pino, and J. McElvey, eds.), p. 83. Plenum Press, New York, 1978.
70. Jarrett, W. F. H., Crighton, G. W., and Pirie, H. M. *Exp. Parasitol. 24*, 9, 1969.
71. Malmquist, W. A., Nyindo, M. B. A., and Brown, C. G. D. *Trop. Anim. Health Prod. 2*, 139, 1970.
72. Irvin, A. D., Brown, C. G. D., and Stagg, D. A. *Exp. Parasitol. 38*, 64, 1975.
73. Hulliger, L., Brown, C. G. D., and Wilde, J. K. H. *Nature 211*, 328, 1966.
74. Cunningham, M. P. *In* "Immunity to Blood Parasites in Animals and Man" (L. Miller, J. Pino, and J. McElvey, eds.). Plenum Press, New York, 1978.
75. Hirumi, H., Doyle, J. J., and Hirumi, K. *Science 196*, 992, 1977.
76. Evans, M., and Levy, L. *Infect. Immun. 7*, 76, 1973.
77. McLeod, R., and Remington, J. S. *Cell Immunol.*, 1977.
78. Friedman, M., and Trager, W. *Am. Soc. Trop. Med. Hyg.*, 1977.
79. McLeod, R., and Remington, J. S. *J. Trop. Med. Hyg.*, 1978.
80. Greenwood, B. M. *Ciba Found. Symp. 25*, 137, 1974.

DISCUSSION

DR. LILLY: Why was Duffy-negativity not selected for in
Europe as it was, apparently, in Africa since vivax malaria
was a grave problem in Europe until relatively recently?
DR. BLOOM: I don't know.
DR. AMOS: Are you sure that it's a very common deficiency?
I thought Duffy-negative was relatively rare, except in some
parts of Africa.
DR. BLOOM: Dr. L. Miller has recently completed a study of
West Africans; he was unable to find a Duffy-positive. The
people are almost universally Duffy-negative.
DR. LILLY: I can confirm that; it's in Race and Sanger.
DR. WYLER: I can confirm it also. There's very little
incidence of Duffy-positive; Duffy-negative is very high.
DR. AMOS: Are these Duffy-negatives doubly negative?
DR. YUNIS: Yes, they're Fy/Fy homozygous double negatives.
DR. DIENER: May I suggest, as an alternative to what you
call "jamming of the immune system by polyclonal activation,"
that the increased background to various red cells and DNP derives from exposure of cryptic red cell autoantigens?
DR. BLOOM: I don't know how to deal with that. In Africa, everybody would have a good background to endotoxin so
that it isn't impossible that it could be an LPS-like phenomenon or it could be some other polyclonal mitogen.
DR. PREHN: I would take mild issue with one of your state-
ments. To do so, I will tell you that in Maine a moose sometimes goes berserk and appears on the main street of Bangor
or Portland. Such moose are inevitably found to be suffering
from infection with "brain worms." The worms cause a marked
inflammatory response that does the damage. Several years
ago, several hundred healthy deer were slain as a population
control measure. It was found that the soft tissues of the
retro-orbital spaces of every deer were loaded with "brain
worms" but there was no histological evidence of any inflammation or any defense mechanism. Both parasites and deer were
healthy. Thus, the statement that, in the absence of some
immunological defense, the parasite will necessarily kill the
host may not always be entirely correct. Sometimes, as in
this instance, it appears that the inflammatory reaction to a
foreign invader is the cause of the morbidity. Numerous
other examples of similar phenomena could be cited.
DR. BLOOM: Your point is well taken. To every simple
and sweeping generalization there will be exceptions. Not
only in their saprophytic interactions, I should point out
that there are exceptions at the other extreme of my generalization. I understand that in lower animals there are para-

sites that must indeed kill their hosts in order to be transmitted. I guess H. L. Mencken had the last word when he said,
"To every complex question, there is a simple answer--and it's
always wrong."

DR. LILLY: Along these lines, it seems that in the mouse
leukemia virus system, the nonimmune genetic mechanisms for
resistance are very frequently not the mechanisms that cause
absolute resistance. Therefore, it is likely that the immune
system actually "mops up," that is, the nonspecific defense
systems have reduced the infection to a point at which the
immune system can cope. Wouldn't you think this is important?

DR. BLOOM: Yes, David Bradley has evidence that, in
Leishmania infections, there is a major autosomal, dominant,
non-H-2-linked, major determinant of resistance. If you compare mouse strains that are normalized for this mechanism,
there is a difference between those that will live and those
that will die. The gene that determines this difference and
functions after the spread of disease is controlled, is H-2
linked. I would guess that it would have the same role here
as that which H-2 has in leukemia.

DR. WYLER: I have a comment. One of the common aspects
of the protozoal diseases that initiate both polyclonal activation and immunosuppression is the presence of tremendous
amounts of particulate antigen in the circulation. In addition, splenomegaly with macrophage hyperplasia occur in these
diseases and the splenic macrophages ingest the parasite
material. In the malaria model, we have found that early in
infection adherent spleen cells elaborate, *in vitro*, increased
amounts of lymphocyte-activating factor. Later in infection,
they elaborate a factor that suppresses T cell responses. By
"feeding" normal macrophages parasitized erythrocytes, we can
reproduce these findings *in vitro*. It therefore seems likely
that the immunomodulating effects of soluble macrophage products on T cells may possibly play a role in mediating polyclonal activation and immunosuppression in these diseases.

DR. SCHWARTZ: I'd like to ask a somewhat simple-minded,
and perhaps heretical, question. We teach our medical students that the purpose and function of the immune system is
to protect against infectious diseases, but I wonder if that
is correct. In thinking about your presentation, the idea
occurred to me that we could have had a similar talk about
bacterial infections if there were no such things as antibiotics. If we go back to the 1920s, people were dying of pneumococcal pneumonia because either the organism had evaded
the immune system or the immune system was inadequate for
dealing with the infection. So, it may be a mistake to believe what we teach the medical students in the first instance.
Of course, if this is correct, then the whole idea of an immu-

nological approach to these infections is wrong. Maybe what you should be seeking is a "penicillin" for schistosomiasis instead of trying to manipulate the immune system.

DR. BLOOM: We teach our students a little differently. In fact, one of the questions we always ask is to have them identify those infectious diseases which, in the absence of antibiotics, medical intervention or prophylaxis, the immune system can handle. My second point is that many people have been looking for effective drugs in these diseases for a long time. In fact, there may well not be any; in Chagas disease, for example, there is no vaccine or drug that can be used. I don't think our objectives are mutually exclusive.

DR. GOOD: I would like first to react to Dr. Schwartz' most provocative question simply by noting the extraordinary contribution that has been made by "the experiments of nature" represented by the patients with the genetically determined immunodeficiency diseases. There is a striking difference between normal children and patients who cannot make antibodies with respect to how pneumococcal and streptococcal infections are handled. The oldest children with Bruton's X-linked agam-maglobulinemia are just the age of penicillin, because with-out their immune system they go on to die of their first in-fection. Thus, I think we should continue to teach medical students the importance of the immune system in normal sub-jects in resistance to bacterial, viral, and fungus infection and to learn about parasitic infections so that we can inter-pret what we are observing appropriately. The importance of immunity in resistance to these parasitic infections is pro-bably best reflected by the complex interfaces that exist be-tween the adaptive parasites and the equally adapted immune system that is revealed in Dr. Bloom's magnificent discussion. I am impressed by many things that Dr. Bloom said, but I must challenge the idea that it is a monoclonal activation of B lymphocytes that accounts for the hypergammaglobulinemia in kala azar, malaria, and other diseases in which the immu-nologic machinery is jammed. A corollary of this view would be that polyclonal activation should not be compatible with very much antigen-antibody complexes in the circulation. The facts are just the opposite; in each of these diseases, there are huge amounts of complexes and they are activating the complement system.

DR. BLOOM: My guess is that with so much immunoglobulin, it is possible to have high levels of complexes and polyclonal immunoglobulin coexisting as well.

DR. LEVY: I'd like to comment. Another interesting ex-ample of adaptive antigenic variation is equine infectious anemia (EIA) virus. Dr. Kono in Japan has demonstrated that this virus, very quickly after infection of horses, changes

its envelope antigen.   The horse develops neutralizing antibodies to the parental strain but a different type emerges in
the horse.   The only mechanism of eliminating the infection
is via cellular immunity against the shared group-specific
antigen.   This variation occurs very rapidly.   Most interestingly, EIA replicates preferably in macrophages.

DR. LILLY: Is it parallel to the variation in influenza
virus?

DR. LEVY: It's much faster.

DR. DOHERTY: With the influenza viruses, very rapid mutational changes can be induced by selecting virus in the presence of monoclonal antibodies derived from B cell hybrid
clones.   These experiments have been done by Drs. W. Gerhard
and R. G. Webster.

DR. MUSHER: I would like to remind you of the lack of analogy between bacterial and parasitic infections.   Most bacterial infections are acute and fulminating, while the parasitic and protozoal infections are chronic.   Streptococcal
sepsis has little to do with infections discussed by Dr.
Bloom.   Mycobacteria, *Brucella abortus,* and *T. pallidum* (if
you consider it a bacterium) are among the few that cause
chronic infection.   *Staphylococcus aureus* occupies an intermediate position.   The chronic infections are the ones that
present the interesting problem of escape from immune surveillance.

DR. GOOD: I'd like to respond.   Don't things really
change when you have an immunodeficiency?   In immunodeficiency
the very low grade pathogens or even intermediate grade pathogens, like staphylococci, induce chronic infections and produce the same kind of things in patients with failure of their
phagocytic mechanisms.   For this reason, I believe that the
bulk of this acute component is due actually to the reactions
of the immune system in one way or another.

GENETIC RESISTANCE TO ECOTROPIC TYPE-C RNA VIRUSES[1]

Philip N. Tsichlis[2]
Susan E. Bear
Henry St. G. Tucker[3]
Robert S. Schwartz

Tufts Cancer Research Center
and the Department of Medicine
Tufts University School of Medicine
Boston, Massachusetts

INTRODUCTION

Genes within the major histocompatibility (H-2) complex of the mouse are known to influence susceptibility or resistance to virus-induced neoplasms (1). These genes exert effects on both spontaneous virus-induced tumors (2) and those that arise after deliberate infection with certain oncogenic viruses (3-9). H-2-linked resistance to virus-induced leukemia is, however, not absolute. In the case of the Gross leukemia virus, the $H-2^b$ haplotype confers dominant resistance, where $H-2^{k/k}$ mice are susceptible. However, as Boyse showed, congenic AKR ($H-2^{k/k}$) and AKR ($H-2^{b/b}$) mice ultimately have the same incidence of leukemia (10), although the disease has a longer latent period in the latter than in the former strain. Genes outside the H-2 complex may also affect viral leukemogenesis. For example, more than a dozen years ago Tennant and Snell implicated several non-H-2 genes in susceptibility to Tennant virus-induced leukemias (11). This was followed by evidence for at least two non-H-2-linked genes (*Fv-1* and *Fv-2*) (12), one of which plays a definitive role in susceptibility

[1]*This investigation was supported by grant #CA 07937 and Contract #NO-1-CP-61046, awarded by the National Cancer Institute, DHEW.*
[2]*Fellow of the American Cancer Society.*
[3]*Damon Runyon Fellow.*

or resistance to almost all mouse leukemia viruses (13-16).
Inferential evidence has also suggested that a non-H-2-linked
gene (*Rgv-2*) is involved in the case of the Gross Passage A
virus (17) and, more recently, a locus that is not linked to
the H-2 complex (*Srlv-1*) has been implicated in susceptibility
to radiation leukemia virus-induced leukemia (18).

Therefore, loci within the H-2 complex are not the sole
factors that determine the outcome of viral leukemogenesis.
Elsewhere, we have delineated the concept that viral leukemogenesis is a multiphasic, complex process (19), each step of
which is under genetic control. The genome of the mouse contains structural genes of potentially oncogenic viruses (20-
24) genes that regulate the expression of these structural
genes (25), additional genes that restrict the replication of
the virions (13-16), genes that influence immunity to the viruses (26), and probably numerous other genes that contribute
to the intricate process of malignant transformation, expansion of the transformed clone, and its ultimate development
into a recognizable neoplasm. In our view, the final outcome
depends on interlocking mechanisms determined by multiple
genes.

Given that multiple genes are involved in the process of
leukemogenesis, the determination of susceptibility or resistance to virus-induced leukemia can be thought of as a "black
box" experiment. Typically, mice naturally expressing virus or
deliberately injected with a leukemogenic virus are observed
for a certain period of time and the number of cases of leukemia are enumerated and correlated with H-2 haplotypes or
other genetic traits. Although this kind of experiment may
provide linkages between leukemia and a particular genetic
locus, nothing is revealed about the mechanism involved.

Our approach, which will be presented here, is to inject
mice with an oncogenic virus, thus bypassing structural viral
genes and regulatory cellular genes, and then to examine the
genetic mechanisms by which resistance (or susceptibility) to
the injected virus is mediated. If we accept that naturally
expressed retroviruses are a necessary requirement in the leukemogenic process (this is supported by extensive literature)
(27-31), an understanding of the mechanisms involved in resistance or susceptibility to the viruses may provide insights
into the process of viral leukemogenesis.

MATERIALS AND METHODS[1]

Mice. All mice used in this work were purchased from the
Jackson Laboratory, Bar Harbor, Maine, except the B10.G
strain, which was kindly provided by Dr. Jack Stimpfling, Mc-
Laughlin Research Institute, Great Falls, Montana, and the
AKR (H-2[b]) strain, kindly provided by Dr. Elizabeth Stockert,
Sloan Kettering Memorial Cancer Research Institute, New York.
The B10.A mice used were provided from an ecotropic virus-
negative colony established in our laboratory (30). All F_1
mice were bred in our laboratory.

Preparation of Virus. A potentially oncogenic, endogenous
ecotropic (B-tropic) virus of B10.A origin was grown in BALB/c
3T3 cells. The cells were cultured in Dulbecco's Modified
Eagle's Medium (Grand Island Biological Company, New York),
which was supplemented with 120 units of penicillin/ml, 120
µg of streptomycin/ml and 10% FCS. Supernatants were pooled,
clarified by centrifugation at 4°C (12062g for 10 minutes),
aliquoted in siliconized vials, and frozen at -70°C. The content of infectious virus was determined by the XC plaque
assay (32). Before injection the virus was diluted in medium
without FCS to a concentration of 10^3 PFU/ml. Each mouse received 200 PFU (0.2 ml) IP. Control animals received 0.2 ml
of medium IP.

Virus Assay. The XC procedure of Rowe *et al.* (32) as
modified by Melief *et al.* (33) was used. MEF were prepared
from 14-17 day old NIH-Swiss and BALB/c embryos. On day 1 the
embryo cells were trypsinized from primary lines and seeded
into 60 × 15 mm plastic Petri dishes (Falcon Plastics, Oxnard,
California) at a concentration of 4×10^5 cells/dish. The
next day, after 1 hour of treatment with 25 µg/ml DEAE-dextran
(Sigma Chemical Co., St. Louis, Missouri) in 2 ml of media
without FCS, the embryo cells were overlaid with ten-fold
serial dilutions of spleen cells in 4 ml of medium using 10^7
viable cells at the most concentrated inoculum. The culture
medium was changed on day 4, and on day 7 after inoculation

---

[1]*Abbreviations used in this paper: Mice: B10 for C57BL/
10 Sn, B10.A for B10.A SgSn, B10.Br for B10.Br SgSn, B10.D2/o
for B10.D2 old Sn and B10.D2/n for B10.D2 new Sn. Other:
anti-VEA antibody, antibody to viral envelope antigens; MEF,
mouse embryo fibroblasts; MuLV, murine leukemia virus; FCS,
fetal calf serum; PFU, plaque-forming unit; IP, intraperitoneally; IV, intravenously; DEAE-dextran, diethylaminoethyl
dextran.*

the medium was aspirated again, the plates were irradiated
with 1000-1500 ergs/mm^2 UV light, and immediately overlaid
with 1×10^6 XC cells/dish. Three days later the plates were
fixed with methanol and stained with Giemsa. A dissecting
microscope was used for enumeration of the plaques. By definition, a plaque is an area where there are at least three
syncytiae and absence of growth of XC cells.

When the virus titer in a fluid preparation was tested,
the semiconfluent MEF monolayer was overlaid with 0.4 ml of
tenfold serial dilutions of virus. After an adsorption time
of 45 minutes and cells were overlaid with 4 ml of media.
The remainder of the procedure was as described above. All
cell cultures were grown in MEM 4X (Grand Island Biological
Co., Grand Island, New York) supplemented with antibiotics and
10% unheated FCS.

Antiviral Envelope Antibody (VEA). The radioimmune precipitation assay of Ihle *et al.* (34) was used. Briefly, test
plasma or serum was serially diluted in TNE (0.05 *M* Tris HCl,
0.10 *M* NaCl, 0.001 *M* EDTA, pH 7.3) and incubated with 0.05 ml
of ^{3}H-leucine-labeled ecotropic virus (26), containing 0.2 µg
of protein ($\doteq$6000 cpm), for 1 hour at 37°C. The virus-antibody complexes were precipitated with a polyspecific rabbit
antimouse gamma-globulin serum (Cappel Laboratories, Downing-
town, Pennsylvania). Radioactivity of the supernatant and
washed precipitates was determined after they were dissolved
in Aquasol. The anti-VEA titer was expressed as the $\log_2$ of
the highest dilution of serum or plasma that caused 50% precipitation of the radiolabeled virus.

Cell-Mediated Cytotoxicity (Table 1). Virus-resistant
and -susceptible animals were tested. The effector cells
(spleen, lymph node, nylon wool column T-enriched spleen cells,
and peritoneal exudate cells) were sensitized against the virus either *in vivo* (virus-injected animals) or *in vitro* by
incubation with infected fibroblasts. Nonsensitized lymphoid
cells were used as controls. Spleen and lymph node cells
were prepared by mincing the organs through a sterile tantalum
screen and peritoneal exudate cells by flushing the peritoneal
cavity with sterile Hanks balanced salt solution (Grand Island
Biological Co., Grand Island, New York).

Virus-infected MEF, PHA (Wellcome Reagents Ltd., Beckenham,
England) -stimulated AKR (H-2^k) and AKR (H-2^b) spleen cells,
and EL-4(H-2^b) tumor cells were used as targets. All target
cells were tested for expression of virus with the XC infectious center assay (33). Effector cells and target cells were
matched for H-2 and comparisons were made between infected
and uninfected mice of the same strain. After labeling with

TABLE I. Methods That Failed to Detect CMI in Virus-Infected Mice[a]

Sensitization	Detection system
Virus inoculation	^{51}Cr release
In vitro incubation	End-labeling
(with infected fibroblasts)	

Effector cells	Strains
Spleen	C57L
Lymph node	C57Bl/10
T-enriched spleen	DBA/2
PEC	Bl0.A

Target cells	Positive control
Fibroblasts	Allogeneic sensitization
Tumor cells	
PHA blasts	

[a] Performed by H. S. Tucker, 1976-1977.)

^{51}Cr, the target cells were washed three times and incubated with effector cells at 37°C in a 5% CO_2 atmosphere at a ratio of $\frac{200}{1}$ to $\frac{5}{1}$ in a volume of 200 µl in RPMI 1640 supplemented with 10% FCS. After 4 hours of incubation the cells were centrifuged at 200 rpm for 10 minutes and 100 µl of the supernatant was counted in a gamma counter. The results were expressed as percentage specific lysis, which was calculated using the following formula:

$$\text{specific lysis (\%)} = \frac{\text{experimental } ^{51}Cr \text{ release} - \text{spontaneous } ^{51}Cr \text{ release}}{\text{maximum } ^{51}Cr \text{ release} - \text{spontaneous } ^{51}Cr \text{ releast}} \times 100$$

In a few experiments using fibroblasts as targets, cytotoxicity was measured using end-labeling of surviving targets with ^{51}Cr (35).

Antibody and Complement-Mediated Cytotoxicity. The same target cells used in cell-mediated cytotoxicity were used here. 50 µl of cell suspension (1 × 10⁵ cells) in RPMI 1640 containing 10% heat-inactivated FCS were incubated with 50 µl of serial dilutions of known heat-inactivated mouse serum known to contain anti-VEA antibodies. After 45 minutes of incubation at 37°C in a 5% CO_2 atmosphere, an optimal concentration of hamster complement was added and the mixture was incubated for 30 more minutes. The degree of cytotoxicity was determined by trypan blue (0.1%) exclusion.

Virus Neutralization Assays. Approximately 100 PFU of virus of the appropriate tropism were incubated in 0.2 ml of MEM 4X containing twofold serial dilutions of anti-VEA antibody-containing serum. After one hour of incubation at 37°C in a 5% CO_2, atmosphere the mixture was diluted to an approximate volume of 0.4 ml and plated on embryo fibroblasts of the appropriate tropism. The XC test procedure was then carried out. The virus was either frozen-thawed or freshly harvested according to the method of Ihle *et al.* (36).

Rabbit Antimouse Lymphocyte Serum (ALS) and Normal Rabbit Serum (NRS). ALS was purchased from Microbiological Associates, Bethesda, Maryland, as Lot No. 13120. The sera was raised by inoculation of Swiss Webster mouse lymph node cells into New Zealand white rabbits. The ALS we used had an endpoint cytotoxicity titer against Swiss Webster lymph node cells of 1:6400 and prolonged skin graft survival of DBA/2 → C57BL/6 to 25.4 ± 2.7 days over a control survival time of 10.4 ± 1.3 days when inoculated in four doses of 0.25 ml IP every other day. The normal rabbit sera (NRS) was also purchased from Microbiological Associates and represents the bleeding of an age-matched uninjected New Zealand white rabbit.

Thymectomy. Thymectomy of young (3-4 week old) B10 mice was performed under a dissecting microscope by suction of the thymus after incision above the sternal notch.

Antithymocyte Serum. Rabbit antimouse thymocyte sera (ATS), lot 15183, was purchased from Microbiological Associates, Bethesda, Maryland. The sera was raised in New Zealand white rabbits by inoculation of Swiss Webster mouse thymocytes and effected a mean survival time of 30.1 ± 1.6 days of skin grafts of DBA/2 on C57BL/6 mice. In our laboratory this ATS was tested in a complement-dependent cytotoxicity assay utilizing B10 spleen, thymus, and bone marrow. At a dilution of 10^{-3}, the ATS killed 96.6% of thymocytes, 38.3% of spleen cells, and 5% of bone marrow cells.

Thymus Reconstitution. Thymectomized and ATS treated mice were reconstituted with a syngeneic, age- and sex-matched subcutaneous thymus graft and 10^8 thymus cells IV.

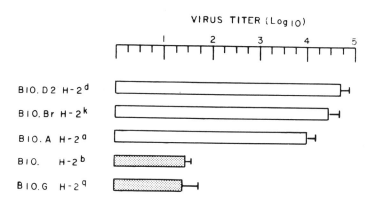

FIGURE 1. *Virus titer in the spleen of five congenic
strains of mice injected with 200 PFU of an ecotropic B-tropic
virus isolated from a healthy old B10.A mouse, 10 weeks after
virus inoculation. The titers are expressed as $\log_{10}$ of the
number of XC plaques/10^7 viable spleen cells. Mean $\pm$ SE. An
average of 25 mice/strain was used.*

RESULTS

*Resistance to Deliberate Infection by B-Tropic Virus in
Congenic Strains of Mice.* The following congenic resistant
strains of mice were injected IP at the age of 6 weeks with
200 PFU of B0tropic virus: B10 ($H-2^b$), B10.A ($H-2^a$), B10.D2/o
($H-2^d$, C5 deficient), B10.D2/n ($H-2^d$, C5 normal), B10.Br
($H-2^k$), and B10.G ($H-2^q$). Ten weeks after virus inoculation,
the virus titer in the spleen of each mouse was examined by
the XC infectious center assay. The results, expressed as
$\log_{10}/10^7$ spleen cells, are shown in Fig. 1. The mice can be
divided into two groups: *virus-susceptible* [B10.Br ($H-2^k$),
B10.D2/o ($H-2^d$), B10.D2/n ($H-2^d$), and B10.A ($H-2^a$)] and *virus-
resistant* [B10 ($H-2^b$) and B10.G ($H-2^q$)]. Since the mice are
congenic, the data suggest that one or more genes within the
H-2 complex are important in the early phases of infection by
the virus. The results in B10.D2/o (C5 deficient) and B10.D2/n
(C5 normal) mice indicate that deficiency of C5 does not lead
to higher levels of virus than in corresponding mice without
the deficiency.
    The reproducibility of the results is shown in Fig. 2,
which demonstrates two separate experiments in C57BL/10 mice
inoculated with different batches of B-tropic virus. The re-

sults obtained in the two experiments are virtually identical.
The virus titers obtained in the B10 strain follow a normal
distribution, and 96% of these mice have a titer less than
$\log_{10}$ 3.5 (mean + 2 SD). This value, 3.5, clearly separates
the resistant B10 from the susceptible B10.D2/o and B10.Br
strains (Fig. 3). We therefore use a mean $\log_{10}$ titer of 3.5
to define resistance and susceptibility: any strain with a

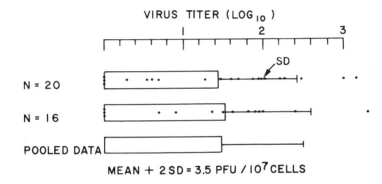

*FIGURE 2. Virus titers in the spleen of individual virus
inoculated B10, B10.Br and B10.D2/o mice 10 weeks after virus
inoculation. Clear-cut difference between resistant and susceptible strains.*

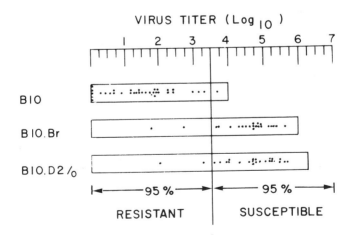

*FIGURE 3. Virus titers in the spleen of virus-inoculated
B10 mice, 10 weeks after virus inoculation. Two experiments
done 1 year apart using two different batches of the same virus.*

mean $\log_{10}$ titer less than 3.5 (when tested 10 weeks after infection) is called *resistant* and any strain with a mean $\log_{10}$
titer of 3.5 or higher (when tested 10 weeks after infection)
is called *susceptible*. This definition applies only to infection by the B-tropic virus we used.

Response to Infection in (Susceptible × Resistant) Crosses.
Six week old (B10 × B10.Br)F_1 mice were injected with 200 PFU
of virus and the titers in their spleens was estimated 10 weeks
later. The results are shown in Fig. 4. All the F_1 hybrids
were resistant, but there was a tendency in these animals
toward slightly higher virus titers than their B10 parents.
This might indicate a gene dosage effect. A similar effect
has been shown by Chesebro *et al*. in their studies of recovery
from Friend virus-induced leukemia (6).

Susceptibility to MEF to In Vitro *Infection by MuLV.* Although all B10 mice are $Fv-1^b$ and the virus we used was B-
tropic, an H-2-related effect on viral replication could not

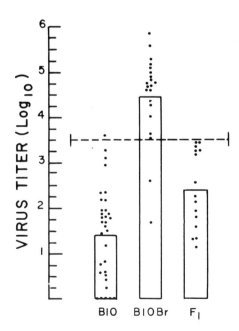

FIGURE 4. *Virus titers in the spleen of individual virus-
inoculated B10, B10.Br, and (B10 × B10.Br)F_1 mice. The results of (B10 × B10.A)F_1 were similar.*

TABLE II. *Susceptibility of MEF to the Same Multiplicity of Infection of MuLV*[a]

Strain	XC Plaques/plate: mean ± SE
B10.D₂/old	70.0 ± 5.4
B10	80.5 ± 6.8
BALB/c	79.2 ± 6.25

[a]*Hitness, 1 hit*

be excluded by the preceding results. Accordingly, embryo fibriblasts from B10, B10.D2/o, and BALB/c mice were infected with tenfold serial dilutions of virus. Six identical 60 mm Petri dishes were inoculated with each dilution of virus and the number of infected cells was determined. The results are given in Table II. There were no differences among susceptible and resistant strains, thus excluding an inherent block to infection or replication as the explanation of the preceding results.

Kinetics of Infection. Groups of 6-week-old B10 and B10.A mice were injected with 200 PFU of virus and then sacrificed every 2 weeks. Virus titers in the spleens of each group are shown in Fig. 5. No virus could be detected in either B10 or B10.A mice 2 weeks after infection. Six weeks after infection virus titers in both strains were similar; however, by 10 weeks relatively high titers persisted in B10.A mice, whereas they declined in B10 mice. Other data (not shown) indicate that relatively high titers of virus persist indefinitely in B10.A mice, whereas in B10 mice the virus continues to be present in low titers.

The results of these experiments again indicate that there is no H-2-related cellular restriction on the replication of the injected virus. The implications of this finding is that differences between resistant and susceptible strains can be attributed to a mechanism that comes into play after infection is established and that eliminates replicating, infectious virions.

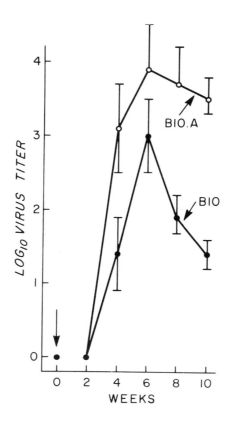

FIGURE 5. Kinetics of infection by the ecotropic B-tropic virus we used, in a resistant (B10) and a susceptible (B10.A) strain of cogenic mice. Each point represents the mean of the titer of an average number of 15 mice. The bars represent SE.

Immune Responses to Virus and to Virus-Infected Cells

Anti-(VEA) Antibody. Anti-VEA antibody levels were determined in the serum of mice 10 weeks after virus inoculation and simultaneously with determination of virus titers. The distribution of antibody titers in one resistant and two susceptible strains, as well as in the F_1 hybrids between a resistant and a susceptible strain, is shown in Fig. 6. Even though the resistant strain tends to have slightly higher antibody titers, the difference in antibody responses is minimal and of questionable significance. Figure 7 shows the correlation between the antibody titer in the serum and the simultan-

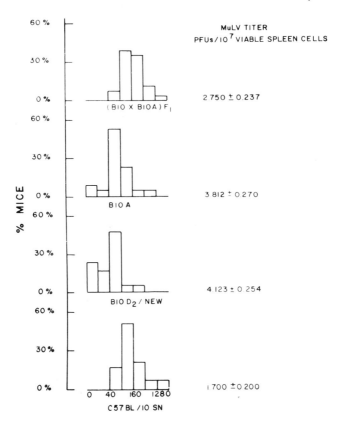

FIGURE 6. *Anti-VEA antibody titer distribution in three congenic strains of mice (B10, B10.D$_2$/o, B10.A) and the F$_1$ between B10 and B10.A, 10 weeks after virus inoculation. The antibody titer represents the dilution of mouse sera, which precipitated 50% of the radiolabeled virus.*

eously tested virus titer in the spleen. Although there was a tendency toward higher titers of antibody in resistant mice, the extreme variability of the data does not permit an association between the two. Figure 8 shows anti-VEA antibody titers in ALS-treated, virus-injected mice and controls. The ALS-treated mice had high titers of virus in their spleens, yet their anti-VEA antibody responses were in the range of those of the control mice.

The protective significance of antiviral antibody in these mice is further questioned by our inability to show any virus-neutralizing activity or cytotoxic activity of serum against virus-infected cells (data not shown).

Cell-Mediated Immune Response. Cell-mediated immune responses against virus-infected cells were examined in several

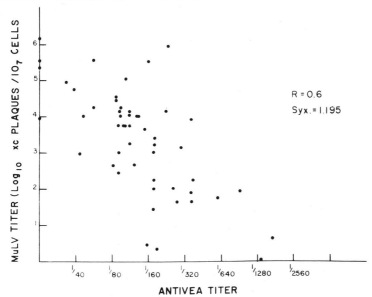

FIGURE 7. Anti-VEA antibody titer in the serum vs. virus
titer in the spleen of individual virus inoculated mice, 10
weeks after virus inoculation. The individual mice in this
figure belong to the B10, B10.D$_2$/o, and B10.A congenic strains.

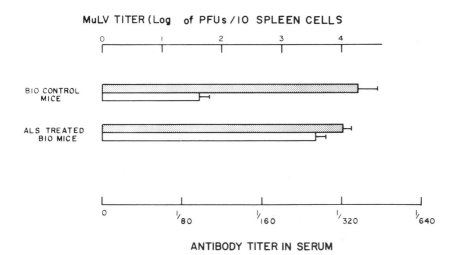

FIGURE 8. Virus (open bars) and antibody (dark bars)
titers in B10 mice treated with antilymphocyte serum (ALS)
and injected with virus, and B10 control mice injected with
virus only. Results at 10 weeks after virus inoculation.

TABLE III. MuLV Titers in the Spleen of B10 Mice Treated with Antilymphocyte Serum (ALS) and Inoculated with 200 PFUs of B-Tropic Ecotropic MuLV, 10 Weeks after Virus Inoculation

Treatment	Viral titer: log_{10} mean $\pm$ SE
ALS + virus	3.625 ± 0.180
ALS alone	0
NRS + virus	2.153 ± 0.311
NRS alone	0

ways (see Methods). Experiments using different sensitization schedules, different effector and target cells, and different detection systems failed to reveal any evidence of cell-mediated cytotoxicity in both susceptible and resistant animals (data not shown).

The Role of the Thymus. Virus-resistant B10 mice were injected IP at the age of 5-6 weeks with rabbit antimouse ALS every other day for four doses. Two days after the last injection of ALS, they were infected with 200 PFU of B-tropic virus. Mice treated with ALS alone, with normal rabbit serum plus virus, or with normal rabbit serum alone were used as controls. Virus titers in these mice are given in Table III. The normally resistant B10 mice were highly susceptible as a result of the ALS treatment. ALS or mouse rabbit serum alone did not stimulate the spontaneous expression of virus. Virus-infected mice treated with normal rabbit serum were not significantly different from mice given only virus.

Next, 3-4 week old mice were thymectomized and, after recovery, they were injected IP with four doses of ATS at 48-hour intervals. Ten days later, half of the mice were reconstituted with a subcutaneous syngeneic thymus graft and 10^8 thymocytes IV. Both thymus grafts and thymocytes were age- and sex-matched with the recipients. Six days later all mice were injected with 200 PFU of virus. A nonmanipulated group of B10 mice of the same age was injected with 200 PFU of virus. Titers of virus are shown in Fig. 9. Thymectomized, ATS-treated mice were highly susceptible to the virus, whereas ATS-treated mice that had been restored by thymus grafting behaved like intact, resistant animals. The results suggest that the thymus is required for H-2-mediated resistance to the B-tropic virus.

In another experiment, 6-week-old B10 mice were injected

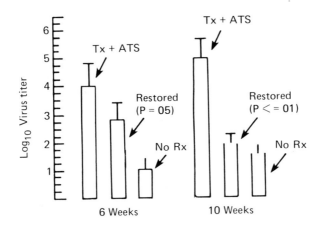

FIGURE 9. *Virus titers in the spleen in thymectomized and antithymocyte serum (ATS) treated vs. thymectomized and ATS treated thymus reconstituted mice. Virus-injected, otherwise unmanipulated B10 control mice were also used. All mice were injected with virus and were tested at 2, 6, and 10 weeks after inoculation.*

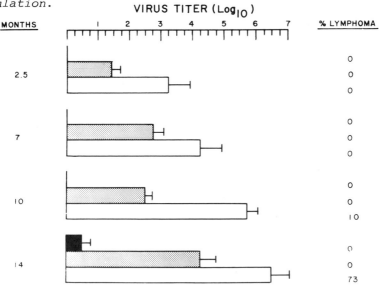

FIGURE 10. *Virus titers (mean ± SE) and incidence of malignancy in B10 mice injected with virus and treated with ALS at the age of 6 weeks (open bars). Control mice injected with virus only (hatched bars) and ALS only (dark bars) are also presented. Each group consisted of 10–15 mice except the group of virus-only mice tested 14 months after virus inoculation, which contained only four mice, three of which had low virus titers, one of which had a high virus titer.*

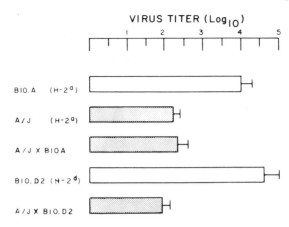

FIGURE 11. Virus titers (mean ± SE) in the spleen of virus-inoculated A/J, B10.A, (A/J × B10.A)F_1, and (A/J × B10.D_2/o)F_1 mice 10 weeks are virus inoculation. The titers in B10.D_2/o mice are shown for comparison. An average number of 25 mice/strain was tested.

with 200 PFU of virus; 3 weeks later, four doses of ALS (0.25 ml every other day) were given. Groups of animals were examined 2.5, 7, 10, and 14 months later. The results are given in Fig. 10. Not only were extremely high titers of virus observed, but 8/11 of the 14-month-old mice had reticulum cell sarcomas. Mice treated with ALS or virus alone failed to develope malignancies and had only low titers of virus.

Non-H-2-Linked Genes and Resistance to Infection. Susceptibility to the B-tropic virus was examined in B10.A and A/J mice, both of which are H-2[a]. Results are shown in Fig. 11. Whereas B10.A mice were susceptible, A/J mice were resistant. Therefore, a gene (or genes) affecting the early phases of infection by the virus must be located outside the H-2 complex. The results on the (A/J × B10.A)F_1 and (A/J × B10.D2/o) F_1 hybrids shown in the same figure indicate that the non-H-2-linked gene(s) act in a dominant fashion. The number and location of the non-H-2-linked gene(2) are unknown. The mechanism of its action is probably similar to the mechanism of action of the H-2-linked gene, in view of the lack of additive effect when the non-H-2 genes are present together with H-2[b], as in the A.BY mice (Fig. 12).

The possible role of immunological mechanisms involved in this phenomenon is also indicated by the high anti-VEA antibody titers seen in virus-injected A/J mice as shown in Fig. 13.

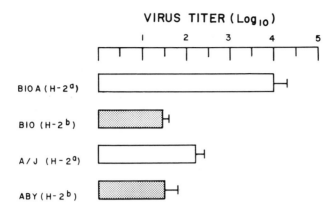

FIGURE 12. *Virus titers (mean ± SE) in the spleen of virus-inoculated A/J, B10.A, A.BY, and B10 mice.*

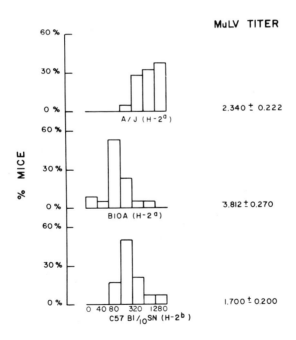

FIGURE 13. *Anti-VEA antibody titer distribution in A/J mice in comparison with the titers observed in B10 and B10.A mice.*

DISCUSSION

The evidence we have presented may be summarized as follows:

(1)   There are in the mouse mechanisms that can eliminate or inhibit the replication of MuLV after infection has been established.

(2)   These mechanisms are genetically controlled. Relevant loci map within the H-2 complex, but powerful resistance mechanisms are specified by a gene (or genes) located elsewhere.

(3)   Resistance conferred by the non-H-2 gene (or genes) is dominant; inheritance of the H-2-linked effect is complex and may be due to gene dosage.

(4)   Inability to control an established infection with the virus we studied was associated with a high risk of malignant lymphomas.

(5)   Thymocytes are essential for expression of H-2-linked resistance to the oncogenic virus. Suppression of thymic function resulted in persistent, chronic, high-grade infection and, ultimately, meoplasia. It is not yet known if thymocytes play any role in the non-H-2 gene(s)-mediated resistance to MuLV.

(6)   It is not clear how thymocytes participate in the process. Differences in levels of antiviral antibodies between susceptible or resistant mice are not decisive. An extensive search for cell-mediated immunity to virus in resistant mice was unrewarding.

The effects of the genes we studied are not absolute; the defense against ecotropic viruses also involves other genes, such as Fv-1 (13-16), and SRV (35), which exert effects on viral replication before infection is established. Although our studies used mice that were deliberately injected with virus, and thus bypassed structural or regulatory genes that control its expression, the results seem relevant to "natural" infection because ecotropic virus can rarely be isolated from mice that are resistant to injected virus (e.g., B10), whereas such virus is relatively common in mice that are susceptible to injected virus (e.g., B10.A) (30). Moreover, Nowinski and Doyle reported that athymic (nu/nu) BALB/c and C57BL/6 mice had high incidences of spontaneous ecotropic expression and significantly lower titers of antiviral antibodies than their intact (nu/+) littermates (37).

Our findings on the role of the thymus in H-2-mediated resistance to infection by ecotropic virus in deliberately infected mice, suggest that the immune system plays an import-

ant role in the early phases of infection with endogenous retroviruses. Anti-VEA titers in our studies of deliberately
infected mice showed some correlation with H-2 haplotype,
higher titers being associated with the resistance-mediating
haplotype H-2^b, but it is difficult to conclude that anti-VEA
antibody was the protective mechanism. There was, for example,
no correlation between the level of anti-VEA antibody and virus titer in individual mice of any strain. Moreover, B10
mice treated with antilymphocyte serum had very high virus
titers, yet the levels of anti-VEA antibody were no different
from mice injected with virus, but not treated with antilymphocyte serum. Furthermore, we could not demonstrate serum-
neutralizing activity against either frozen-thawed or freshly
harvested virus, and no cytotoxic activity against virus-
infected cells was found in the serum of mice with high anti-
VEA antibody titers. The role of humoral immunity in naturally infected mice has been extensively investigated. It has
been shown that all strains of mice spontaneously expressing
ecotropic virus produce antibody directed against the virus
(34,38-43) and, more specifically, against the virus envelope
glycoproteins gp70, gp45, and p15(E) (44-46). The level of
antibody was shown by Nowinski and Doyle to be genetically
controlled by an H-2-linked locus that specifies high antibody
titers in a dominant fashion (47,48). These antibodies can
neutralize freshly harvested infectious virus (36) and they
are cytotoxic against virus-infected cells (49). However, it
remains to be established whether they are protective *in vivo*.
Their constant association with persistent virus infection
suggests that any protective effects they may have are feeble.

There are as yet no convincing data that cell-mediated
immunity participates in the control of natural or deliberate
infection by ecotropic virus. Neither we nor Meruelo *et al.*
(9) have been able to find reproducible evidence *in vitro* of
cell-mediated immunity to the leukemogenic viruses we studied.
The inability to show directly that the immune system participates in H-2-linked resistance against ecotropic virus represents a paradox in view of the evidence that the thymus
plays an essential role in this phenomenon. This might be
explained by the insensitivity of the *in vitro* immunological
methods we used, or by the possible existence of immunological
control mechanisms that are not detected by conventional immunological techniques.

Thus far, our discussion has dealth only with the endogenous retroviruses of mice. Laboratory variants of these
viruses, including members of the Friend-Moloney-Rauscher
(FMR) group, as well as members of the murine sarcoma virus
(MSV) group, induce malignancies that can be highly immunogenic. The demonstration of both humoral and cell-mediated im-

muty against these viruses and the tumors they induce is relatively easy (50-52). The immunogenic properties of these
viruses may be due to modification of their proteins by mutation or recombination (53). Thus, immunological comparisons
between these agents and the endogenous viruses of mice must
be regarded with caution.

The mechanism by which genes of the H-2 system mediate
resistance to infection by exogenous murine retroviruses probably involves selective interaction between virus and H-2
components. Viral antigens, specifically gp70 (54, 55) and
p30 (56-59), are expressed on the cell surface of both productively and nonproductively infected cells. In the murine
sarcoma virus (MSV) and the Friend virus (52,59) systems it
has been shown that viral components expressed on the cell
surface interact selectively with products of the K and/or
D genes of the H-2 complex. Similar interactions were found
in methycholanthrene-induced, ecotropic virus-infected EL-4
leukemia cells (60,61). Thus, in these cases immune responses to viral antigens involve recognition of both viral
antigens and the associated H-2 components. If this applies
to endogenous leukemia viruses, some H-2 products, such as
those specified by H-2^k or H-2^d, may not interact with viral
antigens to form an immunogenic complex, whereas others, such
as H-2^b, might be relatively efficient in this regard. The
role of the H-2 gene products may, however, involve more than
immune recognition. Lilly and Freedman (62) have presented
evidence in the Friend virus system that the major histocompatibility complex seems to modify the expression of viral antigens or infectious virions by infected cells. Suppression
of viral expression by a permissive H-2 haplotype could allow
unchecked proliferation of the transformed cells. Alternatively, the relevant H-2 gene could inhibit expression of
the virus, thereby limiting its spread and reducing the risk
of leukemia.

The significance of our data on the early events of infection by ecotropic virus is indicated by the high incidence
of tumors in resistant B10 mice treated with ALS and injected
with virus. The effects of ALS are short-lived (63), and
the possibility it acts by abrogating an immune defense against
transformed cells is minimal. An important question currently
under investigation relates to virus interactions in the pre-
leukemia stage of these mice. The isolation of ecotropic-
xenotropic (polytropic) recombinant viruses from thymuses of
preleukemic AKR, C58 (64,65), HRS/J (66), and B10.AKM (P.
Tsichlis, unpublished observations) mice, as well as the demonstration of XC-negative ecotropic viruses with oncogenic
potential in spontaneous tumors of the AKR and the C58 strains
(67) indicate that the induction of a malignant clone is pre-

ceded by a change in the genome of the endogenous virus. This
genetic change in the virus could account for its oncogenicity.
High titers of ecotropic virus, as in antilymphocyte serum-
treated mice, could increase the probability of mutation or
recombination with a xenotropic virus in an animal that ex-
presses both agents. Therefore, the ability to suppress replication of even a nononcogenic retrovirus may reduce the
risk of malignancy since the mutational or recombinational
event may also lead to a virus with new antigenic determinants.
In a mouse already immunosuppressed by high titers of ecotropic virus (68-70) any immune response against the new antigens may be inefficient, thereby increasing further the
risk of leukemia.

Genes of the H-2 complex may also influence late steps in
viral leukemogenesis. Lilly *et al.* (31) studied the spontaneous expression of ecotropic virus and the incidence of
malignancy in (BALB/c × AKR)F_1 mice and in the backcross to
AKR. The H-$2^{k/k}$ mice had a higher incidence of malignancy
than the H-$2^{k/d}$ mice, even though there was no difference in
virus expression between them. Zarling *et al.* (71) and
Kiessling *et al.* (72-75) have described a class of killer
lymphocytes that is present in mice independently of retrovirus infection. These cells are cytotoxic both *in vitro* and
in vivo, against certain virus-induced tumor cells. The
presence of these lymphocytes ("natural killer cells") was
shown to be controlled at least by one gene linked to the H-2
complex (76,77). Their role in leukemogenesis might be important after tumor cells have been induced by the virus.

In conclusion, our work deals with the early events of
viral leukemogenesis, and more specifically with the control
over the replication of the virus after infection is established. We consider this as one step in the long series of
events by which endogenous murine retroviruses lead to the
development of leukemia. Each step is controlled by a different gene(s). The resistance or susceptibility to leukemia
conferred by any individual gene is not necessarily absolute
and the outcome is probably due to an interlocking series of
events. In this view, susceptibility to viral leukemia requires
a relatively large number of permissive genes, whereas resistance could be due to possession of relatively few inhibitory
genes. Perhaps this explains why leukemia is a rare disease
in genetically heterogeneous populations.

References

1. Lilly, F., and Pincus, T. *Adv. Cancer Res. 17*, 231, 1973.
2. Lilly, F. *Genetics 53*, 529, 1966.
3. Lilly, F., Boyse, E. A., and Old, L. J. *Lancet 2*, 1207, 1964.
4. Tennant, J. R., and Snell, G. D. *J. Nat. Cancer Inst. 41*, 597, 1968.
5. Lilly, F. *J. Exp. Med. 127*, 465, 1968.
6. Chesebro, B., Wehrly, K., and Stimpfling, J. *J. Exp. Med. 140*, 1457, 1974.
7. Muhlblock, O., and Dux, A. *J. Nat. Cancer Inst. 53*, 993, 1974.
8. Lonai, P., and Haran-Ghera, N. *J. Exp. Med. 146*, 1164, 1977.
9. Meruelo, D., Lieberman, M., Ginzton, N., *et al. J. Exp. Med. 146*, 1079, 1977.
10. Boyse, E. A., Old, L. J., and Stockert, E. *In Proc. Conf. on RNA Viruses and Host Genome in Oncogenesis, Amsterdam, May 12-15 1971* (P. E., Emmelot and P. Bentvelzen, eds.). North-Holland Publ. Co., Amsterdam, 1972.
11. Tennant, J. R., and Snell, G. D. *Nat. Cancer Inst. Monogr. 22*, 61, 1966.
12. Lilly, F. *J. Nat. Cancer Inst. 45*, 163, 1970.
13. Pincus, T., Hartley, J. W., and Rowe, W. P. *J. Exp. Med. 133*, 1219, 1971.
14. Pincus, T., Rowe, W. P., and Lilly, F. *J. Exp. Med. 133*, 1234, 1971.
15. Rowe, W. P., Hartley, J. W., and Lilly, F. *J. Exp. Med. 137*, 850, 1973.
16. Jolicoeur, P., and Baltimore, D. *Proc. Nat. Acad. Sci. USA 73*, 2236, 1976.
17. Lilly, F. *Transplant. Proc. 3*, 1239, 1971.
18. Meruelo, D., Lieberman, M., Deak, B., *et al. J. Exp. Med. 146*, 1088, 1977.
19. Schwartz, R. S., and Datta, S. K. *Blood Cells*, in press.
20. Todaro, G. T., and Huebner, R. J. *Proc. Nat. Acad. Sci. USA 69*, 1009, 1972.
21. Rowe, W. P. *Cancer Res. 33*, 3061, 1973.
22. Chattopadhyay, S. K., Lowy, D. R., Teich, N. M., *et al. Proc. Nat. Acad. Sci. USA 71*, 167, 1974.
23. Chattopadhyay, S. K., Rowe, W. P., Teich, N. M., *et al. Proc. Nat. Acad. Sci. USA 72*, 906, 1975.
24. Gelb, L. D., Milstien, J. B., and Martin, M. A. *Nature New Biol. 244*, 76, 1973.
25. Taylor, B. A., Meier, H., and Huebner, R. J. *Nature New Biol. 241*, 184, 1973.

26. Tucker, H. S. G., Weens, J., Tsichlis, P., *et al.* *J. Immunol. 118*, 1239, 1977.
27. Rowe, W. P., and Pincus, T. *J. Exp. Med. 135*, 429, 1972.
28. Huebner, R. J. *In* "Comparative Leukemia Research" (R. M. Dutcher, ed.), p. 22, Karger, Basel, 1970.
29. Peters, R. L., Hartley, J. W., Spahn, G. J., *et al.* *Int. J. Cancer 10*, 283, 1972.
30. Melief, C. J. M., Louie, S., and Schwartz, R. S. *J. Nat. Cancer Inst. 55*, 691, 1975.
31. Lilly, F., Duran-Reynals, M. L., and Rowe, W. P. *J. Exp. Med. 141*, 882, 1975.
32. Rowe, W. P., Pugh, W. E., and Hartley, J. W. *Virology 42*, 1136, 1970.
33. Melief, C. J. M., Datta, S. K., Louie, S., *et al.* *Proc. Soc. Exp. Biol. Med. 149*, 1015, 1975.
34. Ihle, J. N., Yurconic, M., Jr., and Hanna, M. G., Jr. *J. Exp. Med. 138*, 194, 1973.
35. More, R., Yron, I., BenSasson, S., *et al.* *Cell. Immunol. 15*, 382, 1975.
36. Ihle, J. N., and Lazar, B. *J. Virol. 21*, 974, 1977.
37. Nowinski, R. C., and Doyle, T. *Virology 77*, 429, 1977.
38. Oldstone, M. B. A., Aoki, T., and Dixon, F. J. *Proc. Nat. Acad. Sci. USA 69*, 134, 1972.
39. Hanna, M. G., Jr., Tennant, R. W., Yuhas, J. M., *et al.* *Cancer Res. 32*, 2226, 1972.
40. Batzing, B. L., Yurcovic, M., and Hanna, M. G., Jr. *J. Nat. Cancer Inst. 52*, 117, 1974.
41. Aaronson, S. A., and Stephenson, J. R. *Proc. Nat. Acad. Sci. USA 71*, 1957, 1974.
42. Nowinski, R. C., and Kaeler, S. L. *Science 185*, 869, 1974.
43. Schwartz, R. S., Donnelly, J., Melief, C. J. M., *et al.* *J. Immunol. 116*, 657, 1976.
44. Lee, J. C., and Ihle, J. N. *J. Nat. Cancer Inst. 55*, 831, 1975.
45. Ihle, J. N., Domotor, J. J., Jr., and Bengali, K. M. *J. Virol. 18*, 124, 1976.
46. Nowinski, R. C., Kaeler, S. L., and Baron, J. *Infect. Immun. 13*, 1091, 1976.
47. Nowinski, R. C., and Doyle, T. *J. Immunol. 117*, 350, 1976.
48. Nowinski, R. C. *Infect. Immun. 13*, 1098, 1976.
49. Nowinski, R. C., and Klein, P. A. *J. Immunol. 115*, 1261, 1975.
50. Fefer, A., McCoy, J. L., and Glynn, J. P. *Cancer Res. 27*, 1626, 1967.
51. Law, L. W., Ting, R. C., and Stanton, J. F. *J. Nat. Cancer Inst. 40*, 1101, 1968.
52. Blank, K. J., Freedman, H. A., and Lilly, F. *Nature 260*, 250, 1976.

53. Troxler, D. H., Boyars, J. K., Parks, W. P., *et al.* *J. Virol.* *22*, 361, 1977.

54. Del Villano, B. C., Nave, B., Croker, B. P., *et al.* *J. Exp. Med.* *141*, 172, 1975.

55. Obata, Y., Ikeda, H., Stockert, E., *et al.* *J. Exp. Med.* *141*, 188, 1975.

56. Yoshiki, T., Mellors, R. C., Hardy, W. D., Jr., *et al.* *J. Exp. Med.* *139*, 925, 1974.

57. Ferren, J. F. *Int. J. Cancer* *12*, 378, 1973.

58. Epstein, L. B., and Knight, R. A. *Br. J. Cancer* *31*, 499, 1975.

59. Gomard, E., Duprez, V., Reme, T., *et al.* *J. Exp. Med.* *146*, 909, 1977.

60. Schrader, J. W., Cunningham, B. A., and Edelman, G. M. *Proc. Nat. Acad. Sci. USA* *72*, 5066, 1975.

61. Henning, R., Schrader, J. W., and Edelman, G. M. *Nature* *263*, 689, 1976.

62. Lilly, F., and Freedman, H. A. *In* "Animal Virology" (D. Baltimore, A. S. Huang, and C. F. Fox, eds.), p. 359. Academic Press, New York, 1976.

63. Tursi, A., Greave, M. F., Torrigiani, G., *et al.* *Immunology* *17*, 801, 1969.

64. Hartley, J. W., Wolford, N. K., Old, L. J., *et al.* *Proc. Nat. Acad. Sci. USA* *74*, 789, 1977.

65. Staal, S. P., Hartley, J. W., and Rowe, W. P. *Proc. Nat. Acad. Sci. USA* *74*, 3065, 1977.

66. Hiai, H., Morrissey, P., Khiroya, R., *et al.* *Nature* *270*, 247, 1977.

67. Nowinski, R. C., Hays, E. F., Doyle, T., *et al.* *Virology* *81*, 363, 1977.

68. Peterson, R. D., Hendrickson, A. R., and Good, R. A. *Proc. Soc. Exp. Biol. Med.* *114*, 517, 1963.

69. Shearer, G. M., Mozes, E., Haran-Ghera, N., *et al.* *J. Immunol.* *110*, 736, 1973.

70. Haran-Ghera, N., Ben-Yaakov, M., and Peled, A. J. *Immunology* *118*, 600, 1977.

71. Zarling, J. M., Nowinski, R. C., and Bach, F. H. *Proc. Nat. Acad. Sci. USA* *72*, 2780, 1975.

72. Kiessling, R., Klein, E., and Wigzell, H. *Eur. J. Immunol.* *5*, 112, 1975.

73. Kiessling, R., Klein, E., Pross, H., *et al.* *Eur. J. Immunol.* *5*, 117, 1975.

74. Kiessling, R., Petrányi, G. G., Klein, G., *et al.* *Int. J. Cancer* *17*, 275, 1976.

75. Haller, O., Kiessling, R., Örn, A., *et al.* *J. Exp. Med.* *145*, 1411, 1977.

76. Petrányi, G. G., Kiessling, R., and Kelin, G. *Immunogenetics* *2*, 53, 1975.

77. Petrányi, G. G. Kiessling, R., Povey, S., *et al.* *Immunogenetics* *3*, 15, 1976.

DISCUSSION

DR. LILLY: A good while ago, we were studying the susceptibility to Gross virus leukemogenesis and found the A
strain to be peculiarly resistant, the genetic basis of which
we were not able, at the time, to locate since they have all
the known genes that influence virus susceptibility. They
should have been susceptible; we checked and found that resistance was not H-2 linked in any particular cross. Another
thing I can confirm, which puzzles me both in our work and in
yours, is that in the Friend virus system, we also have never
been able to see cell-mediated cytotoxicity directed against
cells that are merely virus infected. We can readily develop
cell-mediated cytotoxicity against Friend virus tumor cell lines,
but not against spleen cells from primary Friend virus-infected
mice. This has always puzzled and annoyed us to no end. I
also have one question from your slide in which you showed
your preliminary studies of mapping of the H-2 effect on viral
replication; it was not clear on the slide whether you had
eliminated the J region or not.

DR. TSICHLIS: It is not eliminated. Actually, this was
one of the interesting parts of the whole mapping study. The
I-J region is still included and we are planning to test that.
The way we will do that is to test 3R mice, which are identical with 5R except in the I-J region. As you saw in the
slides, the I-J region in the 5R strain is k. The I-J region
in the 3R is b. We have obtained the 3R strain now to specifically test the hypothesis that the resistance-mediating
genetic locus maps specifically within the I-J region.

DR. SCHWARTZ: I am delighted to hear somebody else say
that they cannot find cytotoxicity; Dr. Tucker, who was a research fellow, invested an entire year trying to find this
and failed. I think this is extremely important, if true, because we have all the data on the Doherty-Zinkernagel model
with virus-infected cells, yet it does not seem to be operative in the case of mouse leukemia viruses. It seems to me
that those of us who have been trying to find this ought to
get together and write a negative paper. Whether it will be
published or not is another matter but it seems to me that
it's a very important negative and I just wondered if anyone
else in the audience has attempted to find classic cell-mediated immunity and has been able to do so on a regular basis.
I'm not talking about your tumor cells now, I'm talking about
normal, productively infected cells. Has anybody been successful?

DR. DIENER: Maybe what is needed is a time kinetics study.

DR. SCHWARTZ: Dr. Tucker did at least four or six different time points during the course of infection (early, middle, late) and never found it.

DR. DOHERTY: I don't have an answer, but I can comment. For all the conventional infectious viruses (i.e., nononcornaviruses) that have been investigated, cytotoxic T cells have been shown. The only virus with a somewhat equivocal status in this regard is Herpes Simplex virus. This system requires that suppressor cells first be removed by treatment of the mouse with cyclophosphamide; these experiments originated from H. Wagner's laboratory. CMC has even been shown for the Coxsackie viruses, which are not known to cause serologically detectible changes on cell surfaces (Wong, Woodruff, and Woodruff, *J. Immunol*. 1977).

DR. TSICHLIS: A significant role for the suppressor T cell has been entertained in our system. Normally resistant mice are susceptible to the B-tropic ecotropic virus we used, when injected at birth, at a time when only thymus-dependent suppressor cells have been shown in the mouse using functional assays. Also, the tentative participation of the I-J region of the MHC in the relevant resistance gene further supports the hypothesis that suppressor cells are involved. Experiments to answer this question are now in progress.

DR. LEVY: I can think of two controls that you should do before concluding with your interpretation of the data. (1) The sensitive mouse strain should also be treated with ALS since the increase in virus titers that you see in the resistant strain may not be specific. Mice treated with ALS are known to have higher levels of virus. (2) Aged fibroblast cells from the two strains should be tested for sensitivity and kinetics of virus infection. One could imagine that the embryo cells of the two mice may be similar but the aged cells may differ. With aging, the cells from the resistant strain may place gp70 on the cell surface and block infection. Such a phenomenon has been observed with cat and mouse cells in culture. In essence, you may actually be looking at a gene for gp70 production.

DR. TSICHLIS: Susceptible strains have not been treated with ALS as yet. We are planning to do this control. At this point, in view of the data in newborn susceptible mice who have the same susceptibility at birth and at the adult age, I would expect that treatment with ALS would probably not change their phenotype. In reference to the second control experiment that you suggested, only embryo fibroblasts have been tested at this point. Adult fibroblasts have not been tested and I think this is a very good suggestion to rigorously exclude this possibility. The results of the *in vivo* experiment of the kinetics of virus infection in susceptible and resistant strains indicate that the results will not be different between adult and embryo fibroblasts. I agree though that this should be done.

DR. AMOS: I have one comment and two general questions. Dr. Hsia at Duke and Dr. Haughton at UNC have tried to show syngeneic lymphocyte-mediated cytotoxicity to Rous-induced sarcomas of mice, in vain. The tumors are good targets because they can be killed in alloimmune reactions. Dr. Haughton's group has transferred immunity in a Winn assay. My questions relate to interferon, since interferon could explain your results. Is the control of interferon level H-2 linked? Is interferon production affected by ALS or ALS and thymectomy? I ask these question because I wonder if you are really working with interferon rather than immunity.

DR. LILLY: Can any one answer that question?

DR. TSICHLIS: I do not know about interferon and H-2 at this point.

DR. LILLY: I also have only anecdotal information about interferon. Does anyone have any real information?

DR. SCHWARTZ: Dr. Amos, in view of the fact that we now have four laboratories in which *in vitro* tests for cell-mediated immunity to type C viruses were negative and, in view of the fact that you said that Haughton can transfer immunity with cells, and since Dr. Tsichlis was able to restore immunity with T cells, there must be some T cell mechanism of protective immunity. What is your explanation for this? Is it a technical problem or are we dealing with a novel mechanism of immunity that is waiting to be described?

DR. AMOS: I don't think it's a technical question because any laboratory is relatively good at cell-mediated immunity; it's been a "specialty-of-the-house" for a while. It was Geoff Haughton who did the Winn assays, not my lab. We can see H-2 specificity if we transfer Rous virus-induced tumor in C57 mice to C3H or vice versa; then we can get a very good anti-H-2 associated type of immunity. It isn't that the tumors aren't good targets because they're good targets for allogeneic reactions. However, I would suggest that we're seeing manifestations of natural killing as an immune mechanism *in vivo*, possibly with a relatively long lag phase.

DR. SCHWARTZ: We thought also of natural killers and looked for them *in vitro* and couldn't find them by looking for ADCC.

DR. AMOS: Oh, well, Dr. Koren, Dr. Buckley, and myself have shown that natural killing and ADCC are not the same.

DR. LILLY: In our system, we're presumably looking at the effects of the same virus since the killing that we see of tumor cells (that is, in Friend virus-induced tumor cell lines) is indeed virus specific. The same killer cells do not kill H-2-matched Gross virus-induced tumor cell lines. And we can do the reciprocal of that experiment. So, if the killer cells that work on virus-induced tumor cells do not work on primary virus-infected spleen cells, it must say something about involvement of transformation itself in the specificity of the killing.

DR. NOWINSKI: I'd like to comment on the role of antibody and the levels of virus in a particular animal. To a certain extent, our conclusions have differed here. If you examine my data, especially the C57 Leaden to AKR cross, all the animals that were antibody positive had very high virus titers. When we did these studies two years ago, we believed that there was very little association between antibody and virus titer. It was quite a surprise to us when we ran the $(C57Bl/6 \times AKR)F_1$ hybrid and found a correlation. This was even more striking when we ran the $(PL \times Leaden)F_1$. Since then, I've learned that Dr. Ihle has obtained a very striking correlation between AKR and NIH mice. This brings me back to my original point. Whenever we measure antibody in an infected mouse, we're looking at a situation with an enormous burden of circulating antigen, so that we're really looking at the end result of a very delicate balance. I think the evidence is now slanting toward the fact that antibody does control virus. The actual demonstration of this will be difficult because we must consider the problem of soluble, circulating, viral antigen, which is capable of complexing antibody; the actual virus-antibody balance may not be truly reflected in this situation.

DR. LILLY: I'd like to respond to Dr. Nowinski. The association that you saw between virus titer and leukemia was, according to the probability values you gave, very much stronger than the association that you saw between antibody titer and the development of the disease. I think we might ask if the antibody that is seen there is a cause or an effect of the resistance.

DR. NOWINSKI: The implication of my data is that the virus titer is the most important prognostic event but, in the control of virus, antibody is another important factor. However, there appears to be at least a two-gene requirement for the production of antibody. This becomes slightly less significant when you take a look at it in terms of leukemia mortality.

DR. GOOD: I have a couple of comments and a question. I wonder whether or not the antibody analysis might be made clearer if you look at the subclasses of antibody. It might very well be that what you're analyzing here is perhaps an IgG response or something of that sort. I think that that might be very helpful. Gabriel Ferdandez, Ed Yunis, and I ran into a peculiar situation in correlating the failure of development of mammary adenocarcinoma in our nutritionally deprived mice.

There was a strange form of suppressor cells that suppressed practically any proliferating cell. I wonder whether or not looking at the negative side of the T cell system might be more rewarding than looking at the positive side. We have found, for example, that very powerful suppressor cell effects can be exerted on the porliferation of cells in patients with aplastic anemia. If you were getting the response really before it got started, there might not be an influence on proliferation; there might not be so much need for a killer mechanism. The question really is, Have you done any experiments along that line?

DR. TSICHLIS: No. The data we have would probably advocate that suppressor cells are involved in this system, but experiments like the one you have suggested have not been done as yet.

DR. LILLY: If it were suppression you were looking at, wouldn't you expect nonresponsiveness to be dominant?

DR. TSICHLIS: Possibly yes.

DR. NOWINSKI: I'd like to comment on Dr. Good's remarks. We've looked at immunoglobulin types and have found antibodies present in virtually all the immunoglobulin types.

DR. YUNIS: Have you elicited effective CMI in A/J thymectomized mice challenged with adjuvants using the model of C. Reimisch of the Sydney Farber Cancer Institute of Boston? Immunogenetics of leukemia resistance should be studied in the absence of suppressive phenomena such as T suppressor cells.

DR. TSICHLIS: No, this experiment has not been done.

DR. THEIS: With respect to resistance not related to the H-2 locus in MuLV, have you considered the role of macrophages, since they are known to operate in inherited resistance and susceptibility in other virus disease, such as mouse hepatitis virus and arboviruses?

DR. TSICHLIS: No, not yet; detailed studies on the exact mechanisms by which the thymus mediates resistance to B-tropic ecotropic viruses have not been done. The possible role of the macrophates has been considered, but not investigated as yet.

DR. VAN ROOD: Could the first two speakers indicate whether they expect, on the basis of their experiences in the mouse that human siblings suffering from leukemia would share HLA haplotypes more frequently than expected?

DR. NOWINSKI: It certainly is conceivable, however, with the polygenic nature of the disease, it may not be possible to readily determine such a relationship.

DR. TSICHLIS: If human leukemia is caused by RNA tumor viruses, something which certainly has not been proven as yet. There is a good possibility that HLA might be playing a sig-

nificant role in susceptibility or resistance to the development of disease. It should be made clear, though, that the
role of the H-2, as well as of other genetic loci regulating
the various steps of the process of viral leukemogenesis, is
not absolute and its effect might be overcome by inheritance
of other susceptibility or resistance conferring genes (reference 10 in text of chapter).

Session III
Immunopathology I

OVERVIEW

Robert Good

Sloan-Kettering Institute for Cancer Research
New York

The immunologist has learned much from experiments of nature. One of the most fascinating experiments of nature that
has helped the physician understand biologic processes is immunologic deficiency. The manifestations of this disease--
infections in infancy and occurrence of early death--have led
to a knowledge of the fundamental importance of cellular immunology and, later, to the subdivision of lymphocytes into
functional subsets, each with a role to play in immune function and immunoregulation.

We are beginning to understand, I think, some of the many
aspects of cells that are involved in immunologic functions
and of the molecules involved. We recognize that there are
two major arms of the immunity system. These arms each have
hands and fingers; working together, they utilize both cellular and molecular means. They constitute a finely tuned system for keeping many unwanted substances out of the body,
yet can maintain order within the complicated immunologic system. One interesting aspect of this has recently come to our
attention. Charlotte Cunningham-Rundles, W. Brandeis, and
N. K. Day have studied patients with selective absence of IgA.
These patients not only have antibodies against milk protein,
as Buckley and Dees long ago showed, but they absorb milk protein in an extraordinary way. These individuals are almost
constantly in possession in their serum of large amounts of
antigen-antibody complex against proteins in milk. I think
this observation serves to illustrate how really important
it is both to consider the immunodeficiencies per se and to
consider the immunodeficiencies in the light of the immunologic
capacities that remain. The immunoglobulin-producing apparatus
is being stimulated, but it is being stimulated excessively
by certain food substances, because the local antibody system
is not keeping those food substances out.

I am not going to go into any detail on how sophisticated
our analysis of the cells of the immunity system, especially
in the mouse, has become. The entire system of cell differentiation sequence ananlysed by alloantigens that Old and
Boyse have described and that has been very helpful in dissecting the functions of the cells of the immunologic system,
can be driven by one molecule--thymopoietin--that has been completely defined by Gideon Goldstein. Both the development of
the differentiation alloantigens and the development of function can be achieved with the help of this molecule. A peptide of 49 amino acids, this molecule has been analysed to the
point where it seems clear that its major activity resides in
a much smaller sequence located between the 29th and 42nd amino
acid residues. In that tridecapeptide, almost in the center
of the molecule, can be found the major activity for controlling differentiation of cells of the immunologic system.

We recognize that patients with common variable immunodeficiency frequently have autoantibodies; sometimes almost
all of the gammaglobulin in the serum can be autoantibodies. Also
IgA-deficient patients suffer from autoimmune diseases. This
has been found wherever these patients have been studied a-
round the world. The latest evidence comes from Japan. Patients with other forms of primary immunodeficiency may also
have excessive frequencies of arthritis and a great variety
of manifestations that I will not take time to detail because much has been published on this subject earlier.

The fact that we are beginning to understand the immunologic system well enough to do something about its malfunctions is illustrated by a youngster who is now 11 years of
age. He was cured of his severe combined immunodeficiency disease more than 10 years ago by a bone marrow transplantation
that, incidentally, created an aplastic anemia of which he
could also be cured by receiving a second bone marrow transplantation. He remains absolutely well, has no manifestations
of susceptibility to infection or any other disorders--a
healthy, vigorous youngster now over 10 years after the
initial transplantation that cured a fatal disease.

It has been possible to extend the observation that was
made by using a matched sibling donor, to achieve correction
of SCID, using matched donors other than sibs within the
family, or even matched donors outside the family. Now even
mismatched donors are being used successfully; for instance,
a donor of a fetal liver taken at a stage before there was
any significant lymphoid tissue development in the fetal liver.
So, it has become possible to make major insertions to correct
the immunologic system that has developed defectively. What
looks to me like a very, very exciting and encouraging line
is the experiments that led to these successful fetal liver

transplantations. The basic experiments were carried out in
animals by Edmond Yunis, our associates, and me, following
the lead of Delta Uphoff. If the fetal liver is taken early
in development, you can sometimes transplant fetal liver cells
across major histocompatibility barriers without any evidence whatsoever of graft vs. host reaction. Other experiments have been carried out in a number of laboratories,
e.g. by Dickke and van Bekkum, and their colleagues, with mice.
If lymphocytes are eliminated from the bone marrow, lethal
irradiation can be treated; there is no graft vs. host reaction, and you have a fully functional immunologic system
that is tolerant of the host, tolerant of the donor, but
capable of recognizing everything else and functioning, I
think, very normally, including normally with respect to protection against a variety of virus infections. Müller-Ruch-
holtz did the same thing with rats, but he removed the hazardous GVH-producing cells by treating the marrow with antilymphocyte serum capable of destroying most lymphocytes, not
just T cells. Most dramatic experiments along this line have
been carried out at Notre Dame by Pollard and his co-workers.
Bone marrow cells essentially free of lymphocytes that can
react with the host (by virtue of taking them from the bone
marrow of germ-free donors) are used to cross major histocompatibility barriers. They treated leukemia effectively
and prevented recurrences of leukemia by introducing R genes
in this way. Bone marrow transplants probably can, among
other things, prevent expression of the oncorna virus of AKR
mice, which otherwise develop fatal malignant disease; it can
treat effectively reticulum cell sarcomas of SJL mice, and
it can even treat and prevent malignant adaptions produced by
lymphocytic choriomeningitis virus infection, introduced
early in life. Such treatment leads to a lymphomatous type of
degeneration later in life. These experiments bring to mind
findings Barnes reported. What he did was to take the Tar-
kowski tetraparental mouse model and put cells from CBA mice
together with AKR cells in the approximate eight-cell embryonic stage. The animals, of course, had their virus. Many
of their cells were cells of the AKR parent, and they thus had
the proper genetic makeup. Some animals had maybe only 5% of
cells from the CBA resistant-strain donor, yet these animals
did not develop the AKR leukemia. A very small contribution
from the appropriate genetic host interferred with the development of leukemia. These experiments are not yet fully
understood; maybe they have to be reproduced before they become scientific fact; but they are extraordinarily provocative
with respect to the idea that there can be a major surveillance
mechanism capable of interfering with the development of some
forms of very serious malignant disease. We also see something

of this in patients who are born without certain complement
components. Now that we have the whole complement system
completely defined, at least in immunochemical and functional
terms, we can define diseases that are based on one or
another of these complement components being left out. It
has become increasingly clear that these patients are very
prone to develop infection. They are even more strikingly
prone to develop the diseases that we have always called autoimmune diseases or immunologically based diseases. Some patients with genetically determined deficiencies of C_1r, C_1s,
or C_1 esterase inhibitor, C_2, C_4, C_5, C_6, C_7, and C_8 have
been described with syndromes like lupus erythematosus.
Just prior to my coming here, we saw a patient with a genetically determined C_2 deficiency who had developed so much
antigen-antibody complex and cryoglobulinemia, that his
central nervous system was being destroyed. This patient
had become blind, just as do some patients with macroglobu-
linemia; he also had other manifestations like the butterfly
rash of lupus erythematosus. So these deficiencies that may
develop in the immunologic system, on genetic or on other
grounds, have opened the door to the development of knowledge of a variety of diseases that we have not previously
understood very well. With the complement system, as with
the specific immunity system, we are already beginning to
correct the abnormalities by transplantation, e.g. with marrow.

One other aspect that I would like to focus on briefly is
the problem of aging, and whether we shall be able to manipulate some of the immunologic and other aspects of aging.
It seems very clear now that with aging there is regularly
loss of thymic function. This loss can be quantified through
measurement of the thymic humoral substance of J. F. Bach
and through methods we have developed based on the assays of
Gideon Goldstein. Accompanying the loss of T cell function
there is an appearance of a wide variety of autoantibodies
and associated autoimmune phenomena. One dramatic model, in
my view, is the New Zealand black (NZB) and the $(NZB \times NZW)F_1$
mouse. In these strains one sees an early decline of thymic
activity, a decline of at least some immunologic functions,
and the dramatic appearance of a variety of autoimmune phenomena as evidenced by the immunological assault on vital
organs. These manifestations are very similar to those Yunis
and I produced by thymectomy. In that situation, too, we
observed very early the appearance of a variety of autoimmune
phenomena, evidence of immunologic assault associated with deficiency of one of the immunologic systems.

At present we can almost completely prevent the immunodeficiency, the development of the autoimmune manifestations,
and the development of the immunologic assault on the vital

organs and double the lifespan of the mice, simply by dietary manipulation. If you cut calories from the time of weaning, i.e., reduce the total food intake, you can delay the development of all of these autoimmune manifestations, the involution of the thymus, and the development of the splenomegaly. In this fashion, the animals can be kept free of what I would call the diseases of aging. By the diseases of aging I mean vascular disease, increased susceptibility to infection, renal diseases, malignant diseases, and perhaps development of autoimmune manifestations and immunologic assault. This approach to controlling disease by manipulation of the immunologic system, through diet, is probably most dramatically demonstrated by new evidence indicating that simply by controlling one element in the diet, one can either have severe combined immunodeficiency or not. That element is zinc. If zinc is withheld, or if zinc cannot be absorbed, a profound immunologic disease associated with severe skin and bowel lesions and with central nervous system malfunction develops. If you give appropriate zinc therapy to patients with that genetically determined fault in absorption of zinc (parenterally, or orally in large doses) the combined immunodeficiency is immediately corrected. It looks as though the possibilities of using the immunologic surveillance and protective mechanism are so manifold that we shall be able to make manipulations that are relatively simple and completely controllable. I am extremely optimistic that our understanding of the immunopathologic processes will bring us a wide variety of pharmacological, biological, and even simple dietary means of manipulation that can be widely applied. What I would call cellular engineering, macromolecular engineering, and, more recently, engineering related to block the processes of involution of the immune system, will be increasingly applied to some diseases that have baffled physicians to the present.

AN INTRODUCTION TO HLA AND DISEASE
AND DISEASE SURVEILLANCE*

D. Bernard Amos

Duke University Medical Center
Durham, North Carolina

E. J. Yunis

Sidney Farber Cancer Center
Boston, Massachusetts

INTRODUCTION

This synopsis is intended to set the stage for other
papers in this session dealing with specific aspects of the
relationship between HLA and disease. While not presented in
its present form during the conference it is intended to guide
the reader of this volume. It discusses the organization of
the HLA immunoregulatory system and its possible role in immunosurveillance and the consequences of escape from immunosurveillance, namely, a large variety of diseases of different
pathologies.

I. BACKGROUND

HLA is a composite term for what Ceppellini has called a
"supergene." It includes glycoproteins, which are recognized
through the reactions of selected antisera. It also includes

*Supported by grants from the National Institutes of Health:
CA 20531-01 (E. J. Yunis), GM 10356 (D. B. Amos), and CA 19589-
01 (E. J. Yunis) .

other components, which are recognized by electrophoretic
techniques or through their biologic activity. In 1960 only
a few leucocyte and tissue antigens were known and these few
were defined by serologic techniques of rather poor reprodu-
cibility. In less than 20 years there has been an explosion
of knowledge about antigenic markers of nucleated human cells,
about their biologic attributes including their effects in
tissue and organ transplantation, their association with some
forms of complement deficiency, and their associations with
disease. To a large extent, this explosive growth owes its
nurture to the unique international collaboration that has
developed since the First International Workshop held at Duke
University in 1964 (1). This and the two succeeding workshops
were a combination of practical experimentation with some reagents (cells or sera) being used by all participants, and
data analysis (2,3). As the workshops became more comprehensive, the laboratory procedures were completed before the workshop, so that recent workshops have consisted of a summary analysis of combined data (joint report) and also of presentations
of details of findings from individual laboratories (4,5). The
net result has been a rapid and widespread dissemination of
information published under a series of volumes, all carrying
the title "Histocompatibility Testing" together with the year
the workshop was held, the latest being "Histocompatibility
Testing 1977." Throughout the early evolutionary phase of the
definition of HLA the principle stimulus and source of support
for research was organ transplantation; now disease associations are providing an ever-increasing component of the investigations.

Although investigation of the H-2 alloantigens of the
major histocompatibility system of the mouse (H-2) started 20
years before the discovery of the major histocompatibility
system of man (HLA), during the last 10 years the definition
of the genetics and polymorphism of both mouse and man, in
great part, have developed in parallel. Some of the major
recent developments in the advances of immunogenetics as related to the major histocompatibility complex (MHC) are

(1) the discovery of recombination between four different
regions (A, B, C, and D) and probably with a fifth (DR), of
the major histocompatibility system, HLA, thus showing that
the MHC is truly a genetic complex;

(2) the introduction of techniques of cytogenetics including banding techniques that permit morphological identification of chromosomes and fine structural analysis of seg-
ments of chromosomes, i.e., translocations;

(3) Synteny, based on studies of cell hybrids between human and animal cells, which permits identification of enzymes

and antigens as chromosomal markers in cell hybrids;

(4) discovery of linkage between enzyme, red cell, and complement markers of chromosome 6 of man with the markers of the HLA system;

(5) the development of methods that enrich different subsets of lymphocytes;

(6) methods to produce continuous cultures of pure lymphocyte subsets;

(7) the finding of specific alloantigenic systems restricted to lymphocyte subsets such as the I-region of the mouse and the HLA-DR region in man;

(8) chemical characterization of two different classes of molecules isolated from membrane of cells: HLA (and H-2) antigens and antigens derived from the B lymphocyte subsets (often called Ia antigens);

(9) studies of the genetic control of immune responsiveness (Ir), immune suppression (Is), and other aspects of immune regulation involving interaction of T lymphocytes (helper or suppressor), B lymphocytes and macrophages regulated by the MHC. While these latter have only been clearly documented in the mouse, the close similarity between the mouse and human MHC in other ways leads us to suppose the analogy may extend to these functions.

These discoveries permit a diagrammatic representation of the loci of the HLA system in chromosome 6 of man and the H-2 loci in chromosome 17 of the mouse (Fig. 1). This map shows how comparable the systems are and how our knowledge of the genetics of the system has grown. Hopefully, further knowledge combined with experiments performed with isolated subsets of lymphocytes could lead to understanding of unknown functions of the gene products encoded by the HLA segment of the short arm of chromosome 6 (6-17).

II. GENERAL CHARACTERISTICS OF THE HLA SYSTEM

The region of chromosome 6 associated with the transplantation antigens and with a variety of immunological effectors is called the HLA region. Currently, five principal loci have been recognized: HLA-A, B, C, D, and DR. These loci demonstrate an extraordinary degree of polymorphism. They are usually inherited as a gametic unit on a segment of chromosome called a haplotype. An individual who has the same gene or allele at a given locus on both homologous chromosomes is said to be *homozygous* at that locus; when the two alleles are not the same, the individual is said to be *heterozygous*. Similarly, an individual can be homozygous or heterozygous for the whole complex, true homozygotes being very rare in most popu-

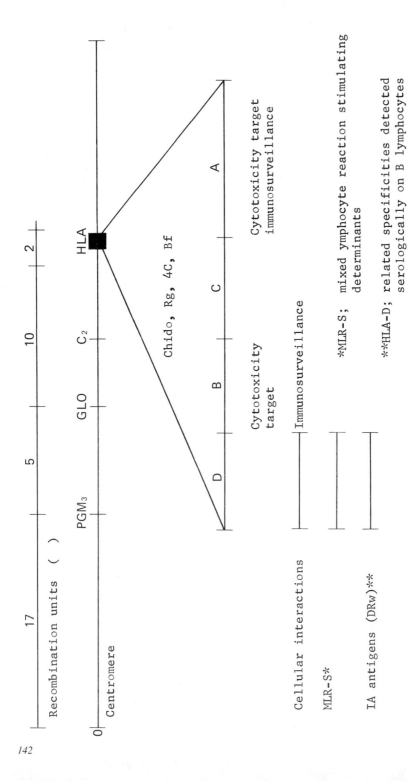

FIGURE 1. HLA: chromosome 6 (short arm).

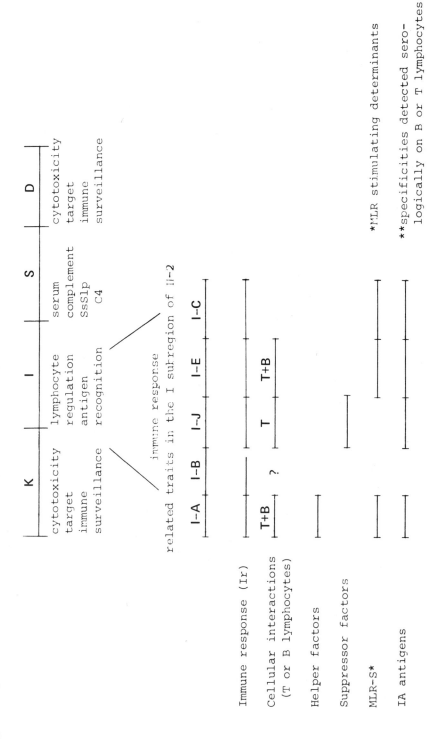

Figure 1. H-2 Complex: general classes of traits controlled by H-2 region. (Modified from reference 17.)

lations. Since both allelic forms of the antigen are expressed,
the alleles are said to be codominant. Chromosome 6 is con-
tributed to the children in a family by each parent; each of
these chromosomes is marked by 5 or more antigens or functions
of the HLA haplotype. If the inheritance of gametes is random,
the different combinations of the four parental haplotypes
should be present in equal numbers among the siblings giving
four possible HLA genotypes to the sibship. During meosis,
homologous chromosomes pair prior to reduction of the number
of chromosomes from 46 (diploid) to 23 (haploid) and recombine
and exchange genetic material by a mechanism called "crossing
over." The five named loci of HLA have all been shown to
separate from each other in recombinants. The frequency of
recombination or crossing over between the five HLA loci is
less than 2%.

Following the 1975 and 1977 International Histocompatibility Workshops, the WHO HLA Nomenclature Committee provided
terminology for 57 HLA-A, B, and C antigens, 11 HLA-D specificities, and 7 HLA-DR antigens (18,19). Other linked loci
code for complement factors (properdin factor B, 2C, and 4C)
two red cell groups, Chido and Rogers (13). Linkage studies
of HLA and other genetic markers together with synteny studies
have established that the enzyme phosphoglucomutase-3 lies
approximately 15 centimorgans and the enzyme glyoxylase, 10
centimorgans from HLA, lying between the HLA region and the
centromere of chromosome 6 (13).

III.   THE HLA-D REGION OF MAN AND THE I-REGION OF H-2 OF THE
       MOUSE

There are many analogies between the HLA-D region of HLA
and the I region of the mouse. For instance, genes of the Ia
subregion of the I region are responsible for expression of
allospecificities on B cells and monocytes that are involved in the allogeneic stimulation of helper T cells
in the mixed-leukocyte reaction. The HLA-D alleles sub-
serve the same function in man. This same I region in
the mouse codes for genes that control the immune response;
some of these genes not only mediate help, but also mediate suppression of the immune response. The same may
be true for HLA. The distinction between lepromatous
and tuberculoid leprosy and the proclivity to develop ragweed
hypersensitivity may both be reflections of Ir gene activity
and are believed closely linked to HLA. The genetics of the
immune response in the mouse is extremely complicated. While
the response to some antigens is thought to be controlled by
a single locus, it has been found that two interacting genes
may be required to develop Ir or Is. In man, the I region has

not been conclusively demonstrated as yet, but since Ir I in
the region of H-2 of the mouse is only one locus out of the
four or more Ir loci, studies in man will go very slowly if
man too has multiple, unlinked Ir genes. Most probably,
knowledge will come from exceptional families, for example,
families in which there is limited polymorphism for an HLA-
linked Ir gene and homozygosity for other, nonlinked, Ir genes.

An interesting degree of complexity remains to be resolved
in the mouse MHC. The I region has been subdivided into several (the exact number is still uncertain) subregions of
which the best known are IA, IC, and IJ. Genes in IA code
for T cell help for B cell responses and for the so-called
Ia cell surface antigens of B cells and of a T cell subset(s).
A number of these Ia antigens have been defined, some (private)
are specific for a single mouse strain and its derivatives,
while others (public) are shared by a number of strains. A
number of determinants that are responsible for the stimulation by B cells of T cell helper cells (MLC specificities or
MLR-S) are also coded for in the IA region, but these do not
necessarily coincide. Indeed, the actual determinants that
are responsible for proliferation in MLC have not been identified whereas the Ia antigens have not only been isolated and
characterized, they have even been partly sequenced. Antibodies to Ia will block MLC responses (20). This would imply
that the mixed lymphocyte reaction stimulator (MLR-S) determinants are Ia antigens. However, in most cases, the strain
distributions of Ia and MLR-S are not identical and antibodies
to β_2-microglobulin (or to HLA) will block MLCs, although the
Ia antigen unlike the H-2 or HLA molecule is not found in association with a β_2-microglobulin molecule, implying the formation of an H-2-Ir macromolecular complex. However, at least
some of the antibodies used in the MLC blocking experiments are
now known to be contaminated with antibodies to H-2-like antigens against specificities (Qa) controlled by genes outside
the IA region (21). This finding may require a redefinition
of the boundaries of H-2 to include Qa or may be an indication
of a separate MHC-like system adjacent to H-2. Alternatively,
many of these antibodies may act in ADCC to lyse the stimulator cell (22).

HLA-D typing involves culturing lymphocytes from the unknown individual with nonreplicating lymphocytes from an individual known to be homozygous for a given HLA-D allele. Thus,
the cell to be typed is exposed in a series of tests to typing
cells (HTC) from donors who are homozygous for HLA-Dw1 or Dw2
or Dw3 and so on. Failure of the unknown to respond indicates
that the cell shares an HLA-D allele in common with the HTC;
fairly representative would be a failure of an unknown to res-

pond to HLA-Dw1 and Dw3 HTC, but with a good response to Dw2, Dw4, and other HTC; this would type the subject as Dw1, Dw3.

HLA-DR typing is performed by separating B lymphocytes by any of several procedures; e.g., rosetting T cells and separation from B cells by sedimentation of rosettes, removal of Ig-bearing cells with affinity-labeled anti-F(ab)'$_2$ etc. The purified B cells are then exposed to anti-B cell antibody. This antibody is usually obtained by absorbing unwanted antibodies to HLA-A, -B, and -C from an anti-HLA serum by absorption with platelets. Complement is added as in HLA typing with the proviso that extensive screening of individual rabbit sera to exclude toxic samples is mandatory. The interpretation of data on B cell antigens is still largely subjective, many antigens have not yet been defined, and the complexities of these antigens and of their genetic control have far to go before they are resolved. There may, for example, be two or more loci for B cell antigens in the HLA-DR region as well as one in the HLA-A region.

IV. THE HLA SYSTEM AND THE GENETICS OF SUSCEPTIBILITY OR RE-
     SISTANCE TO DISEASE

Any discussion of HLA and disease susceptibility should take into account the following facts: nosologic classification of diseases is based partly on knowledge of the consequences of etiologic factors and partly upon grouping of clinical signs and symptoms into syndromes. Additional knowledge of the clinical aspects of the disease such as differences in age of onset, differing prognosis, and new subgroupings of symptoms can lead to new subdivisions of diseases (splitting); the separation of juvenile onset and mature onset as two distinct forms of diabetes would be a typical example. On the other hand, increase of knowledge of the etiology might tend to include in one disease several conditions with varying clinical manifestations (lumping). Many clinicians believe in a link between such diseases as Graves' disease and Addison's disease as polyglandular disease possibly with a common etiology. With this in mind, we also need to point out that from the susceptibility point of view, diseases are the result of many factors that are primarily the result of the genetic composition of the individual interacting with environmental factors such as infections or inflammatory agents. Genetically speaking, diseases may also be caused by a single point mutation that can affect several organs or present several manifestations (pleotrophism); however, one clinical manifestation may be the result of different mutations at different points in the genome (genetic heterogeneity or polygenic factors in diseases). Of course, since environmental factors are important in most diseases and few diseases show complete expression even in monozygotic twins or inbred mice, it is not surprising that even in the purest forms of disease susceptibility, not all members inheriting the abnormal genes are affected. Many geneticists speak about "penetrance" to describe this phenomenon. When environmental factors are important, concordance may be greatest between sibs of the same sex, sharing the same bedroom or even bed.

In this discussion we shall describe some aspects of HLA and disease associations that may illustrate the possible role of HLA markers in the nosology of many diseases. HLA antigens have been found associated with diseases of different specialities of medicine: neurology, psychiatry, infectious diseases, rheumatology, orthopedic surgery, hematology, endocrinology, cancer, dermatology, cardiology. Many of the strongest associations are with autoimmune diseases. A detailed description of these associations has been given in a recent publication of the Proceedings of the First Conference on HLA and Disease (23). In this presentation, we shall only emphasize the salient features of the field as it relates to the present conference.

The relationship between a genetic marker such as HLA and a trait such as a disease susceptibility can be established in either of two ways: by studying a large population of unrelated individuals, or by a study of families. The first method gives the association between HLA and the disease. The second establishes a linkage relationship. Because of the small size of many families and the infrequency with which the same disease is found in two members if a family, the population method is most often employed. This has been very successful in a number of instances and especially when the associated antigen has a rather low frequency in the population. Association is usually expressed as a ratio called the relative risk (RR). For example, HLA-B27 is found in about 6% of Caucasions; ankylosing spondylitis (AS) is an uncommon disease; over 90% of Caucasians with AS have the antigen B27 and the RR is approximately 90. (In Japanese, where B27 is rare, the RR is over 300! As a point of reference the highest relative risk of a blood antigen in disease is blood group O and duodenal ulcer; RR is 1.5-2.0 (23).

Family studies are most rewarding where the expression may be dominant such as with ankylosing spondylitis (24), ragweed hypersensitivity (25), and spina bifida occulta (26), the first being an example of close linkage and the latter two being probably loose linkage. In other family studies the HLA region has served as a genetic marker to detect possible

recessive susceptibility genes in linkage studies: hemochromatosis (27,28), juvenile onset diabetes mellitus (29,30), and
tuberculoid leprosy (31).

In no instance has an HLA region product itself been
shown to be the basis for susceptibility to disease. Some of
the theoretical possibilities for the association or linkage
will be discussed later. For the present, it is convenient
to consider the HLA specificities as markers for genes, not
yet identified, which lie in or near the HLA region, which
are the actual disease-associated loci.

The marker concept for HLA can be exploited in a rather
unusual manner. This is because of a phenomenon known as
linkage disequilibrium, which is known for other genetic
systems but seems to be exceptionally prominent in the HLA
system (32). Alleles of two genes on the same chromosome of
a founder of a population should undergo replacement through
crossing over so that with time, the same combination should
not be found more often than would be expected by chance.
For example, suppose Fletcher Christian introduced the gametic haplotype bearing the HLA alleles A1-B8 into the Polynesian population of Pitcairn, where this haplotype would otherwise be unusual. Two of the most common haplotypes in Poly-
nesia are A11-Bw22 and A9-Bw40, so if this is also true of
Pitcairn, one would expect within a certain number of genera-
tions (readily calculable since the frequency of crossing
over is known) that A1-Bw22 or A1-Bw40 would become as common
as A9-B8 or A11-B8 and that A1-B8 would become rather unusual.
This is probably true, but the time interval required would
be several thousand years! For the first few hundred years
(beyond the time expected to separate them if recombinations
occur randomly), any individual typing as HLA-A1 would almost
certainly carry B8 as the second specificity on the haplotype.
Suppose further that Fletcher Christian had psoriasis and
carried the C-locus allele HLA-Cw6. We would be able to predict with good precision which of his descendants would carry
this specificity (and be susceptible to psoriasis) since
HLA-C maps between HLA-A and HLA-B. With very rare exceptions, all individuals typing as HLA-B8 would also be HLA-Cw6.
Similar "founder effects" will be found in other rapidly expanding populations to a less extreme extent.

The association between HLA and a given disease is not
absolute and, therefore, the HLA system (or genes linked to
it) is only one of the several genetic factors predisposing
to a disease. Since other genetic factors have not yet been
identified and, all of the genes in the HLA region are not
yet fully characterized, it is not possible to determine
whether the exceptions reflect the operation of polygenic
factors or if they are reflections of our inability to detect

some of the loci. It is not expected that all individuals bearing the disease susceptibility gene will manifest disease because other genetic and environmental factors are required to produce clinical detectable disease.

The significance of linkage disequilibrium is obscure. There is a tendency to believe that selection pressure from diseases and genetic drift could explain some of the associations with HLA alleles or with alleles of other genetic systems (33). Selection could also be produced through the formation of the zygote through a mechanism speculated by Bennett *et al.* (34). The T alleles in the mouse and by analogy in man are linked to the major transplantation region and could influence the frequency of recombination within the region or possibly suppress nonviable gametic combinations (35-37). Our bias is toward some selective advantage of certain combinations since the linkage disequilibrium (l.d.) may differ to an extraorindary degree between different alleles of the same two loci, e.g., Bw35 and Cw4 are in extraordinarily high linkage disequilibrium while the disequilibrium between Bwl3 and Cw6 appears to be very much lower.

V. CLINICAL IMPLICATIONS

While at least one disease is associated with alleles of each of the four loci of HLA, most of the associations of diseases described to date have been with antigens of the HLA-D and HLA-DR loci. However, the most detailed knowledge, since it has been accumulated over a longer time, relates to the HLA-A and -B loci. The associations of HLA-B27 with ankylosing spondylitis or of A3 with hemochromatosis (the diseases with the highest relative risk for an HLA antigen) are extraordinarily high, and run about 10 times greater than the associations for most of the other diseases with a particular HLA allele.

Table I lists some of the other diseases, the HLA alleles, and the relative risks for each. Many of the diseases such as Beçets disease or dermatitis herpetiformis are relatively uncommon; some such as hemochromatosis are rare and insidious in onset, while others such as schizophrenia may present a variety of clinical forms making diagnosis somewhat uncertain. To what extent HLA typing can help in diagnosis is being vigorously explored. Perhaps its greatest value will be in identifying family members at risk when one member of the family has been found to be suffering from an insidious onset disease due to the recessive gene. It is also believed that in some instances the prognosis of a disease is better if the patient

TABLE I. Diseases Showing Positive HLA Antigen Association (Caucasians)

Disease	HLA	No. of studies	Patients		Controls		RR[a]	p[b]
			Total	Pos-range(%)	Total	Pos-range(%)		
Rheumatology								
Ankylosing spndylitis	B27	21	967	70-100	7879	3-12	90.1	1E-10
Reiter's disease	B27	21	321	65-100	5517	4-14	36.	1E-10
Yersinia arthritis	B27	8	116	58-78	2293	9-14	18	1E-10
Salmonella arthritis	B27	2	18	60-69	1987	8-10	18	3.1E-10
Psoriatic arthritis	B13	4	86	9-37	996	4-8	408	7.7E-08
	B27	5	97	17-58	1071	4-14	806	1E-10
	Bw38	2	44	17-27	416	3-3	9.09	5.6E-07
	Bw17	4	121	6-35	996	4-9	5.8	1E-10
Acute anterior uveitis	B27	3	291	37-58	1533	7-10	9.4	1E-10
Adult rheumatoid arthritis	Dw4	1	43	72	45	13	16.8	1.5E-08
Neurology								
Multiple sclerosis	Dw2	7	734	47-70	1095	15-31	4.3	1E-10
Myasthenia gravis	B8	5	259	38-65	1881	18-31	4.4	1E-10
Dermatology								
Psoriasis vulgaris	B13	8	688	2-34	5601	2-9	4.67	1E-10
	B17	8	688	12-36	5601	4-11	4.69	1E-10
	Bw37	3	220	4-16	1029	1-3	6.35	7.3E-08
Dermatitis herpetiformis	B8	7	269	58-87	4081	17-33	8.74	1E-10
	Dw3	2	66	62-93	293	19-20	13.5	1E-10
Behcet's disease	B5	5	102	18-86	1360	9-25	7.43	1E-10

							RR[a]	p[b]
Endocrinology								
Juvenile insulin-dependent diabetes	B8	13	1200	19-55	6856	2-29	2.42	1E-10
	Dw3	1	42	50	157	21	3.8	3.0E-04
	Dw4	1	79	42	157	19	3.5	5.6E-05
Thyrotoxicosis	B8	7	550	25-47	5188	16-27	2.34	1E-10
	Dw3	2	112	52-54	202	16-21	4.4	4.9E-09
Subacute thyroditis	Bw35	3	80	63-73	2512	9-14	16.8	1E-10
Idiopathic Addisons' disease	B8	2	52	20-69	2417	18-24	3.9	7.3E-06
	Dw3	1	30	70	157	21	8.8	3.4E-07
Gastroenterology								
Coeliac disease	B8	11	505	45-89	50003	11-29	8.6	1E-10
	Dw3	1	28	96	100	27	73	1E-10
Autoimmune chronic active hepatitis	B8	8	339	98-68	3830	8-24	2.9	1E-10
Idiopathic hemochromatosis	A3	2	80	76-78	299	27-31	8.3	1E-10
	B14	1	51	25	204	3	9.2	3.1E-06
Immunopathology								
Sicca syndrome	B8	4	127	38-58	2637	21-31	3.15	2.5E-10
	Dw3	1	29	69	58	10	19	4.1E-08
Other disease								
Cryptogenic fibrosing alveolitis	B12	1	15	80	616	30	9.4	1.1E-04

[a]RR, Relative risk.

[b]p, Floating-point notation; not multiplied by the number of antigens studied. General cut-off point was a p value of 4×10^4 (corrected p value of 0.01 if 25 antigens were studied).

has a specific HLA allele. Thus it is believed that HLA-B15
may be important in preventing complications of diabetes mellitus (38) or HLA-B12 may improve the outlook in multiple
sclerosis (39). There may also be some important prognostic
associations with cancer: an increased frequency of HLA-B8 has
been reported in long-term survivors of breast cancer (40). A
higher than expected frequency of HLA-A2 in chronic lymphocytic
leukemia was initially believed to represent a similar effect
on survival, but since the raised frequency is also present
at time of first diagnosis, the increase of HLA A2 appears to
represent another example of a weak association with HLA
rather than an effect on the course of the disease (41). Since
this association is with an A locus rather than with a B locus
specificity, it is possible that the strongest association will
be with a locus outside the region we now think of as the HLA
haplotype.

It is becoming apparent that many of the disease associations originally described for HLA-B are much stronger when
the associations are made with HLA-D. Unfortunately, HLA-D
typing is much more expensive and time-consuming than HLA-A
or -B typing, so few of the patients have been HLA-D typed.
HLA-D characterization is also less complete and some alleles
are not yet identified or the appropriate typing cells are not
available. Fortunately, the HLA-DR locus, which can be identified by serological methods, is close to HLA-D and in strong
linkage disequilibrium (a few investigators believe HLA-D and
HLA-DR are the same locus and the same gene product is being
measured in two different procedures). While DR typing is in
its infancy, it will soon greatly facilitate characterization
of the D region of the haplotype (42). There are also very
strong indications that some of the sera to B cell antigens
detect additional products of the haplotype. The authors believe there are at least two DR loci in the D region and another in the A or B region of the haplotype.

Another factor that we believe may be very important in
the future is that some specificities may only be expressed
on the B (or T) lymphocytes of affected subjects, i.e., do not
appear in normals. There are two reasons why this may be true
and why, in future serologic studies, this may help in the
identification of recessive homozygotes or of individuals at
risk.

(1) Some antigens may represent interactions between the
homologous haplotypes. Hybrid or interacting antigens are
well-recognized in the dove and in the rabbit, but have not
yet been described in mouse or man (43,44). An interesting
system with the same implications for population studies as
hybrid antigens are the hybrid or hemopoietic histocompati-

bility antigens, which are postulated to account for F_1 hybrid reactivity against parental bone marrow (45). Recently, it has been found that two complementary genes in the I region of the mouse H-2 are required for both immune responses and immune suppression to specific antigens (46,47). Complementary susceptibility genes may be required, and therefore their exis- tence may explain to some extent penetrance and/or recessive- ness vs. dominant genetic inheritance of HLA-associated dis- eases.

(2) Some antigens may result from the interaction of an etiologic agent and receptors (alloantigens) on the cell sur- face. This is implicit in the extensive studies on altered self following virus infections in the mouse. MHC antigens are implicated in the modification of the surface of affected cells exposed to virus or to hapten; they have also been im- plicated in the response to syngeneic tumors (48-52). Semliki forest virus associates with MHC products on the human lympho- cyte (C. Terhorst, personal communication). A hapten-HLA complex would present new possibilities for antigenic speci- ficity. Such an interaction would explain the report of Mann *et al.* that sera from mothers of children with celiac disease may have antibodies that react only with lymphocytes from the affected child and with other subjects with the same disease (53). This hypothesis may explain why some reports found higher associations of some anti-DRw3 antisera with celiac disease and dermatitis herpetiformis or some anti-DRw2 anti- sera with multiple sclerosis.

During the 7th International Histocompatibility Workshop, this problem was not resolved because the analysis of B cell speci- ficity associations with diseases was not made with single sera.

Furthermore, associations found with some of the markers of the HLA haplotype may not show up with other haplotype mar- kers in population studies, although they would in family studies. An example is rheumatoid arthritis, which has an association with Dw4, but where no association has been found with the A, B, or C antigens. In non-Caucasians, it has been reported that tuberculoid leprosy is associated with HLA-DRw2. In family studies there is evidence that the form of leprosy, tuberculoid or lepromatous, is haplotype related (31).

VI.   ETIOLOGY AND MECHANISMS OF HLA AND DISEASE ASSOCIATIONS

     It is not possible at present to give many concrete exam-
ples of etiologic agents that cause diseases associated with
HLA although there are several hints. Postinfectious arthropathy is one condition in which a high proportion of patients
with B27 develop arthritis, mono- or polyarticular, following
infections with Yersinia, Salmonella, and Chlamydia. Also,
intoxication by Shigella has been reported to be followed by
development of AS. Thirty-nine out of 50 patients examined
were B27 (24). These findings together with the high relative
risk of "classical" ankylosing spondylitis, Reiter's syndrome,
and anterior uveitis suggest a possible relationship between
HLA-B27 and a mutant allele or a genetic locus for a group of
pliotrophic diseases associated with a gene or genes closely
linked to HLA and in linkage disequilibrium with HLA-B27.
This example is one in which it may be possible to think that
patients from these diseases belong to one common etiology.
Mechanistically the pathologic manifestation may involve a
response to altered self, e.g., to cell membranes altered by
exposure to slow virus, and an attempt to eliminate the altered
cells. Disease may thus involve undiscovered immune reactions
in some diseases, including those associated with HLA-B27.
     With respect to diseases to which HLA-D alleles show strong
association, it is possible to suspect viral agents, such as
Coxsackie B type 4 in diabetes and a paramyxovirus in multiple
sclerosis. In these diseases, there is a strong association
between antigens coded by the D locus and disturbed immune reactions, including polyclonal gammopathy, abnormal T cell regulation and increased propensity to develop autoantibodies.
This may imply D locus linked Ir genes as in the I region of
the mouse H-2 system. For example, the increased ability of
B8 and DRw4 (A. H. Johnson, personal communication) diabetics
to make anti-insulin antibodies and antibodies against pan-
creatic islets than diabetics without B8 (54), or the finding
that B8 Addison's possess higher titers of antiadrenal antibodies (55). These findings may provide further clues to
mechanisms of HLA and disease associations. It is impossible
to explain all of the HLA-associated diseases on the basis of
a single etiology. While immunological malfunctions may be
responsible for many of the diseases, it is difficult to see
how hemochromatosis, which has very strong associations with
HLA-A3, can be attributed to immunological factors. However,
since several enzymes and several cell surface glycoproteins
are known to be coded for by the HLA region, it is reasonable
to suppose that some of the HLA associations are due to abnormalities in the enzymes or in receptor functions (including

hormones) of the cell surface glycoproteins (56). This could, of course, relate to iron binding in the case of hemochromatosis.

VII. THE HLA SYSTEM, IMMUNOREGULATION, AND IMMUNOLOGICAL SURVEILLANCE

The two prime requirements of an immune system are that it provide a very powerful defense against the etiologic agents of disease and that it be so modulated that it can discriminate between an invader (nonself) and self and can unleash its power of attack only on the former. At this meeting, many examples have been presented of conditions under which an invader, metazoan, protozoan, or microbial is able to circumvent or subvert the immunological system. In this paper we have alluded to a variety of conditions in which autoaggression appears to be the prime cause of the clinical disease; as an additional example, disease in the compromised or tolerant host to lymphocytic choriomeningitis may actually run a more chronic course or be more benign than in the actively immune host.

Although discussed only briefly at this meeting, the possible failure of the immune system to control neoplastic growth may be one of the most rewarding subjects for discussion and study. The theory as stated by Lewis Thomas and implicit in the philosophy of earlier workers is that one of the fundamental purposes of the immune system is to recognize a neoplastic cell as altered self and to destroy it (57,58). For recognition purposes, the antigens of the MHC would make excellent reference standards. Jerne in his theory of the generation of antigenic diversity used the polymorphism of the MHC as an essential component of the hypothesis (59). While the concept of immunological surveillance for neoplasms is being challenged, perhaps it would be appropriate to restate it as it applied to modified self in the disease state.

Many objections have been raised to the concept of immune surveillance, notably the lack of increase in frequency of solid neoplasms in immunosuppressed or immunodeficient hosts even after exposure to carcinogens, difficulties in demonstration of tumor-specific antigens in some tumors, etc. However, the realization that there are many additional components to the immune system compels continuing evaluation of the possibility of homeostatic or destructive immunological processes at a stage in oncogenesis before the tumor develops. One might cite the studies of Haran-Ghera and others, who have shown an increased frequency of tumors after transfer of thy-

mus to irradiated recipients (60), immunostimulation of tumors
as observed by Gorer (61) and later popularized by Prehn (62),
the finding that natural killer (NK) cells are present in apparently normal numbers in immunodeficient patients (63) or in
nude mice (64), and the growing awareness of the induction of
immune paralysis by products of the tumor (65) are but a few of
the factors. Anyone reading this book will see examples of
other immunosuppressive factors, for example by infectious
agents, (and tumors are very frequently colonized by microbes)
and must realize that there is a constant flux between effector and suppressor components of the immune system.

Reference has already been made to the work of Zinkernagel
and Doherty (48,49), Shearer (50), and others on the recognition of virally or haptenically altered self. Some of the
effective haptens in this system are ring structures comparable to some of the chemical carcinogens. From the work
of McMichael *et al*. (66) and more recently C. Terhorst (personal communication), it is possible to implicate antigens of
the MHC as receptors for viruses in man (50).

In mice, Lilly has shown MHC restriction of immunity to
tumor viruses (51) and Williams *et al*. have demonstrated that
multiple-MHC genes may interact to restrict the growth of
chemically induced tumors transplanted into histocompatible
hosts (52). The MHC is, therefore, a prime candidate as a
repository for oncogenic factors, chemical or viral, and
possibly also as the regulation site for immunoregulation of
the immune response to tumors. Germain and his colleagues
have reported that antibodies to MHC products can block the
cytotoxic effects of immune lymphocytes against syngeneic
tumor cells (67). While this is not quite the same as demonstrating autoimmunity to tumors, it is a close approximation
and implicates the MHC both in syngeneic killing and as a target for blocking the killing process.

In recently reported experiments, Green *et al*. (68) and
Williams and Frelinger (69) were able to control the growth
of syngeneic tumors by treatment of the mice with antiserum
to subregions of the MHC. Both groups decreased tumor size
in hosts treated with anti-I-J serum, and in our case (69) an
anti-D-end serum had equivalent effects. As we increase our
knowledge of the complexity of immune response regulation as
controlled by the MHC, it is possible to produce selective
immunodeficiency in favor of suppression of tumor growth by
eliminating suppressor T cells, e.g., with anti-I-J region
sera. On the other hand, in susceptible individuals or strains
of mice, the same antisera may favor production of autoimmunity.

In conclusion, we believe that the MHC represents a unique
cluster of genes, some regulatory of immunity and some invol-

ved in self-recognition. Perverting or subverting the positive
and fundamental effects of the MHC leads directly to a variety of diseases, or to a failure to regulate and react against
disease.

It is possible that there are many mechanisms underlying
the HLA and disease associations, as well as other mechanisms
independent of the HLA loci. The knowledge of HLA is incomplete, especially of HLA-D and DR. Therefore, it is not
possible to type yet for some alleles with disease susceptibility. The present knowledge has served primarily to assist
the pathologist and the clinician to classify and subclassi-
fy diseases.

The studies of HLA and disease will help to increase the
knowledge of the HLA system, which will lead to understanding
of the functions of these gene products, to include immune
response and immune suppression. The relationship of the HLA
system and immune response and suppression is not yet elucidated. Less understood are the mechanisms of HLA and disease
associations. However, the HLA system may give important
clues to understand normal surveillance as well as the mechanisms (immune) involved in production of alteration of regulation of immune response that are involved in escape mechanisms
of immune surveillance and disease.

VIII. SUMMARY

The general features of the major histocompatibility system
have been discussed. The glycoproteins of the HLA-A, -B, and
-C loci exist as a complex series of commonly encountered
alleles. HLA therefore provides a useful indicator of indivi-
duality both in the population and in the family. The HLA region also includes genes having other functions, including
the control of complement components and of specificities
(HLA-D) responsible for the stimulation of allogeneic lymphocytes and possibly important for the discrimination between
self and nonself. Many diseases have an association with a
particular allele of an HLA antigen. While most of the early
descriptions of the associations were with B locus alleles,
these associations are often greater with HLA-D alleles. In
addition, a few diseases are now known to be most closely
linked to HLA-A or -C. It is unlikely that the HLA antigen
itself is involved in the disease process but because of its
extreme polymorphism HLA provides a very convenient series of
markers for the important 6th chromosome. The article includes speculation about the nature of the disease associations
and also on the role of the MHC in immune surveillance.

Acknowledgments

Our thanks are due to Dr. R. Michael Williams and Ms.
Donna Kostyu for their reading of this manuscript and to Ms.
Janice Kerber for its preparation.

References

1. Workshop on Histocompatibility Testing, Amos, D. B. (ed.)
   In "Histocompatibility Testing" (P. S. Russell, H. J. Winn,
   and D. B. Amos, eds.), p. 147. Publication 1229, National
   Academy Sciences--National Research Council, Washington,
   D.C., 1965.
2. Workshop on Histocompatibility Testing, a Preliminary
   Report, Bruning, J. W., van Leeuwen, A., and van Rood,
   J. J. (eds.) *In* "Histocompatibility Testing 1965" (H.
   Balner, F. J. Cleton, and E. J. Eernisse, eds.), p. 275.
   Munksgaard, Copenhagen, 1965.
3. The Workshop Data, Curtoni, E. S., Mattiuz, P. L., and
   Tosi, R. M. (eds.) *In* "Histocompatibility Testing 1967"
   (H. Blaner, F. J. Cleton, and E. J. Eernisse, eds.).
   Munksgaard, Copenhagen, 1967.
4. Allen, F., Amos, D. B., Batchelor, R., *et al.* *In* "Histocompatibility Testing 1970" (P. I. Terasaki, ed.), p. 17.
   Munksgaard, Copenhagen, 1970.
5. Joint Report, Bodmer, J. G., Rocques, P., Bodmer, W. F.,
   Colombani, J., Degos, L., Dausset, J., and Piazza, A.
   (eds.) *In* "Histocompatibility Testing 1972" (P. Terasaki,
   ed.), p. 620. Munksgaard, Copenhagen, 1972.
6. Amos, D. B., and Ward, F. E. *Physiol. Rev. 55*, 206, 1975.
7. Bach, F. H., and Amos, D. B. *Science 156*, 1506, 1967.
8. Yunis, E. J., and Amos, D. B. *Proc. Nat. Acad. Sci. (USA)
   68*, 3031, 1971.
9. McKusick, V., and Ruddle, W. F. *Science 196*, 340, 1977.
10. Snell, G. D., Dausset, J., and Nathenson, S. *In* "Histo-
    compatibility," p. 212. Academic Press, New York, 1976.
11. Benacerraf, B. *Transplant. Proc. 9*, 825, 1977.
12. Dupont, B., Hansen, J., and Yunis, E. J. *In* "Advances in
    Immunology," Vol. 23 (F. Dixon and H. Kunkel, eds.). p.
    188, Academic Press, New York, 1976.
13. Bodmer, W. F. *In* "Third International Workshop on Gene
    Mapping," p. 24. Karger, Basel, 1976.
14. Murphy, D. B., Herzenberg, L. A., Okumura, K., Herzenberg,
    L. A., and McDevitt, H. O. *J. Exp. Med. 144*, 699, 1976.
15. Okumura, K., Herzenberg, L. A., Murphy, D. B., McDevitt,
    H. O., and Herzenberg, L. A. *J. Exp. Med. 144*, 685, 1976.

16. Katz, D. H., and Benacerraf, B. (eds.) "The Role of Products of the Histocompatibility Gene Complex in Immune Responses," p. 780. Academic Press, New York, 1976.

17. Schreffler, D. C. *In* "HLA and Disease" (J. Dausset and A. Svejgaard, eds.), p. 32. Munksgaard, Copenhagen; Williams & Wilkins, Baltimore, 1977.

18. WHO-IUIS Terminology Committee. *In* "Histocompatibility Testing 1975" (Kissmeyer-Nielsen, ed.), p. 5. Munksgaard, Copenhagen, 1975.

19. WHO-IUIS Terminology Committee. *In* "Histocompatibility Testing 1977" (W. F. Bodmer, J. R. Batchelor, J. G. Bodmer, H. Festenstein, and P. J. Morris, eds.), p. 14. Munksgaard, Copenhagen, 1977.

20. Cresswell, P., and Geier, S. S. *Nature 157*, 147, 1975.

21. Flaherty, L., Stanton, T. H., and Boyse, E. A. *Immunogenetics 4*, 101, 1977.

22. Geier, S. S., and Cresswell, P. *Cell. Immunol. 35*, 392, 1978.

23. Dausset, J., and Svejgaard, A. (eds.). "HLA and Disease." Munksgaard, Copenhagen; Williams & Wilkins, Baltimore, 1977.

24. Brewerton, D. A., and Albert, E. *In* "HLA and Disease" (J. Dausset and Svejgaard, A., eds.), p. 94. Munksgaard, Copenhagen; Williams & Wilkins, Baltimore, 1977.

25. Blumenthal, M. N., Amos, D. B., Noreen, H., Mendell, N. R., and Yunis, E. J. *Science 181*, 1301, 1974.

26. Amos, D. B., Ruderman, R., Mendell, N. R., and Johnson, A. H. *Transplant. Proc. 7*, 93, 1975.

27. Simon, M., Bourel, M., Genetet, B., and Fauchet, R. *N. Engl. J. Med. 197*, 1017, 1976.

28. Kravitz, K., Skolnick, M., Edwards, C., Cartwright, G., Cannings, C., Amos, B., Carmelli, D., and Baty, B. *In Proc. Conf. Genet. Epidemiol.* (N. E. Morton, and C. S. Chung, eds.). Academic Press, New York, 1978.

29. Barbosa, J., King, R., Noreen, H., and Yunis, E. J. *J. Clin. Invest. 60*, 989, 1977.

30. Rubinstein, P., Suciu-Foca, N., and Nicholson, J. B. *N. Engl. J. Med. 297*, 1036, 1977.

31. deVries, R. R. P., Fat, L. A., Nigenhuis, L. E., and van Rood, J. J. *Lancet ii*, 1328, 1976.

32. Bodmer, J., and Bodmer, W. F. *In Proc. Sheba Int. Symp. Genetic Polymorphisms and Diseases in Man* (B. Ramot, ed.), p. 131. Academic Press, New York, 1973.

33. Mi, M. P., and Morton, N. E. *Vox, Sang. 11*, 434, 1966.

34. Bennett, D., Boyse, E. A., and Old, L. J. *In* "Cell Interactions" (L. G. Silvestri, ed.), p. 247. Elsevier, New York, 1972.

35. Mattiuz, P. L., Ihide, D., Piazza, A., Ceppellini, R., and Bodmer, W. _In_ "Histocompatibility Testing 1970" (P. I. Terasaki, ed.), p. 193. Munksgaard, Copenhagen, 1970.

36. Amos, D. B. _In_ "Immunological Approaches to Fertility Control" (E. Diczfalusy, ed.). Karolinska Institute, Stockholm. 1974.

37. Lindblom, J. B., Friberg, J., Hogman, C. F., and Gemzell, C. _Tissue Antigens 2_, 352, 1978.

38. Barbosa, J., Noreen, H., Goetz, F. C., Simmons, R., Deleiva, A., Najarian, J., and Yunis, E. J. _Tissue Antigens 7_, 283, 1976.

39. Jersild, C., Dupont, B., Fog, T., Platz, P. J., and Svej-gaard, A. _Transplant. Rev. 22_, 148, 1975.

40. Falk, J., and Osoba, D. _In_ "HLA and Malignancy" (G. P. Murphy, ed.), p. 205. Munksgaard, Copenhagen, 1977.

41. Dausset, J. _In_ "HLA and Malignancy" (G. P. Murphy, ed.), p. 131. Munksgaard, Copenhagen, 1977.

42. Ward, F. E., Johnson, A. H., Amos, D. B., and Zmijewski, C. M. _In_ "Histocompatibility Testing 1977" (W. F. Bodmer, ed.). Munksgaard, Copenhagen, 1977.

43. Shaw, D. H. _Ann. N. Y. Acad. Sci. 97_, 153, 1962.

44. Cohen, C. _J. Immunol. 84_, 501, 1960.

45. Bennett, M. _Transplantation 14_, 289, 1972.

46. Dorf, M. E., Stimpfling, J. H., and Benacerraf, B. _J. Exp. Med. 1_, 1459, 1974.

47. Debre, P., Waltenbaugh, C., Dorf, M., and Benacerraf, B. _J. Exp. Med. 144_, 272, 1976.

48. Zinkernagel, R. M., and Doherty, P. C. _Nature 248_, 701, 1974.

49. Doherty, P. C., Blanden, R. V., and Zinkernagel, R. M. _Transplant. Rev. 29_, 89, 1976.

50. Shearer, M., Reha, T. G., and Schmitt-Verhulst, A. _Transplant. Rev. 29_, 222, 1976.

51. Lilly, F. _J. Exp. Med. 127_, 465, 1968.

52. Williams, R. M., Dorf, M. E., and Benacerraf, B. _Cancer Res. 35_, 1586, 1975.

53. Mann, D. L., Katz, S. I., Nelson, D. L., Abelson, L. D., and Strober, W. _Lancet i_, 110, 1976.

54. Bertrams, J., Jansen, F. L., Gruneklee, D., Reiss, H. E., Drost, H., Beyer, J., Gries, F. A., and Kunert, E. _Tissue Antigens 8_, 13, 1976.

55. Schernthaner, G., Mayr, W. R., and Ludwig, H. L. _In_ "HLA and Disease," Vol. 58, IV-24. INSERM, Paris, 1976.

56. Ivanyi, P., Hampl, R., Starka, L., and Mickova, M. _Nature New Biol. 283_, 280, 1972.

57. Thomas, L. _In_ "Cellular and Humoral Aspects of the Hyper-sensitivity States" (J. Lawrence, ed.), p. 529. Hoeber-Harper, New York, 1961.

58. Burnet, F. M. "Immunological Surveillance." Pergamon Press, New York, 1970.
59. Jerne, N. K. *Ann. Immunol. (Paris) 124C*, 171, 1974.
60. Haran-Ghera, N., and Peled, A. *Nature 241*, 396, 1973.
61. Gorer, P. A. *Adv. Immunol. 1*, 345, 1961.
62. Prehn, R. T. *Transplant. Rev. 28*, 34, 1976.
63. Koren, H. S., Amos, D. B., and Buckley, R. H. *J. Immunol. 120*, 796, 1976.
64. Herberman, R. B., Nunn, M. E., Holden, H. T., and Lavrin, D. H. *Int. J. Cancer 16*, 230, 1975.
65. Fauve, R., Hevin, B., Jakob, H., Gaillard, J., and Jacob, F. *Proc. Nat. Acad. Sci. 71*, 4052, 1974.
66. McMichael, A. J., Ting, A., Sweerink, H. J., and Askonas, B. A. *Nature 270*, 524, 1977.
67. Germain, R., Dorf, M., and Benacerraf, B. *J. Exp. Med. 142*, 1023, 1975.
68. Green, M. I., Dorf, M. E., Pierres, M., and Benacerraf, B. *Proc. Nat. Acad. Sci.*
69. Williams, R. M., and Frelinger, J. F. *Cancer Res. 38*, in press.

Ia-LIKE ANTIGENS IN HUMAN AUTOIMMUNE
DISEASES: HLA AND DRw ANTIGENS
IN CHRONIC ACTIVE HEPATITIS AND DIABETES MELLITUS*

R. Michael Williams

Division of Tumor Immunology
Sidney Farber Cancer Institute
and
Department of Medicine
Peter Bent Brigham Hospital
Boston, Massachusetts

Kenneth R. Falchuk
Charles Trey

Departments of Medicine,
New England Deaconess
and
Peter Bent Brigham Hospital
Boston, Massachusetts

Harriet Noreen
Jose Barbosa

University of Minnesota
Minneapolis, Minnesota

Devendra P. Dubey
William G. Cannady
Donna Fitzpatrick
Sharon Martin
Edmond J. Yunis

Division of Immunogenetics
Sidney Farber Cancer Institute
Boston, Massachusetts

Bo Dupont

Memorial Sloan-Kettering Cancer
Institute
New York, New York

*This research was supported in part by NIH CA 19791 and
NS 14387 (RMW), CA 20531 (EJY), CA 19589 (EJY), ACS #IM-149
(RMW), and CA 17404 (BD).*

INTRODUCTION

A study of the genetic correlates of autoimmune disease
must consider the accumulating evidence from basic immunobiology that the immune response is regulated by multiple intricate positive- and negative-feedback loops (1). By focusing
on the major histocompatibility complex (MHC) further insight
regarding precise mechanisms of autoimmune disease may be
generated. There is no doubt that in this genetic system alone,
there will be multiple interacting genes participating to produce a single recognized pathological entity (2). The importance of various subregions of the MHC has been emphasized in
detail. In particular, the I region of the mouse MHC (H-2)
seems to control many of the cell interactions that are involved in the regulation of host responsiveness (3). In the
mouse and the rat, this region also seems to play the dominant role in the induction of specific unresponsiveness to
allogeneic transplanted tissues (4,5). In man, the HLA-D
region is the equivalent of the mouse I region and the rat
mixed-lymphocyte interaction defined locus.
Since the HLA-D locus lies outside the HLA-B locus, the
overwhelming predominance of B locus antigen associations
with disease has frequently been attributed to likely linkage
disequilibrium between B-locus antigens and some more directly responsible genes in the D-region, which are thought to
produce disease through abnormal immunoregulation. Indeed,
the most popular hypothesis to explain the mechanisms of HLA-
associated disease is that there are immunoregulatory genes
in the HLA-D region and that these genes are functioning abnormally. However, the extensive studies of the role of the
serologically defined antigens themselves as initiated by the
work of Zinkernagel and Doherty also show how these antigens
may participate specifically in immunopathology, particularly
where virus infection is involved (6).
Abnormally functioning immunoregulatory genes and the
ability of the individual to respond to altered self through
the Zinkernagel-Doherty phenomenon are but two of the means
whereby the MHC may be involved in the pathogenesis of disease.
The finding that multiple MHC-linked genes may influence the
immune response even to simple antigens (7), or be involved
in model autoimmune disease (8) or the resistance to histoincompatible tumors (9), adds to the complexity of the problem
and makes us reflect that we really have little solid information about the involvement of HLA-linked genes with disease.
Many of the possibilities have been discussed elsewhere (10).
It is now possible to explore the HLA-D region through
serologic techniques based on B-cell antigens. These antigens,

called HLA-DR antigens (see preceding chapter), are thought to be analogous to mouse Ia antigens. They are called HLA-DR because they correlate closely with the HLA-D specificities. We can therefore expect to find a plethora of studies appearing that relate specific D region alleles to human disease. Good candidates for initial studies would be those diseases in which there has been a suggestion of B locus association and/or HLA-D locus association as determined by MLC typing. In most cases it is likely that the D and B locus associations demonstrated may be difficult to interpret because of the known linkage disequilibrium between many D locus antigens and corresponding B locus antigens, which may, of course, also affect other genes in these regions. While it is possible that the strongest associations will reflect genetic distance whenever absolute linkage studies are possible, we must bear in mind the fact that the explanation of linkage disequilibrium in terms of mechanism cannot be made with certainty nor can we be confident that there is but a single etiology for any observed disequilibrium.

In the context of the discussion above, it is interesting to note that one disease of abnormal immunoregulation, rheumatoid arthritis, became one of the first diseases to be assocaited in populations with a D locus allele in the absence of any known B locus associations (11). In the present study we have sought to investigate two other chronic diseases, diabetes and chronic active hepatitis (CAH), with the consideration that categorization of these diseases may be improved through HLA-DR typing. Preliminary data from 22 patients with diabetes mellitus and 17 patients with adult onset chronic active hepatitis (CAH) have been analyzed. No increase in HLA-Al, B8, or DRw3 was observed in CAH, whereas the anticipated increases in B8, DRw3, and DRw4 in diabetes were found. There was, however, a significant increase in DRw4 in CAH. Since abnormalities of cell-mediated immune function may underlie these diseases, we also present preliminary data on the only assay of cell-mediated immunity in man, which we believe can be quantitated adequately now, i.e., natural killer cell activity. The limited results available at this time do not show dramatic abnormalities among patients with liver disease compared to controls matched in part for DRw specificities.

MATERIALS AND METHODS

Seventeen adult patients carrying the diagnosis of chronic active hepatitis based on previous liver biopsy were included. This population contained 15 females and 2 males ranging in age from 20-75 years with a median age of 57 years. Only 3 of 13 patients tested had significant levels of antinuclear antibodies and these patients had the following HLA phenotypes: A2, A5, B7, Cw3; Al, A3, B8, Bl8; and A2, A9, Bw35, Cw4. All three had onset of disease during the fourth decade and the single HLA-B8 positive patient also had diabetes. HLA-A, -B, and -C typing was done by the Amos method (12) and HLA-DRw typing methodology and criteria for assignment were based on the 7th International Histocompatibility Typing Workshop Procedures. Data from 22 diabetes patients included in a study to be published elsewhere (1) have been reanalyzed for the purpose of this presentation, and the CAH data was in ref. 14.

Natural killer cell activity was determined by the routine method developed in our laboratory. The K562 chronic myelogenous leukemia cell line was used as the target, and a 4-hour assay was conducted at up to five effector-to-target ratios of 3.125 to 50:1 utilizing a constant number of 25,000 ^{51}Cr-labeled targets and 0.2 ml total reaction volume. After a 5-minute prespin to optimize effector-target conjugation, the plates were incubated at 37°C for 4 hours. Data were analyzed by constructing a log-log plot of percentage corrected chromium release vs. effector-to-target ratio--all done mathematically by computer. The r value given in Table II represents a correlation coefficient for a least-squares regression line that usually contained five experimental data points. Therefore, the "one-hit" nature of the system (15) can be considered to be roughly equivalent to the nearness of r to 1.000. The lytic unit (L.U.) ratio and lytic units were determined at 25% specific cytolysis.

We compare populations of cells utilizing the killer unit (K.U.) that is equivalent to lytic units per 156.25 million cells. This is a more convenient number to work with than is L.U./10^6 cells since most cell preparations have activity in the range of 10-1000 K.U. The lytic unit has dimensions of cells and the K.U. has dimensions of cells^{-1}. The size of K.U. was chosen to be equivalent to 6250 (25% of 25,000) when there was 25% lysis at a lymphocyte to target ratio of 1. The units themselves have no intrinsic meaning beyond that of lytic units per a fixed number of cells.

The distribution of killer unit measurements for normal individuals ranges from 0.001 to over 8000. The value zero is assigned when there is no lysis at any tested effector to target ratio. The distribution of these values is approximately normal and is made almost precisely so by taking the natural logarithm of the killer unit value for each mononuclear cell preparation. The relationship of killer units and lytic units is defined by the formula

$$L.U. \times K.U. = 156.25 \times 10^6$$

so either can be caluculated from the other.

We did not know the blood volume collected, the differential count, or the mononuclear cell recovery, so we could not calculate the number of lytic units per milliliter of whole blood. Very few samples from hepatitis patients were large enough to allow complete analysis for natural killer cell activity. Control cells were selected from among panel members that shared the DRw specificities with the patients studied. They were not matched for any other characteristic.

RESULTS

A comparison of HLA and DR frequencies in normal controls from a combination (MSFCI) of Minnesota (M), Sidney Farber Cancer Institute (SFCI) panels together with the donor panel typed by U.S. Region 7 during the 1977 Histocompatibility Testing Workshop is presented in Table I. Also included in this table are the frequencies of HLA-Al, -B8, and -DR among the 22 diabetes patients and the 17 chronic active hepatitis patients described. Several interesting observations are documented in these data.

In the 22 diabetes patients, a recalculation of relative risk for HLA-DRw3 gives 4.20 and for HLA-DRw4 gives 5.06. Both these results are significant at the $p < 0.005$ level, although correction for the number of DRw specificities ananlyzed would result in a p value of only <0.04.

The relative risk calculation for HLA-Al, -B8, and -B15 show no significant differences among the chronic active hepatitis patients tested and the MSFCI or U.S. 7 workshop control panel. The only DR specificity found to be increased in the chronic active hepatitis patients was DRw4; the relative risk calculation results in 8.4 compared to the MSFCI control panel and 8.8 compared to the U.S. 7 Region control panel. Both of these relative risk values are significant at the 0.005 level, and therefore would be significant at the 0.04 level after corrections for the seven DR specificities examined. There are no other significant differences among the chronic active hepatitis patients compared to either control panel.

TABLE I. Comparison of HLA-A1, -B8, and -B15 and DRw Frequencies among Control Populations and in Patients with Diabetes and Chronic Active Hepatitis

| | Normal individuals (%) | | Diabetes (22) | | | | | CAH (17) | | | | |
	(1) MSFCI (81)	(2) US7 (255)[a]	%	(1) RR[b]	p[c]	(2) RR	p	%	(1) RR	p	(2) RR	p
HLA-A1	24.7	24.1	31.8	1.32	>0.1	1.47	>0.1	35.3	1.66	>0.1	1.27	>0.1
HLA-B8	23.5	18.1	36.4	1.86	<0.05	2.59	<0.05	17.6	0.70	>0.1	0.91	>0.1
HLA-B15	11.1	6.5	9.1	0.80	>0.1	1.44	>0.1	5.9	0.44	>0.1	0.90	>0.1
HLA-DRw1	22.2	16.1	9.0	0.35	>0.1	0.62	>0.1	11.7	0.47	>0.1	0.82	>0.1
HLA-DRw2	28.4	27.1	18.0	0.56	>0.1	0.88	>0.1	23.5	0.78	>0.1	1.22	>0.1
HLA-DRw3	22.2	22.0	54.5	4.20	<0.005	5.10	<0.005	23.5	1.08	>0.1	1.31	>0.1
HLA-DRw4	22.2	24.7	59.0	5.06	<0.005	5.30	<0.005	70.6	8.40	<0.005	8.80	<0.005
HLA-DRw5	21.0	18.0	4.0	0.18	>0.1	0.26	>0.1	17.6	0.81	>0.1	1.16	>0.1
HLA-DRw6	14.8	6.3	4.0	0.27	>0.1	0.83	>0.1	17.6	1.23	>0.1	3.72	>0.1
HLA-DRw7	30.9	23.1	4.0	0.11	<0.05	0.19	<0.1	17.6	0.48	>0.1	0.85	>0.1

[a] Data in "Histocompatibility Testing 1977," Munksgaard, Copenhagen, in press, by Dupont, B., Yunis, E. J., Duquesnoy, R., Pollack, M., Noreen, H., Hansen, J. A., Reinsmoen, N., Annen, K., Greenberg, L., Lee, T. D., WHitsett, C., Antonelli, P., and Braun, D.: HLA-D and Ia-like alloantigens in North American Caucasians, U.S. Region 7.

[b] The formula for relative risk (RR) is $RR = \dfrac{ad}{bc}$, where a is number of antigen (+) patients, b is number of antigen (−) patients, c is number of antigen (+) normal population, d is number of antigen (−) normal population.

[c] p value evaluated using χ^2 calculated with Yates correction.

TABLE II. *Natural Killer Cell Activity in Patients with Liver Disease and Panel Members Partially Matched for DRw Specificities*

Patient I.D. and diagnosis[a]	r	KU[b]	DRw typing result	Anti-ln of ln(KU)[c] (mean ± S.D.)
Patient I.D. and diagnosis[a]				
IH Chronic persistent hepatitis	d	59.8	4,7,5	
9H Acute hepatitis-recovered	0.9092	79.2	4,7	
12H Chronic active hepatitis, × 2 years	0.7936	8.4	4,7,6	64.2 ± 3.6 KU
14H Chronic active hepatitis, × 4 years	0.9897	139.0	4,7	
38H Fatty liver with inflammation	0.9933	35.0	5,7	
44H Acute hepatitis	0.9303	362.5	3,4,7	
Normal Panel I.D.				
3	0.9318	630.1	4,7	
4	0.9295	11.5	4,7,6	
5	0.9958	126.5	4,7, (6)	115.8 ± 4.3 KU
11	0.9957	390.3	5,7	
13	0.9812	149.1	3,5	
14	0.9997	45.1	2,7	

[a] All patients were HBsAG negative.

[b] Killer unit (KU) is unit of cytotoxicity defined in the text.

[c] Natural logarithm of KU [ln(KU)] was used to calculate means, then this value was converted to KU by taking the anti-ln (i.e. $e^{ln(KU)}$). The difference between means is not significant (p > 0.1).

[d] Not calculated because only two effector/target ratios were tested.

The natural killer cell activity in six patients with liver disease compared to panel members partially matched for DR specificities is described in Table II. The mean results demonstrate that the natural killer cell activity of these patients did not differ significantly from that of the partially DR matched panel. The r values for linear regression correlation of log-log transformed data are slightly less than ideal among most of the hepatitis patients. This results in part from the fact that the samples available for testing were very small and could not be studied at all five effector-to-target ratios usually employed in these studies. However, we cannot rule out the possibility that the kinetics of activity by these patients fails to follow log-log linear kinetics, as it does in nearly all normal healthy individuals.

DISCUSSION

Studies of HLA and chronic active hepatitis have generally included cases where autoimmune features such as antinuclear and antismooth muscle antibodies were also present. This corresponds to the CAH-A category of MacKay (16). Hepatitis B antigen (HBsAg) positive cases or CAH-B are usually included as a control group and not considered to be immunological in any form. Cryptogenic hepatitis (CAH-C) refers to a category with no identifying characteristics, being negative for autoantibodies and HBsAg. The third type is drug-associated or CAH-D. This is but one scheme for categorization and therefore is subject to the same difficulties that plague all attempts to "split" or "lump" diseases through overlapping clinical or pathological characteristics. Nevertheless, all these diseases have the common characteristic of liver disease. They each have the positive biopsy findings of chronic active or aggressive hepatitis including perivascular and perilobular round cell infiltrates, which are destructive and frequently progress to cirrhosis and/or liver failure. In the autoimmune type, the increase of HLA-B8 and of the A1,B8 combination has been observed repeatedly (17). We previously showed in a retrospective study of a pediatric population that the A1,B8 haplotype as well as B8, was increased (18). These patients were those who had responded to therapy and thus were available for study. At the time of the first HLA and disease workshop in 1976, there were five reports of an increased frequency of HLA-B8 (19-22). The frequency of B8 in CAH patients was between 61 and 68% compared to 23-27% in control subjects. A single study that reported a normal frequency of HLA-B8 in chronic hepatitis was included as part of a study on celiac disease (23). These patients had fewer of the characteristics of autoimmune type presentation; for example, only five were younger than 40 years of age at presentation. A combination of these data with some additional earlier studies gives a total of 233 subjects with HLA-B8 and a relative risk for chronic active hepatitis in B8 positive subjects of 3.04. A few additional studies containing both old and new subjects have appeared recently and they each confirm an increase in HLA-B8 in CAH of the apparent autoimmune type (24,26).

The earlier study by Page *et al.* demonstrated a true increase in the Al,B8 haplotype through genotyping families (18). A family study recently reported by Dumble and MacKay has been interpreted to suggest that the MLC reaction of a HLA-B8 patient who happens to be phenotypically HLA identical to four normal siblings suggests the existence of a different non-HLA-linked determinant in the patient (27). No extensive studies including HLA-D typing were reported on chronic active hepatitis patients in the last histocompatibility workshop, except for the contribution of Opelz *et al.* (28), which reported an increased frequency of HLA-Dw3 (69%) among 38 cases of chronic liver disease compared to 91 controls (24% HLA-Dw3+). The HLA-B8 associated B cell antigen HLA-DRw3 was also found to be increased. Although the incidence of DRw3 gave a relative risk lower than that calculated for HLA-B8, the general conclusion of this study (28) was that the increased frequency of HLA-B8 in chronic active liver disease was an indirect result of an increase in the frequency of certain HLA-D associated genes. The combined results of all available studies, and making allowance for the observed increased frequency of B8 homozygosity seem to us, however, to indicate a closer association of CAH or CAH-A susceptibility with the HLA-B locus than with the HLA-D locus or an HLA-DR locus.

The present study was on a new group of patients from the practice of adult gastroenterologists in the Boston area. It therefore differs from the previous population that we studied, at least on the basis of age at onset. It also differs in that the only criterion for inclusion was the biopsy diagnosis of chronic active hepatitis with no consideration of the presence or absence of symptoms associated with autoimmune disorders. No increase of HLA-Al,B8 or DRw3 was observed in this group, although there was a significant increase in DRw4. The limited diabetes data confirm the previously described increases in B8 and Bw15. The increases in DRw3 and DRw4 could have been predicted from the increase of Dw3 and Dw4 found previously (29).

It is of interest that the DRw4 specificity is also increased in rheumatoid arthritis, another disease of abnormal immunoregulation. While studies of the biology of the immune

response in experimental animals would support the notion that
B cell antigens or Ia molecules may play an important role in
cell interactions, possibly including the orientation of antigenic specificities in the macrophage membrane (30), we
certainly cannot infer any specific mechanistic considerations
from these population associations with particular DR specificities. One generalization that can, however, be made is
that association of any disease with a particular B, D, or
DR specificity does not necessarily imply that another type
of categorization of the disease would yield the same specific associations. The point is made clearly in the case of
chronic active hepatitis where one approach to categorizing
the disease based on immunological autoimmune features led to
clear predominance of HLA-B8, even to the extent that it appeared that B8 was more closely associated than those HLA-D
or -DR antigens in high linkage disequilibrium with B8. However, a recategorization of the disease based on the presence
of chronic active hepatitis by biopsy led not only to the loss
of the significant associations noted for the autoimmune sub-
category, but the appearance of a completely new association
based on another D locus related specificity.

All these intricacies of the data on the association of
HLA with disease serve to reemphasize the fact that the mechanism of disease may depend on numerous interacting genes of
the major histocompatibility complex in addition to the obvious role of environment and other non-MHC genes. Given this
level of complexity it is fortunate that there are many models
of experimental autoimmune disease that can be applied to
specific or general categories of human disease. Even with
the advantage of these models, it will be necessary to investigate the parameters of immune function that can be accurately
quantified in patients and control populations. Since natural
levels of cell-mediated cytotoxicity, termed natural killer
cell activity, can be identified in normal as well as in dis-
eased individuals, the activity of these cells represents one
starting point for baseline studies of host cell-mediated immune function. If for no other reason, it will be necessary
to consider natural cell-mediated immunity as part of the
"background" in studies of specific cell-mediated cytotoxicity
in autoimmune disease. Perhaps with increasing understanding
of the human MHC, better experimental models for human diseases, and more precise quantitation of the human cell-mediated
immune response, a new set of tools for disease categorization
may become available.

References

1. Eardley, D. D., Shen, F. W., Cantor, H., et al. *In* "ICN-UCLA Symposia on Molecular and Cellular Biology," Vol. 8. Academic Press, New York, 1978.
2. Williams, R. M. *In* "HLA and Malignancy" (G. P. Murphy, ed.), p. 21. Alan R. Liss, Inc., 1977.
3. Paul, W. E., and Benacerraf, B. *Science 195*, 1293, 1977.
4. Staines, N. A., Guy, K., and Davies, D. A. L. *Transplantation 18*, 192, 1974.
5. Catto, G. R. D., Carpenter, C. B., Strom, T. B., et al. *Transplant. Proc. 9*, 957, 1977.
6. Doherty, P. C., Blanden, R. V., and Zinkernagel, R. M. *Transplant. Rev. 29*, 89, 1976.
7. Benacerraf, B., and Dorf, M. E. *Cold Spring Harbor Symp. Quant. Biol. 41*, 465, 1976.
8. Moore, M. J., and Williams, R. M. *Fed. Proc. 34*, 949, 1975.
9. Williams, R. M., Dorf, M. E., and Benacerraf, B. *Cancer Res. 35*, 1586, 1975.
10. Zinkernagel, R. M., and Doherty, P. C. *In* "HLA and Disease," p. 256. Munksgaard, Copenhagen, 1977.
11. Stasny, P. *In* "Histocompatibility Testing 1975," p. 797, Munksgaard, Copenhagen, 1977.
12. Amos, D. B., Bashir, H., Boyle, W., et al. *Transplantation 7*, 220, 1969.
13. Barbosa, J., et al. (in preparation)
14. Williams, R. M., Martin, S., Falchuk, K. R., et al. *Vox Sanguinis 35*, 366, 1978.
15. Mayer, M. M. *J. Immunol. 119*, 1195, 1977.
16. MacKay, I. R. *In* "Immunological Diseases," 3rd Ed. (Samster, ed.). Little Brown & Co., Boston, 1976.
17. MacKay, I. R. *In* "Nationale de la Sante et de la Recordue Medicale" (J. Dausset and A. Svwgaard, eds.), p. 186. Paris, 1977.
18. Page, A. R., Sharp, H. L., Greenberg, L. J., et al. *J. Clin. Invest. 56*, 530, 1975.
19. MacKay, I. R., and Morris, P. J. *Lancet ii*, 793, 1972.
20. Freudenberg, J., Erdmann, K., Meyer zum Buschenfelde, K. H., et al. *Lin. Wschr. 51*, 1075, 1973.
21. Galbraith, R. M., Eddleston, A. L. W. F., Smith, M. G. M., et al. *Br. Med. J. 3*, 604, 1974.
22. Lindberg, J., Lindholm, A., Lundin, P., et al. *Br. Med. J. 4*, 77, 1977.
23. Scott, B. B., Swinburne, M. L., Rajah, S. M., et al. *Lancet ii*, 374, 1974.
24. Morris, P. J., Vaughan, H., Tait, B. D., et al. *Aust. N.Z.J. Med.* (submitted for publication).
25. Freudenberg, J., Baumann, W., Arnold, W., et al. (submitted for publication).

26. Salaspuro, M., Makkonen, H., Sipponen, P., *et al.* (submitted for publication).
27. Dumble, L. J., and MacKay, I. R. *Digestion,* 1976.
28. Opelz, G., Vogten, A. J. M., Summerskill, W. H. J., *et al.* (submitted for publication).
29. Thomsen, M., Platz, P., and Ortved Anderson, O., *et al. Transplant. Rev. 22,* 120, 1975.
30. Rosenthal, A. S., and Shevach, E. M. *J. Exp. Med. 138,* 1194, 1973.

DISCUSSION

DR. VAN ROOD: Is the increased homozygosity of A_1 and B_8 in juvenile chronic hepatitis due to a recessive gene predisposing for the disease?

DR. YUNIS: Our studies published by Page *et al.*, cited in the manuscript, did not include families with more than one case of CAH-A. However, we studied the inheritance of HLA antigens in the families of these patients to establish the increased incidence of HLA-A_1-B_8 homozygotes in our patients. I believe that the increased relative risk in homozygous HLA-B_8 subjects is consistent with dosage effect of the HLA-8 associated antigen involved in disease susceptibility. However, we cannot rule out recessive transmission.

DR. KIRKPATRICK: With respect to the possible mechanisms that you presented in your last slide, is there any direct evidence of cross reactivity between microbial antigens and HLA antigens or that HLA antigens may serve as receptors for viruses?

DR. YUNIS: Yes, McMichael in W. Bodmer's laboratory has recently described the *in vitro* generation of cytotoxic cells against lymphocytes infected with influenza virus. The HLA restriction was produced by HLA-B7 antigen. Similar data have been obtained by Dick Miess in Svejgaard's laboratory in experiments using dinitrofluorobenzene. The HLA restriction was related to HLA-A2.

DR. AMOS: Will you comment on the reported association of B27 and Friedlander's bacillus? We became interested in this partly because Dick Postlethwait at Duke found that some colonies of Friedlander organisms from rat feces could absorb the natural antibody to thymocytes present in adult rat serum.

DR. YUNIS: There is at least one reference to the cross reactivity with B27 in the literature but I do not think the chemical basis for any such cross reaction is known.

DR. KIRKPATRICK: I'd like to ask Dr. Doherty if the genetic restrictions that he has found in the mouse system have been shown to apply to human cells as far as cytotoxicity of virus infected cells is concerned.

DR. DOHERTY: I think that Dr. Yunis or Dr. van Rood can give a more authoritative statement. However, in addition to Andrew McMichael, whom Dr. Yunis cited, there is evidence from Askona's laboratory of an HLA linkage with influenza but I do not know its exact nature. There also is evidence emerging from Dr. Shearer's laboratory with the TNP cytotoxicity system that there also is HLA linkage, but again, I'm not clear on the details.

DR. VAN ROOD: To the best of my knowledge, the information concerning influenza is indeed true; the dual recognition involves HLA-A2. There is also the unpublished work by Zinkernagel and Balner in which dual recognition has been established using vaccinia virus in rhesus monkeys. Our group also has described dual recognition of H-Y in man with HLA-A2 antigen; we have three cases, the most recent is not only A2 but also B7. It is of interest that of the 30 or so people studied to date, the three positive cases were aplastic anemia patients.

DR. SACHS: I wonder whether, if ankylosing spondylitis is one disease entity, the existence of HLA B27 negative cases doesn't imply that the association must be with a gene in high linkage disequilibrium with B27 rather than with B27 itself. In such cases, have any family studies been performed, and, if so, has linkage to the HLA-C locus been detected?

DR. YUNIS: You are correct. The presence of B27 negative patients with ankylosing spondylitis suggests that there are different forms of this disease. The great majority are associated with B27; the remaining cases are associated with HLA-Cw2 and Cw3. It is also possible that susceptibility to ankylosing spondylitis involves several genetic factors; the low frequency of B27 negative cases is probably related to non HLA-factors. Evidence for this was presented by van Rood and associates in family studies where they could suggest the existence of non-HLA recessive genes, as well as B27. So, the studies of HLA in ankylosing spondylitis illustrate both pleotropic and genetic heterogeneity, as well as the role of environmental factors.

DR. GOOD: I think that, even though ankylosing spondylitis seems so homogeneous, there's a very good possibility that there may very well be heterogeneity in the disease.

DR. VAN ROOD: We have specifically studied B27 negative cases by all the known criteria and found no differences. There was one very interesting family in this study. A male patient suffering from ankylosing spondylitis was B27 negative and was married to a B27-positive woman. Of their 11 children five were B27 positive males, of which four suffered from ankylosing spondylitis. It is of interest that the father was the offspring of a cousin marriage. These findings could be compatible with the assumption that the predisposition to ankylosing spondylitis is present either when B27, as a closely linked gene, together with a non-HLA gene in a single dose is carried by the individual or when this non-HLA gene is present in a double dose in the absence of B27.

DR. AMOS: Ward and Biegel have reported that North American Blacks with ankylosing spondylitis are frequently B27 negative. This might be a useful population to look at for a different disease form.

DR. YUNIS: That is true. Ankylosing spondylitis in Blacks should be studied now with the objective of finding other HLA antigens (non-B27) in the B27-negative patients. Of course, HLA-DRw antigens should also be investigated. Let me also comment on the fact that HLA antigens have different frequencies in different ethnic groups. Myasthenia gravis is associated with B12 and Bw35 in Japanese, while it is associated with B8 in Caucasians. Two interesting examples that have relevance to the subject of genetic linkage disequilibrium (nonrandom association) are (1) the specificity HLA-DHO (Japanese HLA-D) is in disequilibrium with A9-Bw35, is absent in Caucasians, and is found associated with myasthenia gravis and Graves' disease among Japanese; HLA-DYT found in linkage disequilibrium with A9-Bw22 is absent in Caucasians, but is found in association with juvenile onset diabetes mellitus in Japanese; (2) in the case of ankylosing spondylitis, studies of frequency of HLA associations suggest that Japanese patients have a higher frequency of HLA-A2,B27, rather than A1 or A3, which are Caucasian antigens. So, linkage disequilibrium in this case may be useful to show the possible origin of a disease mutation and its transmission as a hitchhiker on a haplotype. Non-B27s may reflect a different disease or the same hitchhiker on different haplotypes.

DR. GOOD: I wonder if you would comment on the relationship between complement deficiencies and the major histocompatibility complex. It is of great interest that each of the complement components is linked to HLA; 2C, 4C, and factor B are complement components that address 3C. In this case it is of importance to mention the recent work of Pablo Rubenstein and N. K. Day, who have found 3C to be associated with the seventeenth chromosome of the mouse, about 10 centimorgans from the H-2 histocompatibility region.

DR. YUNIS: The only evidence I can recall from the literature is that of Festenstein's group, who found that an antibody against HLA-Bw4 and -Bw6 activates a 3C receptor. Perhaps Dr. Rosen has a comment.

DR. ROSEN: Although Nussenzweig has shown control of 3C levels by the S region of mouse H-2, I know of no evidence for HLA linkage with 3C polymorphism or deficiency in man.

IDIOPATHIC POLYNEURITIS AS AN AUTOIMMUNE DISEASE

Barry Arnason

Department of Neurology
Pritzker School of Medicine
University of Chicago
Chicago, Illinois

INTRODUCTION

Idiopathic polyneuritis (Landry-Guillain-Barré-Strohl syn-drome) is a relatively rare disease. It occurs in all parts of the world and at all ages. The condition has been esti-mated to have an annual incidence of 1.6 cases per 100,000 population in Olmsted County, Minnesota (1), and of approxi-mately 2 cases per 100,000 population per year on the west coast of Norway (2). These figures may be compared with in-cidences for multiple sclerosis of 3.6 per 100,000 population per year in Olmsted County, Minnesota (3) and 1.9 per year in Norway (4).

Epidemiologic studies from other locales are not avail-able for idiopathic polyneuritis (IP) but there is a consensus among neurologists that the marked differences in incidence seen in different geographical locations in, for example, mul-tiple sclerosis, do not occur. Fragmentary data exist to suggest that IP may be less common among Blacks in the United States than among Caucasians but this point is disputed (5). Histocompatibility studies of IP patients have failed, to date, to show any link between susceptibility to disease and any histocompatibility antigen (6).

The cause or causes of IP remain unknown but there is agreement that the disease is inflammatory in nature and that immune mechanisms have an essential role in the pathogenesis of the process. A case can be made for considering IP as an autoallergic process. A presentation of this case forms the

central theme for the present communication. The autoallergic
thesis of causation of IP rests on several lines of evidence,
which will be developed sequentially.

EXPERIMENTAL ALLERGIC NEURITIS (EAN)

This animal disease was described by Waksman and Adams in
1955 (7) in animals immunized with crude peripheral nerve homo-
genate in complete Freund's adjuvant (CFA) although it was subsequently established that CFA is not essential for disease induction (8). EAN has been produced in essentially all mammalian and avian species in which disease induction has been attempted. EAN is an inflammatory cytodestructive disease of
PNS myelin.

Recent work has pointed strongly to a basic protein of
peripheral nerve myelin (PNS-BP) as the responsible antigen.
The protein has a molecular weight of approximately 12,000 and
has been designated as P_1L in Israel (9), P_2 in America (10),
and BF in Japan (11). PNS-BP is found exclusively in PNS myelin and should not be confused with the basic protein of central nervous system myelin (CNS-BP). Immunization with CNS-BP
induces experimental allergic encephalomyelitis (EAE), an
autoallergic demyelinating disease of the CNS that provides,
in many ways, the CNS counterpart for EAN. CNS-BP is found
in peripheral nerves in varying quantity depending on species.
CNS-BP when isolated from the PNS has been designed P_2 in
Israel (9), P_1 in America (10), and BM in Japan (11). CNS-BP
of PNS origin will induce EAE and in some species, e.g., guinea pigs, lesions in peripheral nerve indistinguishable on
histologic grounds from those of EAN can be induced by immunization with crude CNS white matter or with CNS-BP derived
from either CNS or PNS, although in these circumstances the
typical CNS lesions of EAE are present as well. Immunization
with PNS-BP, in contrast, induces lesions confined to the PNS.

The clinical characteristics of EAN differ to some extent
from species to species but there is, in general, after an
interval of 2 weeks or thereabouts following immunization, a
loss of reflexes, flaccid weakness, ataxia, and a variable degree of sensory impairment. EAN may progress to frank paralysis and death, but if the animal survives the acute phase of
the illness, which endures for from 1 to 3 weeks, clinical
recovery gradually ensues. In monkeys the clinical picture
bears a remarkable resemblance to that of IP in man. Spontaneous relapses are exceptional in EAN. A chronic form of
the disease has been developed in rabbits (12).

Substantial agreement exists as to the pathologic features of EAN (13-18). The earliest discernible event is an attachment of activated lymphocytes to the walls of venules in nerves, followed by passage of these cells through or between the endothelial cells to gain the nerve parenchyma. Within the parenchyma the cells enlarge and proliferate although some proliferative activity is also manifest by intravascular cells. Monocytes accompany or follow the lymphocytes into the nerve parenchyma where they transform into macrophages. Plasma cells and neutrophils are rarely encountered in early EAN lesions. Cellular infiltration precedes the onset of any discernible cytodestruction by 48 to 72 hours. Cytodestructive lesions are confined to regions of cellular infiltration. Primary damage is confined to PNS myelin; Schwann cells show reactive changes only and are not killed by the autoallergic process.

Three types of myelinodestructive change have been recognized in EAN:

(1) Widening of the intralamellar periodicity of myelin consequent to splitting of myelin at the intraperiod lines. This abnormality is seen in some instances only, and resembles the change observed when sera from "selected" EAN animals are added to myelinated peripheral nerve tissue cultures.

(2) Vesicular disruption of external myelin lamellae. This invariably occurs in close proximity to lymphocytes, although direct contact between invading lymphocytes and myelin does not appear to be necessary.

(3) Direct destruction of myelin by macrophages. This last is by far the predominant pattern of myelin breakdown.

Tongue processes of macrophages pierce the Schwann cell basal lamina and the outer myelin lamellae and then extend for substantial distances between lamellae so as to effectively sequester myelin fragments. A bubbly disintegration of myelin in direct contact with the macrophages ensues and the myelin fragments are ultimately ingested and digested. The macrophage tongue processes are remarkably free of organelles such as lysosomes but do contain uniformly dispersed intracytoplasmic fine granules. Extracellular proteolysis prior to ingestion may be occurring but this is not proven and the mechanism by which macrophages become "educated" is completely unknown. The net final result of this remarkable process is to segmentally denude the axon of its investing myelin.

At times when the inflammatory process is particularly intense, axonal interruption may be superimposed on the segmental demyelinating process, which constitutes the hallmark

of EAN. The axon distal to its point of interruption dies and
its investing myelin disintegrates--a process known as Wal-
lerian degeneration.

EAN is ordinarily a monophasic illness and myelin destruction is followed by remyelination, a relatively rapid process.
Axonal interruption is followed by axonal regrowth, and this is
a slow process. Schwann cell proliferation precedes remyelination and is first evident 10 days after disease onset (19).
In recovered animals, areas where remyelination has occurred
can be recognized by their shortened internodal distances and
the thinness of the new myelin that is laid down.

When lymph node or peripheral blood lymphocytes from rats
about to come down with EAN are added to myelinated peripheral nerve cultures, myelin destruction with axonal sparing ensues (20,21). A latent period of 48 hours precedes the onset
of myelin breakdown *in vitro*. It should be noted that myelinated peripheral nerve cultures invariably contain macrophages.
The demyelinative effect is at least relatively specific--
lymphocytes from rats with EAE do not demyelinate peripheral
nerve cultures.

Lymphocytes from EAN animals exposed to crude peripheral
nerve homogenates or to PNS-BP *in vitro* undergo a proliferative response of the type usually associated with the presence
of cell-mediated immunity (CMI) (22,23). Sensitivity of lymph
node cells is first evident several days prior to onset of
clinical disease and positive skin tests of delayed hypersensitivity type first become demonstrable at this same time (23).
EAN can be passively transferred with lymphoid cells either administered systemically (23,24) or injected directly into the
nerves of recipient animals (25).

The role of circulating antibody in EAN is unclear. Attempts to passively transfer EAN with serum administered systemically have failed, and although antinerve antibodies do
develop in EAN animals there is no correlation between disease onset and appearance of antibody or between antibody
titer and disease severity (26).

Pretreatment of rats with nerve in saline prior to attempted
induction of EAN with nerve in CFA blocks development of disease (27). Partial protection from EAN can be passively transferred to virgin recipient rats with sera from rats protected
in this manner (28). Serum from protected rats will also block
myelin destruction *in vitro* by sensitized lymphocytes from EAN
rats (27). These findings suggest that antinerve antibodies
may sometimes exert a protective influence in EAN. The possibility that a circulating suppressive factor may account for
the results just described is made less likely by the finding
that serum from rats immunized with brain in saline, a tech-

nique that partially prevents induction of EAE, fails to block myelin destruction by lymphocytes from rats *in vitro* (27).

This conclusion is reinforced by studies in Marek's disease (see below), a herpes virus induced myelinodestructive disease of peripheral nerves in chickens, the morphologic features of which are indistinguishable from those of EAN. Bursectomy in birds blocks antibody production while leaving CMI responses intact and heightens the severity of Marek's disease neuritis (29). In mammals, antibody responses can be suppressed by surgical destruction of the posterior hypothalamus, a technique that leaves CMI responses intact. In animals so treated, EAN occurs earlier after immunization with nerve in CFA and is of increased severity (30).

Complement probably has no role in lesion induction in EAN, at least in rats. Rats treated with cobra venom to deplete them of C_3 develop EAN of severity comparable to that observed in controls.

Serum from EAN rats sometimes demyelinates rat gasserian ganglion cultures, however (20,31). Three of 23 cultures tested with sera drawn 10 to 12 days postimmunization in our studies were demyelinated as were 9 of 29 cultures tested with sera drawn 13 to 15 days postimmunization. These results may be contrasted with those obtained with lymph node cells. Using cells taken 4 to 6 days postimmunization, a time at which serum is totally ineffectual, 6 of 24 cultures demyelinated, and when cells taken at 7 to 9 days were used 27 of 38 cultures demyelinated. In rats then, demyelination by serum *in vitro* is late appearing and infrequent, whereas demyelination by cells appears early and is present in the majority of instances.

Others have found demyelinating antibodies in the sera of guinea pigs and rabbits with EAN with a greater frequency than has been my experience in rats (31). In recent work serum samples from EAN rabbits that had been preselected for their high titer of *in vitro* demyelinating activity were injected directly into the sciatic nerves of recipient rats. Within a few hours of serum injection a mononuclear infiltrate appeared at the site of injection and myelin stripping by activated macrophages was subsequently observed (32). The antibody was felt to be directed against galactocerebroside. The physiologic relevance of these provocative observations is uncertain at present.

In EAN animals the cerebrospinal fluid (CSF) protein level is markedly elevated but few cells are to be found in the CSF. Electrophysiologic studies demonstrate the decreased conduction velocity characteristic of a demyelinative process.

Coonhound Paralysis

This remarkable disease provides a naturally occurring
canine model for IP in man. Certain dogs develop a subacutely
evolving paralytic illness 1 to 2 weeks after being bitten by
a raccoon. Coonhound paralysis may progress to death but most
dogs ultimately recover (33). The disease is uncommon even
among dogs bitten frequently, but a dog that has recovered
from coonhound paralysis may relapse if bitten again. Relapses may also be induced by injection of centrifuged raccoon
saliva. Severe EAN can be induced in littermates of dogs
that have developed coonhound paralysis by an immunization
schedule that induces only mild disease in other dogs (34).
This finding suggests that there may be a genetically determined predisposition to develop EAN in dogs and that this may
be linked to a predisposition to develop coonhound paralysis.
A genetically determined predisposition to develop EAN exists
in other species--Lewis rats, for example, are particularly
susceptible to EAN. The clinical and pathologic features of
coonhound paralysis are indistinguishable from those of EAN in
dogs (33,34).

Marek's Disease

Marek's disease (MD) occurs in chickens infected with
Marek's disease virus (MDV), an oncogenic herpes virus. Weakness and paralysis develop within a few weeks of infection
with associated lymphocytic infiltrates, enlargement, and
edema of peripheral nerves. The peripheral nerve lesions are
sometimes accompanied by encephalomyelitis. Virus cannot be
recovered from nerve, and virions are not seen when nerve
material from birds with frank neuritis is examined with the
electron microscope.

MDV also induces lymphoid tumors. In MD lymphomas *in vivo,*
a small proportion of cells are productively infected, but MD
lymphoblastoid cell lines maintained *in vitro* do not contain
virions or viral antigen (35). They do contain Marek agent
genome in multiple copies as determined by hybridization
studies (36) and do express a MDV-associated tumor-specific
surface antigen (MATSA) (37).

In vivo Marek's lymphomas are infiltrated with activated
T cells that, it is believed, are reacting against the tumor
cells and possibly against MATSA (38). The tumor cells are
themselves of T cell derivation (39).

The basis for the sequence of events that leads to MD
lymphoma is imperfectly understood. Good evidence pointing
to an early CMI response directed against tumor antigens has

been brought forward using *in vitro* techniques (38). This is followed in birds that develop tumors, though not in resistant birds, by a profound anergy for T-cell-mediated responses, which seems to relate to heightened suppressor lymphocyte activity (39-41). The tumor cells themselves may release suppressor factors. Similar T on T suppressor activity has been demonstrated in primates with T cell lymphomas induced by herpes virus saimiri (42).

The initial lesions in Marek's neuritis consist of activated T cell infiltrates plus macrophages and can be seen at a time when lymphoid tumor cells are not found in nerve (16, 43). This early infiltrate is associated with myelin destruction. The pattern of myelin destruction with sequestration and ingestion of myelin fragments by macrophages is indistinguishable from that of EAN induced in chickens by immunization with peripheral nerve in CFA.

Later, tumor cells begin to infiltrate the peripheral nerves so that the lesions come to contain a mixed population of T-lymphocyte-derived tumor cells, activated T lymphocytes reacting against the tumor cells (and/or nerve), plus macrophages. As the later lesions evolve, the nerves enlarge, as can be seen on gross inspection, become edematous, and axonal destruction is engrafted onto the basic demyelinative process.

Marek's neuritis is T cell dependent. Thymectomy, anti-lymphocyte serum, glucocorticoids, and immunosuppressive agents will all prevent the disease (44). The role of antibody in Marek's neuritis is uncertain. Antibody titers do not differ in susceptible and resistant birds. Neuritis in bursecto-mized birds is of enhanced severity, suggesting that antibody exerts, if anything, a protective role (29,45).

Marek's neuritis, like Marek's lymphoma, can be prevented by immunization with an antigenically related herpes virus of turkeys. Bursectomized birds can be successfully immunized, suggesting that protection from disease depends on CMI. It is possible to prevent Marek's lymphoma development with the membrane fraction of turkey virus infected cells, suggesting that the response is directed against a virus-associated cell surface antigen, such as MATSA (46). How such an antigen might predispose to neuritis is completely unknown.

Idiopathic Polyneuritis

Several parallels exist between the human disease and the model diseases discussed above:

1. *Antecedent Event.* In the model systems disease follows injection of nerve antigen (EAN), foreign protein (coonhound paralysis), or viral infection (Marek's neuritis).

In IP approximately half the patients give a history of
an antecedent infectious illness, most commonly respiratory in
nature. This illness has usually, though by no means invariably, resolved by the time neuritic symptoms begin. The interval between the onset of the prodromal event and onset of IP
is variable; most commonly it is 1 to 3 weeks.

An array of different infectious agents has been linked to
IP (reviewed in reference 47). These include the common en-
veloped virus pathogens of man, measles, rubella, mumps, varicella-zoster, smallpox-vaccinia, cytomegalovirus, Epstein-
Barr (EB) virus, and possibly B virus (a herpes virus of monkeys), when man is accidentally infected with this agent.
Other viruses linked to IP include influenza (both A and B)
(48,49) and infectious hepatitis. IP may also be associated
with mycoplasma pneumoniae infection, and with typhus and
bacterial infections (such as typhoid, listeriosis, brucello-
sis and tularemia) in which the bacillus survives intracellularly.

It is difficult to envisage how so many agents each with
its distinct clinicopathologic manifestations could all cause
the relatively stereotyped syndrome of IP by any directly invasive mechanism. Further, in those uncommon cases where the
disease takes on a recurrent form, individual recurrences may
be preceded by different antecedent infections.

From 5 to 10% of cases of IP follow a surgical procedure
(50), not necessarily complicated by infection. Cases have
followed general and spinal anesthesia and intracranial, thor-
acic, abdominal, urologic, and orthopedic procedures among
others. Recurrent cases are on record in which the initial
attack followed an infection and a recurrence followed surgery, sometimes very rapidly (51) and vice versa. Formerly IP
was seen as a rare complication of fever therapy--in several
such instances a herpetic eruption preceded the onset of the
neuritis.

It has become increasingly clear in recent years that IP
may complicate the course of lymphomatous disease, particularly Hodgkin's disease (52,54). As is well known, anergy is
frequently encountered in lymphoma patients and indeed has
been found in IP patients with underlying lymphomatous disease (54). The clinical and pathologic features of IP complicating lymphoma are indistinguishable from IP occurring under other circumstances. The complication is frequently mis-
taken for vincristine neuropathy, and may in fact be superimposed on vincristine neuropathy, but was known to occur before vincristine therapy was introduced.

The potential similarities between this situation in man

and Marek's neuritis in chickens are noteworthy. Anergy can be demonstrated in both conditions at a time when a putative autoallergic process is occurring. It is also worth noting that IP can complicate Epstein-Barr (EB) virus infection in man. EB virus is both an oncogenic agent and the cause of infectious mononucleosis. Anergy, sometimes of profound degree, is regularly observed in infectious mononucleosis (55).

IP has been encountered in renal transplant patients at times of effective immunosuppression (56). Whether a mild uremic neuropathy sets the stage for this remarkable event is uncertain. A clinical syndrome similar to if not identical with IP is also recognized as a rare but defined complication of lupus erythematosis but pathologic confirmation as to the precise nature of the neuritic process in lupus patients is lacking. One case of IP has been described in an agammaglobulinemic child (57).

IP as a complication of vaccination has received attention recently with the report that approximately one in 100,000 persons given swine flu vaccine during the mass vaccination program embarked upon in the United States during the fall of 1976 developed polyneuritis over the following 6 weeks (58). This translates into a six- to eightfold increase over the expected incidence for this time period. IP cases after swine flu vaccination have tended to show low back pain as a prominent early complaint. Sensory loss has seemed more prominent and motor involvement less severe than in nonvaccinated patients with IP (58). In normal volunteers given swine flu vaccine, an augmented natural killer cell activity was observed 2 weeks after immunization. Possibly an alteration in immune regulation followed swine flu vaccination. Such a postulate will not account for the rarity of polyneuritis after swine flu vaccination unless some second and rarer factor was also in play.

IP has been recognized as a rare but real hazard of vaccination procedures for many years. IP after smallpox vaccination has been amply documented (59). Interestingly this complication is commoner after revaccination, a finding that contrasts with postvaccinal encephalomyelitis, an inflammatory demyelinative disease of the CNS that serves as the CNS counterpoint for postvaccinal IP. Postvaccinal encephalomyelitis almost invariably follows primary vaccination. Instances of IP have been reported after typhoid and paratyphoid vaccination and even after tetanus toxoid. Perhaps related are those IP cases that follow a sting from a venomous insect. Rarely IP has been observed in heroin addicts (60).

IP is a recognized hazard of antirabies prophylaxis with Semple type vaccines prepared from neural tissue. With the introduction of vaccines prepared by growing attenuated rabies

virus in chicken or duck embryos this neurologic complication
appears to have been eliminated, but unfortunately such vaccines tend to be of low potency. A vaccine prepared from
rabies virus infected suckling mouse or rat brain continues
to be widely employed in Latin America. This technique of
vaccine preparation was introduced in an attempt to prevent
rabies vaccination induced emcephalomyelitis, an autoallergic
disease in which an anti-CNS myelin response is induced. Newborn mouse brain is not myelinated and administration of vaccines prepared in suckling mice is not complicated by encephalomyelitis. However, numerous cases of rabies vaccination induced polyneuritis continue to be reported following treatment
with this improved vaccine (61). Some years ago I attempted
to induce EAN in rats and guinea pigs using the Latin American rabies vaccine as antigen but the attempt failed. Cases
of IP have also been reported after administration of the
Margoulis-Choubladze neurovaccine introduced by Russian physicians as a treatment for multiple sclerosis.

As already mentioned IP occurs at all ages, though it is
less common and milder in childhood than in early and middle
adult years. Rabies vaccination induced neuritis is rare in
children. Only 2 of 125 cases in the series of Remlinger were
under 10 years of age (62). Whether these epidemiologic data
tie to age related alterations in immune competence is unclear.

2. Cerebrospinal Fluid. An increase in cerebrospinal
fluid (CSF) protein with few cells is observed in the majority of cases of IP. At the onset of IP the CSF protein is almost invariably normal, but in most instances will be found to
be increased at the end of the first week and thereafter. The
CSF findings are exactly comparable to those observed in EAN.
Oligoclonal banding in the CSF in IP has been reported by Link
(63). In my experience oligoclonal bands are uncommon in the
CSF in IP.

3. Clinical Course. IP evolves subacutely and progression
of illness has ceased at the end of 2 to 3 weeks in the vast
majority of cases. This tempo of evolution is roughly comparable to that observed in EAN, and as with the experimental
disease IP is monophasic in the vast majority of instances.
More chronic forms of the disease are recognized in man, as
in animals, and recurrences are observed in a small proportion
of instances, a circumstance that invites comparison with coonhound paralysis in dogs.

4. Pathology. The pathologic features of IP are indistinguishable in their essentials from those of EAN (52,64-66).

Lymphocytic infiltrates are found throughout the PNS neuraxis
in IP and stripping of myelin lamellae by macrophage tongue
processes with subsequent ingestion and digestion of myelin
fragments has been amply documented in the human as in the
experimental disease. Lesions in IP are confined to the PNS.
In the extensive pathologic material that I have examined,
only reactive changes have been seen in the CNS, with the exception of cases of IP complicating infectious mononucleosis.
Schwann cell proliferation begins 9 to 10 days after onset of
disease exactly as in EAN (52).

IP is a disease of the entire PNS. Motor and sensory
roots, dorsal root ganglia, peripheral nerves down to the
finest myelinated terminal twigs, and the sympathetic ganglia
and nerves may all be involved. The brunt of the process
falls on different parts of the neuraxis in individual cases.

Slowly evolving forms of motor and of mixed motor and
sensory neuropathy often show inflammatory infiltrates and a
pattern of demyelination and remyelination indistinguishable,
save for minor differences, from that seen in acutely evolving
IP (reviewed in reference 49). I believe that most cases of
sporadically occurring neuropathy represent variants of the IP
syndrome. In recurrent polyneuropathies as well, the pathologic features do not differ in their essentials from those
encountered in acute monophasic IP.

Interestingly, in all recovered cases of IP where they
have been assiduously sought, mild but definite inflammatory
infiltrates have been demonstrated in nerve months to years
after seemingly complete clinical recovery (49). This finding
suggests that the disease may normally smolder in subclinical
form. Perhaps indolent subclinical disease activity provides
the substratum for recurrences of disease should immune surveillance become defective for whatever reason.

In herpes simplex virus immunized rats that have recovered
from EAE, an injection of herpes simplex virus can provoke a
recrudescence of disease, perhaps by temporarily damping normal suppressive mechanisms (67). In multiple sclerosis (MS),
a human disease for which EAE has been proposed as a model,
a loss of nonspecific T on T suppressor activity coincident
with flareups of disease can be shown (68). Attacks of MS
ordinarily last 2 to 3 weeks and in this sense are comparable
to attacks of IP. As recovery from an attack of MS begins
there is a rebound of suppressor activity to high normal
levels. Such data are not available for EAN or for IP, but
the notion that a nascent sensitivity to PNS-BP can only be
expressed when the suppressor activity that normally holds
the process in check is abrogated by, for example, an infectious illness, seems a plausible working hypothesis to account
for recurrences of IP. Perhaps in the initial or only attack

of IP, nascent sensitivity flares when immune surveillance is abrogated. Such a formulation of course begs the question of how the nascent sensitivity developed in the first instance.

    5. *Immunologic Studies.* Peripheral blood lymphocytes (PBL) from IP patients will attack and destroy myelin in cultures of rat gasserian ganglion in 80% of cases (20,21). As is the case with cells from EAN a latent period of 48 hours elapses between addition of cells from IP patients and onset of demyelination. The effect is specific for IP and is not seen when cells from patients with other diseases of brain, nerve, or muscle are added to the cultures. In our hands sera or CSF from IP patients have, with occasional exceptions, failed to demyelinate rat nerve cultures, but other workers have reported positive results with serum (69,70). IP sera have also been reported to exert a cytotoxic effect on mouse but not human neuroblastoma cells (71).

    PBL from acute IP patients respond *in vitro* to crude nerve antigen or to PNS-BP as judged by lymphocyte stimulation or macrophage migration inhibition (MIF) assays (72-74). *In vitro* MIF activity correlates with disease activity in acutely evolving cases and has also been observed in cases of more slowly evolving neuropathy. CMI as measured by *in vitro* techniques is specific for IP among diseases of brain, nerve, and muscle. No CMI studies of PBL from IP patients with underlying anergy have been performed to date but would be of paramount interest.

    Antinerve antibodies can be demonstrated in IP by complement fixation and fluorescence techniques. IgM, IgA, and IgG antibodies have all been found in various combinations, which vary from patient to patient (75-76). The role of these antibodies in disease has not been established. The fluorescent antibodies react with both CNS and PNS myelin and can be mutually cross-absorbed (68) yet the disease itself is confined to the PNS. Low levels of immune complexes in serum have also been found in IP (77) but their meaning remains obscure. Deposition of immune complexes in the renal glomeruli has been noted in isolated instances if IP (78). Again, the significance of this observation is uncertain.

    Peripheral blood T cell levels fall as an attack of IP is beginning and rise as it is ending (2). In contrast increased numbers of T cells appear in the CSF during the active phase of the disease (2).

TABLE I. Experimental Allergic Neuritis (EAN) Compared with Idiopathic Polyneuritis (IP)

	EAN	IP
Inducing event	*Immunization with PNS-BP or crude nerve*	*Infection, surgery, vaccination*
Latency	*2-3 weeks*	*1-6 weeks*
Clinical forms		
subacute	*yes*	*yes*
monophasic	*yes*	*yes*
recurrent	*yes*	*yes*
chronic	*yes*	*yes*
Pathology		
lymphocytic infiltrates	*yes*	*yes*
macrophage stripping of myelin	*yes*	*yes*
segmental demyelination	*yes*	*yes*
lesions confined to PNS	*yes*[a]	*yes*
Schwann cell proliferation	*yes*	*yes*
CSF		
increased portein	*yes*	*yes*
lymphocytes	*few*	*few*
Nerve conduction	*slowed*	*slowed*
Lymphocytes destroy myelin in culture	*yes*	*yes*
CMI to PNS-BP	*yes*	*yes*

[a]*If immunized with PNS-BP.*

CONCLUSION

There is compelling evidence to indicate that in IP in man, as in EAN in animals, intense sensitivity to PNS-BP is present when disease is active. For this reason alone I conclude that EAN in animals provides a reasonable working model for the human disease. The similarities that exist between IP and EAN are listed in Table I.

Understanding of IP remains incomplete. The details of

the mechanism by which "educated" macrophages strip myelin without destroying the Schwann cell are not yet worked out. It is by no means clear why the pathologic process in IP, once initiated, should abruptly terminate after 2 to 3 weeks of progression. Study of suppressor cell function in progressing and recovering IP patients may well prove fruitful in this regard.

There is substantial, although admittedly indirect, evidence to suggest that an abrogation of immune surveillance may precede the onset of IP. Disordered immune regulation triggered by infection, by nonspecific stresses such as surgery, or occurring on a background of anergy, as in Hodgkin's disease, may all act to permit development of IP. The antecedent events mentioned above, when taken in sum, are common in the population at large, yet IP itself is rare. A second factor or event would appear necessary therefore to account for the occurrence of IP. The rarity of IP might then be ascribed to the chance coming together of two more common events. The nature of this putative second determinant, which in my view is likely to be development of nascent sensitivity to PNS-BP, remains totally unknown.

References

1. Lesser, R. P., Hauser, W. A., Kurland, L. T., *et al.* *Neurology 23*, 1269, 1973.
2. Nyland, H.--Personal communication.
3. Percy, A. K., Nobrega, F. T., Okazabi, H., *et al.* *Arch. Neurol. 25*, 105, 1971.
4. Presthus, J. *Acta Neurol. Scand. 42 (Suppl. 19)*, 12, 1966.
5. Masucci, E. F., and Kurtzke, J. F. *J. Neurol Sci. 13*, 483, 1971.
6. Hughes, R.--Personal communication.
7. Waksman, B. H., and Adams, R. D. *J. Exp. Med. 102*, 213, 1955.
8. Levine, S., and Wenk, E. J. *Proc. Soc. Exp. Biol. Med. 113*, 898, 1963.
9. London, Y. *Biochem. Biophys. Acta 249*, 188, 1971.
10. Brostoff, S., Burnett, P., Lampert, P., *et al.* *Nature New Biol. 235*, 210, 1972.
11. Kiyota, K., and Egami, S. *J. Neurochem. 19*, 857, 1972.
12. Sherwin, A. L. *Arch. Neurol. 15*, 289, 1966.
13. Åström, K.-E., Webster, H., de F., and Arnason, B. G. W. *J. Exp. Med. 128*, 469, 1968.
14. Lampert, P. W. *Lab. Invest. 20*, 127, 1969.
15. Ballin, R. H. M., and Thomas, P. K. *J. Neurol. Sci. 8*, 1, 1969.

16. Lampert, P., Garrett, R., and Powell, H. *Acta Neuropathol.* *40*, 103, 1977.
17. Schröder, J. M., and Krücke, W. *Acta Neuropathol. 14*, 261, 1970.
18. Wisniewski, H., Prineas, J., and Raine, C. S. *Lab. Invest. 21*, 105, 1969.
19. Asbury, A. K., and Arnason, B. G. W. *J. Neuropathol. 27*, 581, 1968.
20. Arnason, B. G. W., Winkler, G. F., and Hadler, N. M. *Lab. Invest. 21*, 1, 1969.
21. Arnason, B. G. W. *Res. Publ. Assoc. Res. Nerv. Ment. Dis. 49*, 156, 1971.
22. Behan, P. O., Lamarche, J. B., Feldman, R. G., et al. *Lancet i*, 421, 1970.
23. Abramsky, O., Teitelbaum, D., and Arnon, R. *Eur. J. Immunol. 7*, 213, 1977.
24. Åström, K.- E., and Waksman, B. H. *J. Pathol. Bacteriol. 83*, 89, 1962.
25. Arnason, B. G. W., and Chelmicka-Szorc, E. *Acta Neuropathol. 22*, 1, 1972.
26. Waksman, B. H., and Adams, R. D. *J. Neuropathol. Exp. Neurol. 15*, 293, 1956.
27. Lehrich, J. R., and Arnason, B. G. W. *Acta Neuropathol. 18*, 144, 1971.
28. Arnason, B. G. W. "Multiple Sclerosis, Immunology, Virology and Ultrastructure," ICN-UCLA Symposia, Vol. 16, p. 487. Academic Press, New York, 1972.
29. Payne, L. N., and Rennie, M. *J. Nat. Cancer Inst. 45*, 387, 1970.
30. Konovalov, G. V., Korneva, E. A., and Khai, L. M. *Brain Res. 29*, 383, 1971.
31. Yonezawa, T., Ishihara, Y., and Matsuyama, H. *J. Neuropathol. 27*, 453, 1968.
32. Saida, K., Saida, T., Brown, M. J., et al. *J. Neuropathol. Exp. Neurol.* in press.
33. Cummings, J. F., and Haas, D. C. *J. Neurol. Sci. 4*, 51, 1967.
34. Holmes, D. F., and de La Hunta, A. *Acta Neuropathol. 30*, 329, 1974.
35. Powell, P. C., Payne, L. N., Frazier, J. A., et al. *Nature 251*, 79, 1974.
36. Stephens, E. A., Witter, R. L., Lee, L. F., et al. *J. Nat. Cancer Inst. 57*, 865, 1976.
37. Witter, R. L., Stephens, E. A., Sharma, J. M., et al. *J. Immunol. 115*, 177, 1975.
38. Sharma, J. M., and Coulson, B. D. *J. Nat. Cancer Inst. 58*, 1647, 1977.

39. Theis, G. A., McBride, R. A., and Schierman, L. W. *J. Immunol.* *115*, 848, 1975.
40. Theis, G. A. *J. Immunol.* *118*, 887, 1977.
41. Rouse, B. T., and Warner, N. L. *J. Immunol.* *113*, 904, 1974.
42. Wallen, W. C., Neubauer, R. H., and Rabin, H. *Clin. Exp. Immunol.* *22*, 468, 1975.
43. Prineas, J. W., and Wright, R. G. *Lab. Invest. 26*, 548, 1972.
44. Sharma, J. M., Nazerian, K., and Witter, R. L. *J. Nat. Cancer Inst. 58*, 689, 1977.
45. Cotter, P. F., Jakowski, F. M., Frederickson, T. N., *et al. J. Nat. Cancer Inst. 54*, 969, 1975.
46. Nazerian, K., Lee, L. F., and Sharma, J. M. *Progr. Med. Virol. 22*, 123, 1976.
47. Arnason, B. G. W. *In* "Peripheral Neuropathy" (P. T. Dyck, P. K. Thomas, and E. H. Lambert, eds.), p. 1110. W. B. Saunders, Philadelphia, 1976.
48. Wells, C. E. C. *Br. Med. J. 1*, 369, 1971.
49. Stevens, D., Burman, D., Clarke, S. K. R., *et al. Lancet ii*, 1354, 1975.
50. Arnason, B. G. W., and Asbury, A. K. *Arch. Neurol. 18*, 500, 1968.
51. Borit, A., and Altrocchi, P. H. *Arch. Neurol. 24*, 40, 1971.
52. Asbury, A. K., Arnason, B. G. W., and Adams, R. D. *Medicine 48*, 173, 1969.
53. Turinese, A., and Battistin, L. *Riv. Patol. Nerv. Ment. 87*, 580, 1966.
54. Lisak, R. P., Mitchell, M., Zweiman, B., *et al. Trans. Am. Neurol. Assoc. 100*, 140, 1975.
55. Twomey, J. J. *J. Immunol. 112*, 2278, 1974.
56. Drachman, D. A., Paterson, P. Y., Berlin, B. S., *et al. Arch. Neurol. 23*, 385, 1970.
57. Peterman, A. F., Daly, D. D., Dion, F. R., *et al. Neurology 9*, 533, 1959.
58. Hourr, S. A., Wallen, W. C., Madden, D. L., *et al. Ann. Neurol. 1*, 505, 1977.
59. Cambier, J., and Schott, B. *Rev. Neurol. (Paris) 115*, 811, 1966.
60. Smith, W. R., and Wilson, A. F. *J. Am. Med. Assoc. 231*, 1367, 1975.
61. Lopez-Adaros, H., and Held, J. R. *Res. Publ. Assoc. Res. Nerv. Ment. Dis. 49*, 178, 1971.
62. Remlinger, P. *Ann. Inst. Pasteur 42*, 71, 1928.
63. Link, H. *Acta Neurol. Scand. 52*, 111, 1975.
64. Wisniewski, H., Terry, R. D., Whitaker, J. N., *et al. Arch. Neurol. 21*, 269, 1969.

65. Prineas, J. W. *Lab. Invest.* *26*, 133, 1972.
66. Carpenter, S. *J. Neurol. Sci. 15*, 125, 1972.
67. Hochberg, F. H., Lehrich, J. R., and Arnason, B. G. W. *Neurology 27*, 584, 1977.
68. Arnason, B. G. W., and Antel, J. *Ann. Immunol. (Inst. Pasteur) 129C*, 159, 1978.
69. Dubois-Dalcq, M., Buyse, M., Buyse, G., *et al.* *J. Neurol. Sci. 13*, 67, 1971.
70. Cook, S. D., Dowling, P. C., Murray, M. R., *et al.* *Arch. Neurol. 24*, 136, 1971.
71. Rosenberg, R. N., Aung, M. H., and Tindall, R. S. A. *Neurology 25*, 1101, 1975.
72. Rocklin, R. E., Sheremata, W. A., Feldman, R. G., *et al.* *N. Engl. J. Med. 284*, 803, 1971.
73. Sheremata, W., Colby, S., Karkhanis, Y., *et al.* *Can. J. Neurol. Sci. 2*, 87, 1975.
74. Abramsky, O., Webb, C., Teitelbaum, D., *et al.* *Neurology 25*, 1154, 1975.
75. Luijten, J. A. F. M., and Baart de la Faille-Kuyper, E. H. *J. Neurol. Sci. 15*, 219, 1972.
76. Tse, K. S., Arbesman, C. E., Tomasi, T. B., Jr., *et al.* *Clin. Exp. Immunol. 8*, 881, 1971.
77. Tachovsky, T. G., Lisak, R. P., Koprowski, H., *et al.* *Nature 2*, 997, 1976.
78. Whitaker, J. N., Dowling, P. C., and Cook, S. D. *J. Neuropathol. Exp. Neurol. 30*, 129, 1971.

DISCUSSION

DR. COHEN: In the *in vitro* myelin destruction experiments, is the effect mediated by lymphocytes or macrophages?

DR. ARNASON: I don't know. We have not done electron-microscopic studies of our cultures. Myelinated cultures always contain macrophages that act as scavengers to keep the cultures healthy.

DR. BLOOM: I'd like to comment; one possible mechanism to explain how macrophages can produce demyelination has emerged from studies in our laboratory on products of activated macrophages (Commer, W., Bloom, B. R., Norton, W., and Gordon, S., *Proc. Nat. Acad. Sci.*, in press). Supernates of activated macrophages contain a number of neutral proteases. When intact myelin is exposed to supernates of normal, resident mouse peritoneal macrophages, no effect is seen. However, when exposed to supernates of thioglycollate-activated macrophages, degradation is seen, particularly if plasminogen is added. We believe there are two enzymes involved, which degrade primarily, if not exclusively, the basic protein in myelin. One is plasminogen independent and inhibitable by EDTA. The stronger is a plasminogen activator that converts plasminogen to plasmin and can be inhibited by *p*-nitrophenylguanidinobenzoate (NPGB). Serum contains large amounts of potential protease in the form of plasminogen, which can be activated locally by the secreted plasminogen activator of activated macrophages, and which can serve as an amplification of a small amount of macrophage-secreted protease.

DR. EDELMAN: Did you state that lymphocytes from patients with polyneuropathy do or do not respond to basic protein *in vitro* by transforming?

DR. ARNASON: Yes, lymphocytes do transform when exposed to basic protein *in vitro*. Several groups have demonstrated this.

DR. EDELMAN: Was saliva rather than basic protein used in lymphocyte cultures from dogs with coonhound paralysis?

DR. ARNASON: We haven't tried that yet.

DR. EDELMAN: Can you confirm that tick paralysis in man, unlike venomous insect stings, is not an allergic reaction?

DR. ARNASON: Yes, tick paralysis is not an "allergic" disease insofar as we know.

DR. LEVY: I would suggest that some of these autoimmune sequellae result from a virus infection. For instance:

(1) *Herpes virus*: Zualzer has noted autoimmune hemolytic anemia recurring after expression of cytomegalovirus. Mot-

kins and his associates have shown activation of herpes virus in experimental mice following surgery.

(2) *C type*: Gardner reported neurologic disease in wild mice; this was caused by a type C virus, which also causes lymphoma. RNA viruses have been reported associated with Marek's disease. Could such a virus, if present, be leading to the neuritis reported early in the course of Marek's disease?

(3) *Papovavirus*: Multifocal leukoencephalitis is associated with papovavirus in the brain and has peripheral signs. While the disease is not known to go into remission, couldn't such a virus be involved in some of these neurologic disorders?

(4) Finally, couldn't the coonhound disease be caused by virus in the saliva? Centrifugation of the saliva would not necessarily remove the agent.

DR. ARNASON: Herpes virus, of course, persists in human gasserian ganglia and can be demonstrated by electron microscopy but no herpes virus has been found in polyneuritis lesions despite diligent search. I have been impressed by the fact that herpes infections, such as gingivitis or cold sores, do not provide an antecedent for polyneuritis. Gardner's mice have anterior horn cell disease, which is totally different from polyneuritis. The association of Marek's disease with a second virus was reported 4 or 5 years ago and has not yet been confirmed. Papovaviruses are associated with anergy and an absence of inflammation in brain and nerve. The pathologic features are distinct from those of polyneuritis. In reference to the coonhound disease, saliva may very well contain virus and other microbial agents. The major point I hoped to make centers on the genetic predisposition to develop allergic neuritis in blood relatives of the animals with coonhound paralysis.

DR. GOOD: Although herpes simplex infections are not often accompanied by polyneuritis isn't it true that herpes simplex II infections frequently produce polyneuritis?

DR. ARNASON: Yes, this is true for herpes II.

DR. SCHWARTZ: Is the neuropathy of Old Lyme disease a form of polyneuropathy and, if so, have the lesions been examined?

DR. ARNASON: I have no information on this.

DR. SCHWARTZ: What is the role of B cells that can bind basic protein? These cells have been reported in the blood of normal persons.

DR. ARNASON: I'm not sure. Because of its basic nature, this protein is naturally "sticky" to cells. This complicates the interpretation of such observations.

DR. DIENER: With reference to Dr. Schwartz's questions concerning the ability of B cells to bind basic protein, we have shown this binding to be due to IgM receptors and to be specific for basic protein (Young, McPherson, and Diener, *J. Immunol.*). Thus, Dr. Arnason's implication that such binding is nonspecific may not apply here.

DR. J. SANFORD: Since coonhounds hunt possums as regularly as they do coons, is the precipitating factor present in the saliva of possums?

DR. ARNASON: I don't know, but it is clear that a racoon bite, rather than a possum bite, precipitates the disease.

DR. BRITTON: In polyneuritis there is usually an emormous increase of CSF protein in the absence of increased cellularity. Have you looked into the nature of these proteins?

DR. ARNASON: The CSF protein is normal for the first few days of disease; it then rises and stays elevated for several weeks. The protein is chiefly exudative; increased IgA levels are sometimes seen. Dr. Link in Sweden has reported the presence of oligoclonal IgG bands in a substantial number of patients. In my experience, however, oligoclonal bands are seen only in a minor proportion of patients.

DR. EDELMAN: Dr. Athasit, professor of neurology at the Ramathibodhi Medical School in Banghah, Thailand, points out that there seems to be an unusually high prevalence of Guillain-Barre type neuropathy in Thailand. Have similar high prevalences of idiopathic polyneuropathy been found in other countries or population groups?

DR. ARNASON: The syndrome has been described from all areas of the world, but no one has reported unusually high prevalence. I was not previously aware of the anecdotally high prevalence in Thailand.

DR. J. SANFORD: To comment on the Guillain-Barre syndrome following swine influenza vaccine, the only other experience with wide-scale immunization of adults was with tetanus toxoid during World War II. An apparent increase in Guillain-Barre perhaps to the rate of 1 per 100,000 was seen with tetanus toxoid.

DR. ARNASON: I was aware of that; it's mentioned in my manuscript.

ARTHRITIDES ASSOCIATED WITH INFECTION:
PROTECTIVE IMMUNITY VERSUS
IMMUNOLOGICALLY MEDIATED TISSUE DAMAGE

Jay P. Sanford

Uniformed Services University
School of Medicine
Bethesda, Maryland

INTRODUCTION

Clinical arthritis is an important manifestation in a
large number of infections both in man and in animals (Table
I). In addition, there are at least four rheumatic syndromes
in man for which there is cogent evidence of a close association with infection: rheumatic fever, polyarteritis nodosa
due to hepatitis B antigen, Reiter's syndrome, and Whipple's
disease. Ziff has gone so far as to conclude at a World
Health Organization Symposium held in 1974 that "the connective tissue diseases are infectious diseases with a significant genetic component and that the autoantibodies present,
though injurious are secondary to infection" (1).
The mechanisms underlying the occurrence of an inflammatory response of the synovium involve not only the direct effects of the microorganism and failure or delay in immune elimination but perhaps equally important involve the inflammation and damage that result from the immunological reaction(s)
aimed at elimination of the agent or residual antigens. To
introduce the discussion, I have attempted a categorization
based upon that of Dumonde (2) (Table II). This categorization can be further modified to include an assessment of the
role of host response in the process (Table III) (3).

TABLE I. *Systemic Infections Associated with Acute*
Arthritis[a]

Viruses

  Arboviruses: Chikungunya, Onyong-nyong, Ross River,
    Sindbis (R)
  Enteroviruses: Coxsackie virus (R), echovirus (R),
    poliovirus (R)
  Hepatitis B virus
  Herpes viruses: EB virus (R)
  Myxoviruses: influenza (R), mumps (R), rubella
  Pox viruses: variola, vaccinia (R), varicella (R)
  Presumed: erythema infectiosum

Chlamydia: lymphogranuloma venereum (R)

Bacteria (virtually all bacterial species pathogenic for
  man have been associated with septic arthritis)

  Neisseria: meningitidis, gonorrheae
  Yersinia enterocolitica
  Streptobacillus moniliformis
  Mycobacterium leprae

[a]*(R) rare, occurring in less than 1% of patients.*

CATEGORIZATION

Infective Arthritides

     The basis for tropism of organisms for synovial membranes
remains unknown and to my knowledge has received relatively
little investigative attention. Once an organism lodges in
the synovium a cellular response is evoked. The synovial
lining, A cells, is phagocytic, resembling macrophages (4).
The initial inflammatory response is then amplified through
the action of a neutrophil-derived chemotactic glycoprotein
(5). This chemotactic factor can be demonstrated independently of complement activation, kinin generation, and Hageman
factor activity; it cannot be elicited in neutropenic animals.
Many of the mediators of an inflammatory response, including
Hageman factor, prekallikrein, kininogen, and complement, are
present in synovial fluid (6). Provided with the stimulus,
activation of the interrelated pathways that lead to generation of the mediators of inflammation--histamine, serotonin,
kinins, prostaglandins, lysosomal enzymes, permeability factors, and complement activation products--can occur within the

TABLE II. A Categorization of Infection and Associated Arthritides

Arthritis syndrome	Infection known	Organisms in joint	Antigen in joint	Examples
Infective	+	+	+	Gonococcal, small pox
Postinfective	+	−	+	Meningococcal, rubella
Reactive	+	−	−	Yersinia enterocolitica (?), Chikungunya
Inflammatory	−	−	−	Reiter's syndrome

TABLE III. Factors Involved in the Pathogenesis of Infection-Associated Arthritides

Host immune response important?	Organism and/or antigen important?	
	Yes	No
No	Gonococcus Vaccinia	(?) Arbovirus
Yes	Meningococcus Rubella Hepatitis B	Yersinia enterocolitica

synovium. Cartilage erosion with residual damage is usually
the result of the action of lysosomal enzymes released from
neutrophil leucocytes. In the infective arthritides the host
response and/or therapy is critical to recovery with or without residual damage. Whether or not the host immune response
also contributes to prolongation or accentuation of the inflammatory response has not been clarified, but in view of
the rapidity of response, it would appear that the inflammation subsides along with termination of the infection.

Postinfective Arthritides

     There are several clinical situations in which a systemic
infection may be resolved at which time a sterile arthritis
develops. In these clinical situations, effective antimicrobial therapy has not prevented the occurrence of this
delayed type of arthritis. This pattern of postinfectious
arthritis with the meningococcus was described by Herrick and
Parkhurst in 1919 (7). They reported its prevalence to be
8.7%. Subsequently, despite the introduction of effective
antimicrobial agents, the prevalence has remained 2 to 10%.
The arthritis occurs more frequently in adults than in children. It usually begins with the occurrence of severe pain at
an average of 6 days after onset of illness. There is often
an associated febrile response and in about one-quarter of the
patients there are associated skin lesions (typically becoming
bullous, then ulcerating). In 47 patients followed by Whittle
et al., two-thirds had multiple joints involved, with the
following distribution: knee, 31; wrist, 28; elbow, 18; ankle,
17; finger, 9; hip, 4; shoulder, 2; toe, 2 (8). Cultures of
synovial fluid at this stage are characteristically sterile.
In excellent studies by Whittle *et al.*, group A meningococcal
antigen (*n*-acetyl mannosamine phosphate) was detected in the

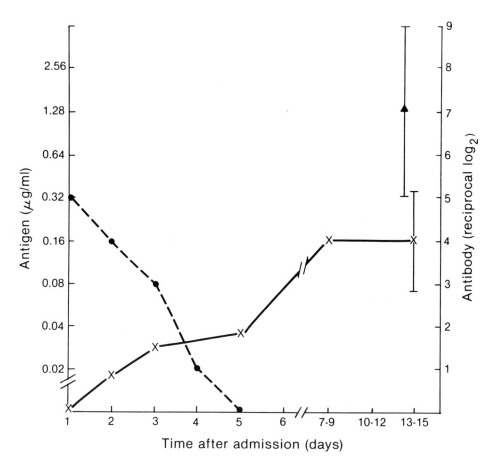

FIGURE 1. Serum antigen (●—●) and antibody (x—x) levels in 13 patients with meningococcal antigenemia and mean antibody level (▲) in 25 serum-antigen-negative patients with meningococcal meningitis.

serum of 13.5% of patients (9). Arthritis developed in 7 of 27 (26%) of patients in whom antigenemia was demonstrated on admission, in contrast with a prevalence of 8.7% in 173 patients who did not have antigenemia (10). Serial studies of antigen and antibody levels were performed on 13 patients (Fig. 1). Suitable conditions for an antigen-antibody reaction with complex formation occur about the fifth day. Detailed studies in two patients suggested the presence of meningococcal IgM antimeningococcal complexes in synovium and synovial fluid white cells (11). The presence of meningococcal

antigen-antibody complexes in synovium clearly supports the
role for an immunologically, probably B cell, mediated process but does not allow one to distinguish between deposition
of preformed circulating complexes or the development of an
Arthus-type reaction to antigen fixed in the tissues.

In an epidemic of rubella in any Army camp occurring in
1917, Geiger noted the occurrence of acute arthritis as a
manifestation of rubella in 36 patients (12). The prevalence
of arthritis in epidemic rubella was most accurately recorded
by Fry et al., who saw 355 patients with presumed rubella.
Seventy-four of the patients were adults, of whom 11 (15%)
had joint swelling with overlying erythema and pain on motion (13). Subsequent reports have summarized the features:
occurring most often in postpubertal women, with the onset of
arthritis either with the rash or within 3 days after eruption.
The duration of arthritis varied from 2 to 14 days and was
self-limited. The small joints of the hands were most frequently involved (85%) followed by involvement of knees,
wrists, and ankles (14). With the introduction of live attenuated rubella vaccine, arthralgia and arthritis became recognized as relatively common side-effects, noted particularly
in postpubertal vaccinees and mostly in women. The arthralgia
generally occurred 2 to 3 weeks following vaccination, an interval that is similar to the incubation period for natural
rubella and consistent with the arthritis occurring about the
time of appearance of the rash. The prevalence varied with
the type of vaccine but ranged from 2 to 10%. Again, the
joint symptoms after vaccination are not associated with per-
manent sequelae but occasional patients have had recurrences
or have shown manifestations beyond several months (15).

The pathogenesis of rubella-associated arthropathy is
poorly understood. Several investigators have isolated rubella virus from joint fluid or synovial biopsy. Other investigators have suggested that these patients have an excessive antibody response. Chiba et al. performed immunological studies on 15 patients who had had rubella vaccine arthropathy 2 to 3 years earlier and compared the responses with
those observed in 18 age-matched subjects who had not had
arthropathy after rubella vaccine (15). Antibody titers (HAI)--
range, mean, and median--were similar in both groups as were
C_3 and C_4 levels. However, peripheral blood lymphocytes from
the arthropathy patients demonstrated less responsiveness to
rubella vaccine as measured by less incorporation of ^3H thymidine into DNA than did the controls ($p < 0.01$). Yet responses
to PHA and mumps vaccine did not differ significantly between
the groups. The number of E rosettes also was decreased in the
arthropathy group ($p < 0.01$). Thus, individuals who have had
rubella vaccine arthropathy demonstrate a selective depression

of cell-mediated immunity to rubella virus. The possibility
exists that individuals who develop arthropathy do so because
they lack the ability to clear rubella virus effectively and
have an antigenic overload.

Arthritis has recently been emphasized as part of the pro-
drome of hepatitis B infection. Clinically the arthritis is
transient and migratory and is often associated with urticaria
or other rashes. The arthritis usually terminates with or
shortly after the onset of clinically apparent hepatitis. Examination of synovial fluid reveals decreased CH50 levels, especially C_4 and C_1q, indicating activation of the classical
pathway (16). Examination of synovium suggests the presence
of hepatitis B antigen. These findings suggest that the arthropathy associated with hepatitis B depends both upon the organism (antigen) and the host response (Table III). However,
the localization of immune complexes with joints may not require the presence of antigen in the synovium (17). This observation assists in the explanation of arthritis complicating
a variety of chronic infections such as leprosy or acne con-
globata (18,19).

One of the best experimental models is that of Dumonde
and Glynn, in which rabbits are immunized with antigen in complete Freund's adjuvant. Several weeks later, the animals
are challenged with intraarticular antigen. Subsequently the
animals develop a rather persistent arthritis (20). In this
model it has been shown that the persistence of arthritis depends upon the persistence of antigen (21). It is attractive
to postulate that the duration of either postmeningococcal,
rubella or hepatitis B arthritis is determined by the persistence of antigen, which is usually of limited duration.

Reactive Arthritides

This category of infection associated with arthritis is
distinct clinically but the pathogenic mechanisms remain to
be elucidated. The syndrome of fever, rash, and arthralgia/
arthritis associated with several of the arboviruses is well
recognized: Chikungunya virus, Onyong-nyong virus in East
Africa, and Ross River virus in Australia. These entities
appear not to be associated with the presence of virus or antigen in the affected joints; however, the data are scanty
(22).

Yersinia enterocolitica, a gram-negative bacillus, has only
recently been recognized as an important cause of acute arthritis in parts of Europe, where Yersinia arthritis is far
more frequent than rheumatic fever (23). The clinical features

include occurrence in young adults, mean age 31 years, no sex predominance, polyarthritis with five or more joints often involved. Associated features include carditis (10%) and urological findings (26%), which include chronic prostatitis, sterile pyuria, and hematuria. In many patients symptoms persist for more than 3 months. Laitinen and associates studied 74 patients with Yersinia arthritis and found that 66% were HLA B-27 positive (24). Furthermore, joint symptoms were more severe in those patients who were HLA B-27 positive. Iritis, conjunctivitis, carditis, and urological involvement occurred only in those patients who were HLA B-27 positive. However, erythema nodosum was most common in the HLA B-27 negative group. Acute synovial lesions and synovial fluid do not contain Yersinia by cultivation techniques or by immunofluorescence (25). Thus, Yersinia arthritis offers another example, along with ankylosing spondylitis and Reiter's syndrome, where the histocompatibility gene B-27 appears linked to the occurrence of rheumatologic disease. There are two hypotheses to account for these observations. One, the antigenic determinants of a particular histocompatibility antigen are so similar to those of the invading organisms that the host cannot produce a suitable immune response. The other, an aberrant Ir gene closely related on the chromosome to the histocompatibility gene may facilitate the immune response (1).

Inflammatory Arthritides

Discussion of this category is beyond the scope of this analysis since I have limited the discussion to infections in man in which the occurrence of arthritis is a usual and integral part of the clinical manifestations.

The interrelationships between these four categories of arthritides are depicted in yet another way in Fig. 2.

SUMMARY

Arthritis is a major clinical feature in a number of infections. Multiple pathogenetic mechanisms appear to be involved in the synovial inflammation. In some, the inflammation may reflect a defective immune response, while in others the immune response may be responsible for the inflammatory changes.

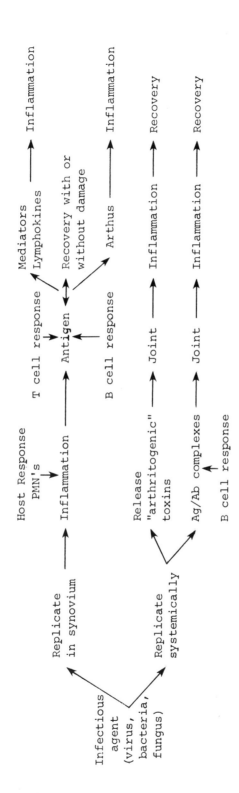

FIGURE 2. *Immunopathological mechanisms in infection-associated arthritides: a hypothesis.*

References

1. Ziff, M.   *In* "Infection and Immunity in Rheumatic Diseases" (D. C. Dumonde, ed.), p. 627.   Blackwell Scientific Publ., Oxford, 1976.

2. Dumonde, D. C.   *In* "Infection and Immunity in Rheumatic Diseases (D. C. Dumonde, ed.), p. 95.   Blackwell Scientific Publ., Oxford, 1976.

3. Phillips, P. E.   *In* "Infection and Immunity in Rheumatic Diseases (D. C. Dumonde, ed.), p. 205.   Blackwell Scientific Publ., Oxford, 1976.

4. Denman, A. M.   *Med. Biol. 53*, 61, 1975.

5. Spilberg, I., Rosenberg, D., and Mandall, B.   *J. Clin. Invest. 59*, 582, 1977.

6. Zeitlin, I. J., and Grennan, D. M.   *In* "Recent Advances in Rheumatology" (W. W. Buchanan and W. C. Dick, eds.), p. 171.   Churchill Livingstone, Edinburgh, 1976.

7. Herrick, W. W., and Parkhurst, G. M.   *Am. J. Med. Sci. 158*, 473, 1919.

8. Whittle, H. C., Abdullahi, M. T., Fakule, F. A., *et al.* *Br. Med. J. 2*, 733, 1973.

9. Whittle, H. C., Greenwood, B. M., Davidson, N. McD., *et al.* *Am. J. Med. 58*, 823, 1973.

10. Greenwood, B. M., Whittle, H. C., and Bryceson, A. D. M. *Br. Med. J. 2*, 737, 1973.

11. Greenwood, B. M., and Whittle, H. C.   *In* "Infection and Immunity in Rheumatic Diseases" (D. C. Dumonde, ed.), p. 119.   Blackwell Scientific Publ., Oxford, 1976.

12. Geiger, J. C.   *JAMA 70*, 1818, 1918.

13. Fry, J., Dillane, J. B., and Fry, L.   *Br. Med. J. 2*, 833, 1962.

14. Lee, P. R., Barnett, A. F., Scholer, J. F., *et al. Cal. Med. 93*, 125, 1960.

15. Chiba, Y., Sadeghi, E., and Ogra, P. L.   *J. Immunol. 117*, 1684, 1976.

16. Schumaker, H. R., and Gall, E. P.   *Am. J. Med. 57*, 655, 1974.

17. Cooke, T. D., Hurd, E. H., Ziff, M., and Jasin, H. E.   *J. Exp. Med. 135*, 323, 1972.

18. Iverson, J. M. I., McDougall, A. C., Leathem, A. J., and Harris, H. J.   *Br. Med. J. 3*, 619, 1975.

19. Windom, R. E., Sanford, J. P., and Ziff, M.   *Arth. Rheum. 4*, 632, 1961.

20. Dumonde, D., and Glynn, L. E.   *Br. J. Exp. Pathol. 43*, 373, 1962.

21. Cooke, T. D., and Jasin, H. E.   *Arth. Rheum. 15*, 327, 1972.

22. Smith, J. W., and Sanford, J. P.   *Ann. Intern. Med. 67*, 651, 1967.

23. Ahvonen, P. *Ann. Clin. Res. 4*, 39, 1972.
24. Laitinen, O., Lierisalo, M., and Skylr, G. *Arth. Rheum. 20*, 1121, 1977.
25. Larson, J. H. *In* :Infection and Immunity in Rheumatic Diseases" (D. C. Dumonde, ed.), p. 133. Blackwell Scientific Publ., Oxford, 1976.

DISCUSSION

DR. LEVY: I have two questions. Are mycoplasmas involved
in the human arthritides, for instance, the "T strain"? Also,
is there streptococcal antigen in the joints in rheumatic
fever?

DR. SANFORD: *Mycoplasma pneumoniae* is not involved to any
extent in the human arthritides. I did not mention it because
of its extreme rarity in human disease; it is involved in
urethritis but not in Reiter's disease. In reference to your
second question, to my knowledge streptococcal antigens have
not been detected in the synovial fluids of rheumatic fever
patients.

DR. YUNIS: As far as I am aware, no evidence exists of
abnormality in immune function in patients with ankylosing
spondylitis. Do you know of the existence of immune dysfunc-
tions in B27 arthritis associated with infections such as
Yersinia?

DR. SANFORD: No. In the course of my review for the presentation, I did not find such data.

DR. PREHN: Please tell us something further about the
nature of Yersinia and its epidemiology. Is its prevalence in
Finland unique or is it a matter of lack of detection elsewhere?

DR. SANFORD: *Yersinia enterocolitica* is a small gram-nega-
tive organism that is difficult to isolate and grow; its
growth requirements are such that it normally would not be
isolated in routine culture media. Most studies, therefore,
have relied on detection of specific antibody for diagnosis.
There is no doubt that there is a prediliction in northern
European countries. It clearly does occur in the United
States and Canada, although it is considerably less frequent.
We are just beginning to determine its real prevalence here.
I believe that we will detect it in two clinical manifestations;
the most important is in patients with acute or recurring abdominal lymphadenitis. The other situation will be in some
patients who we believe have rheumatic fever; to date, how-
ever, studies of these situations are quite preliminary.

DR. LEVY: Is there any example of antigenic mimicry with
these infectious agents?

DR. SANFORD: Antigenic mimicry has been postulated in
Yersinia but, as far as I know, no experimental evidence for
this exists.

DR. LEVY: Do any of these agents uncover normal components
of cells and, through some type of carrier-hapten mechanism,
induce antibody reactions to normal tissue? Such a phenomenon
would explain the persistent fashion of some of these arthritides.

DR. SANFORD: I'm not aware of any available data that would shed light on this question. I do not think anyone can say "no" to this question but I'm not certain that we can really say anything better than "we don't know."

Session IV
Immunopathology II

FILARIAL INFECTION AND THE HOST RESPONSE IN MAN:
PARADOXES AND INSIGHTS

Eric A. Ottesen

Laboratory of Parasitic Diseases
National Institute of Allergy and Infectious Diseases
National Institutes of Health
Bethesda, Maryland

THE PROBLEMS

The filariases are a group of chronic parasitic infections
caused by tissue-dwelling nematodes of the family *Filarioidea*.
While more than 90 species of parasitic filariae can be found
in nature, only about half a dozen commonly infect man, and of
those three produce most of the significant disease. One of
these inhabits the subcutaneous tissue (*Onchocerca volvulus*,
the agent leading to "river blindness" in much of Africa and
elsewhere) and two are lymphatic dwelling (*Wuchereria bancrofti*
and *Brugia malayi*, causing elephantiasis, lymphangitis, and
pulmonary complications throughout much of the tropics and
subtropics). Because of the variety and severity of the pathology they produce and because of the disappointing therapeutic
results with available antiparasitic agents, together they are
responsible for significant health problems for many of the
nearly 200 million individuals estimated to be infected worldwide (1). While information about the immune responses of
these filaria-infected individuals is unfortunately still
rather scant, recent studies in our laboratory together with
earlier investigations of others have yielded certain intriguing observations that lend insight into possible pathogenetic mechanisms in this chronic helminth infection.
    Before discussing these observations, however, it is
important that one review certain features of parasitic hel-
minths--filaria in particular--that often present special, if
not unique, problems for the immune system of the host as it
tries to generate an appropriate response following exposure

to these organisms. First, all such organisms are extremely
large in comparison to the host's inflammatory cells. For
example, adult filariae (*W. bancrofti*), being 4-8 cm in
length, are more than 5000 times the size of a lymphocyte,
and even their offsrping, the circulating prelarval forms
(microfilariae), are 25 times larger than these cells. Second,
and partly resulting from this large size, they are endowed
with extreme antigenic complexity. Third, during infection
the host is confronted with not just one form of the parasite
but rather with multiple forms (e.g., in bancroftian filariasis, infective third-stage larvae carried by mosquitoes, adult
worms residing in the lymph nodes and lymphatic channels, and
microfilariae shed by adult females into the circulation or
surrounding tissues), and each of these forms is morphologically, biochemically, and antigenically distinct from the
others. Furthermore, because of the migration of the parasites during the different stages in their life cycle, the
host's immune system must confront each of these forms at
multiple and varying sites throughout the body. Finally, an
element of chronicity pervades most aspects of these infec-
tions--from the initial period of exposure to infective organisms, which in endemic areas is generally both repeated
and prolonged over years, to the established infections themselves, which often persist for decades. Clearly, then, such
infectious agents present a formidable challenge to the host's
capacity to mount an effective and appropriate immunologic
response!

Three issues are fundamental to understanding the role of
the immune response (or, in the language of this symposium,
the role of the "immunologic surveillance" system) in filarial
infections. One concerns the response of the host at its initial interface with the parasite, i.e., at the penetration
stage of infection where effective defense mechanisms could
be expected to result in protective immunity. A second relates to the inability of the host to rid itself of these infecting organisms, i.e., to the mechanisms involved in the
persistence of the parasites within the host. And the third
major issue deals with the *pathology* generated within the
host as concomitant of the struggle between the parasite and
the immunologic mechanisms directed against it.

THE OBSERVATIONS

In order to investigate the relevant immunologic parameters associated with these three fundamental aspects of the
interface between host and parasite in man, our laboratory

has undertaken collaborative studies with investigators in two
areas endemic for bancroftian filariasis. One study has involved about 400 Polynesian residents of a South Pacific island
(Mauke, Cook Islands) where infection is established in between
1/3 and 1/2 of the population (2). As described elsewhere
(2,3) clinical features of disease in these individuals included elephantiasis, hydrocoele, recurrent "filarial fevers"
(i.e., episodes of fever, lymphangitis, and lymphadenitis),
and asymptomatic microfilaremia. The second study population
was located in South India (Madras), where in addition to the
presentations of filarial disease found in the Cook Islands,
certain patients also exhibited the tropical pulmonary eosinophilia syndrome, a condition characterized by astham, pulmonary infiltrates, high-grade eosinophilia, and elevated filarial antibody titers. Because previous information regarding the immune response in human filariasis had been restricted almost exclusively to studies of serologic responses
(1,4) and skin tests (5,6) much of the data collected thus
far in our immunologic studies have been of a very explora-
tory nature. Even so, certain observations have proved intriguing, and for the remainder of the discussion I have
tried to group our findings, albeit arbitrarily, in a "prob-
lem-oriented" fashion focused upon the major issues of penetration, persistence, and pathology outlined above.

Penetration

Obviously one of the most basic questions that can be
raised about filarial infections (as well as virtually all
other diseases) is why some people in a given region acquire
the infection yet others do not. More specifically, are
differences in the immunologic surveillance mechanisms of individuals responsible for the differences found in susceptibility to infection? If so, can they be readily identified?
In the absence of relevant background information our straight-
forward approach to the problem has been first to study and
compare as many parameters of the host response as we can in
groups of infected and noninfected individuals from endemic
areas. These parameters have included leukocyte dynamics,
lymphocyte responses to filarial and other antigens, antibody titers to various filarial antigens, complement levels,
and immunoglobulin levels. Patients have been drawn from all
of the major clinical categories of bancroftian filariasis
and the "control" populations have consisted of age- and sex-
matched individuals from the same localities as the patients.
Thus--and this is an important point--our control populations
in these studies are not "negative controls" but rather indi-

Eric A. Ottesen

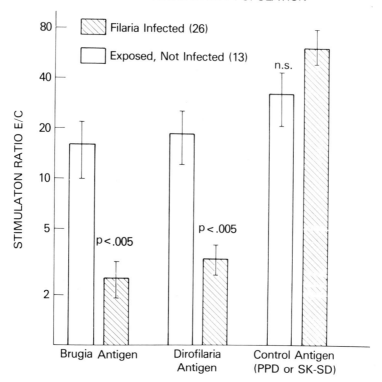

— *FIGURE 1. Lymphocyte responsiveness of study population to filarial and nonparasite antigens. The responses of patients with filariasis are compared to those of individuals living in the same environment but having no clinical or parasitologic evidence of infection. Columns define the arithmetic means of the stimulation ratios in each group and the error bars record one standard error on each side of the mean. Lymphocytes from all individuals were challenged with both PPD and SK-SD, and the higher of the two stimulation ratios elicited by these antigens was used in calculating the average responses shown in the "control antigen" columns.*

viduals *exposed to but not infected with* these parasitic filariae. From the studies three aspects of the host response (i.e., lymphocyte reactivity, antibody titers, and immunoglobulin E levels) have yielded interesting findings, which might well relate to the issue of *penetration* at the host-parasite interface.

In Fig. 1 the lymphocyte blastogenic responses to filarial and nonfilarial antigens are compared in infected and noninfected individuals from the Cook Islands population. While both groups responded to nonfilarial antigens (and in other experimenta to mitogens) in an equivalent and normal fashion, only lymphocytes from the exposed-but-not-infected control group responded with significant blastogenic reactivity when filarial antigens were used as a stimulus. Lymphocytes from infected individuals were essentially unresponsive to filarial antigens. These observations were both surprising and intriguing, but in the absence of additional data it was impossible to decide whether this poor lymphocyte responsiveness to filarial antigens was a cause or an effect of the established infections in this group of individuals. By themselves, therefore, these findings were suggestive but not conclusive in defining a role for lymphocytes in the host's resistance to filarial penetration.

Interestingly, in looking in detail at the serologic responses of infected and noninfected individuals, we've seen similar results. IgG antibody titers to three different filarial antigens (as tested in a sensitive enzyme-linked immunosorbent assay; ELISA) were all at least twice as high in the noninfected control populations as they were in the individuals with filariasis, these differences being significant at the $p < 0.05$ level for all three antigens (7). Furthermore, when immunoglobulin E levels were studied in these populations, the mean values for the exposed-but-not-infected individuals were significantly higher than those of the group harboring filarial infection (7). These significant differences were seen only for the E-class of immunoglobulin, not for IgG, IgA IgM, or IgD.

Thus, just as with the parameters of cellular immune reactivity seen in Fig. 1, both serologic responses to filarial antigens and total IgE production were significantly less vigorous in patients with filariasis than they were in individuals remaining uninfected despite their repeated exposure to these organisms. Again, however, from these single-point-in-time data it is impossible to discern whether these differences in responsiveness were the result of established infection or whether they helped to determined an individual's initial susceptibility to infection.

Observations in an experimental animal model developed in our laboratory suggest that the latter might be the case (8). In this model inbred Lewis rats were infected with filaria of the *Brugia pahangi* species. These filaria are lymphatic dwellers closely related to those which infect man. The experimental schedules of infection were varied to include single large inocula, multiple small frequent inocula, and combinations of both. Regardless of the infecting schedule, about 3/4 of the animals in each group developed microfilaremia

after a prepatent period of about 2-1/2 to 3-1/2 months.
The remaining animals never became microfilaremic and all
available data suggested that the infection never established
itself successfully in these animals. When the immunologic
parameters of the host response in these infected and noninfected groups were compared, there was one striking difference
between the two groups. Those in whom infection was never successfully established all developed filaria-specific IgE antibodies 4-5 weeks after initial exposure to the infecting
organisms, whereas none of those which subsequently became
microfilaremic had an IgE antibody response during that early
period. Later, at 10-15 weeks when microfilaremia appeared
in the infected animals, IgE antibodies could of course be
readily demonstrated, but these observations suggest the
existence of a critical period during the early, prepatent
phase of infection when IgE antibodies might play an important
role in protecting these animals from the establishment of
infection. If such observations are coupled with the single-
point-in-time findings from man, one can reasonably speculate
that the ability to respond to infective filarial organisms
in an immunologically vigorous manner decreases the likelihood that these parasites will successfully penetrate the
host's immunologic surveillance system and establish patent
infection.

Persistence

The mechanisms underlying the persistence of filarial
worms within the host is a subject touching on the most fundamental aspect of parasitism itself, namely, the stand-off between the physiologic responses of the host on the one hand
and those of the invading parasite on the other. As it is
clear that infected hosts in general are immunocompetent,
there must be mechanisms that exist to modify or modulate the
immunologic responsiveness of infected individuals with enough specificity to permit them to tolerate the presence of
these invasive helminths without at the same time subjecting
themselves to a state of broad immune suppression.
We have seen above that patients with filariasis have
lower lymphocyte and antibody responses to filarial antigens
and lower IgE levels than noninfected individuals living in
the same area, and we have speculated on the basis of these
data and the results of animal studies that the serologic differences may imply a role for antibodies in protection of individuals from infection. The meaning of the differences in
cellular reactivity found between infected and noninfected
groups, however, has remained unresolved. Do these differences

represent a cause or an effect of established filarial infection? One hint relating to thise which-came-first question
has come from analyzing the data in Fig. 1 according to the
age of the patients (3). When the responses of children and
adults were analyzed separately, it was seen that though sta-
tistically significant differences in lymphocyte responses to
filarial antigens could be demonstrated between infected and
noninfected individuals of both age groups, the greatest differences were found among children. Indeed, the group of
exposed-but-not-infected children reacted far more vigorously
to filarial antigens than did any of the other experimental
groups (*p* < 0.01). While certainly not definitive, these
findings suggest that early in the course of exposure to filarial infection one may develop vigorous cellular immune reactivity, but with time, repeated exposure to antigen, and
even the establishment of infection, modulating mechanisms
come into play to diminish this cellular responsiveness to
parasite antigens without at the same time significantly affecting the response to mitogens and other antigens.

The mechanisms involved in this modulation of cellular
responsiveness are not yet understood. Recent unpublished
work from our laboratory has sought to define in patients
with filariasis potential cellular and serum inhibitory factors responsible for altering the proliferative responses of
lymphocytes exposed *in vitro* to filarial antigens. Lymphocytes from 12 patients with chronic bancroftian filariasis
(nine with elephantiasis and filarial fevers and three with
microfilaremia) have been cultured in the presence of autologous or homologous normal AB serum and their responses to
mitogens or antigens compared. In these studies it was clear
that while blastogenic responses of unstimulated cultures or
cultures stimulated with phytohemagglutinin or pokeweed mitogen were either unchanged or decreased in the presence of the
AB serum, responses to filarial antigens were greatly enhanced
when the patient's own serum was replaced with the normal serum. On the average there was a three- to fourfold increase
in the proliferative response to filarial antigens, and significant enhancement was seen in all of the patients studied.
Thus, it was evident that inhibitory factors could be demonstrated in the sera of all infected patients.

The question, however, of how specific was this enhanced
antigen responsiveness in the presence of normal serum remains moot. In 6 of the 12 patients, responses to nonfilarial
antigens (PPD and SK-SD) were also enhanced by replacement of
the patient's own serum with clean AB serum. While this 50%
improvement rate certainly contrasts with the 100% rate found
with filarial antigens, still it is not at all clear what
this serum-related defect found in the sequence of antigen

processing, lymphocyte stimulation, and lymphocyte proliferation implies in mechanistic terms. Furthermore, the roles
played by the various lymphocyte and other mononuclear cell
types in modulating the responsiveness of the proliferating
subpopulations of cells also remain undefined at this time,
though recent reports suggest from animal studies that
suppressor lymphocytes can be found in the spleens of filaria-
infected rodents (9).

Turning from these more focused mechanistic considerations
of modulated responsiveness in infected individuals, one might
ask the larger question, "Does the host really recognize these
parasites during chronic infection or is it in some way functionally blinded toward them?" Just as a number of laboratories have found in studying both patients and animals with
chronic schistosomiasis (10-12), our observations in bancroftian filariasis suggest that there is no single answer to this
question; by some parameters there is evidence that the host
recognizes and responds to the parasite, and by others evidence that it does not. In fact, the term *concomitant immunity* has been borrowed from the tumor immunologists to describe the situation in chronic schistosomiasis, where one can
demonstrate protective immunity in animals that at the same
time are found to be harboring numerous adult parasites in an
apparently balanced equilibrium (13).

In filariasis the situation is not yet so well defined but
certainly one can cite numerous striking examples of modulated
host responsiveness in instances in which by other parameters
it is clear that the host is recognizing the presence of the
invading organisms. For example, the very localization of
adult worms in the lymph nodes and adjacent lymphatics provides just such a paradoxical situation. Despite the evidence that antibodies and cellular reactivity have been stimulated by infecting filariae, these parasites choose to reside not in some immunologically protected environment within
the host but rather at the very heart of the peripheral immune
system, the lymphoid tissue, which should be the hotbed of
immunologic reactivity. Yet, by and large, these adult worms
appear to elicit little immunologic response from their host.
The same might also be said of the circulating microfilariae,
which, during their life-span of several months, course freely
through the blood stream--alongside specific antibodies of
all classes, basophils sensitized with antifilarial IgE antibodies, lymphocytes, and mononuclear phagocytes. Despite the
potential for enormous immunologic reactivity, the host usually appears to tolerate these parasites well. Both of these
examples of parasite persistence within the host require that
there exist specific modulating mechanisms acting to restrain
the full potential of the host's immunologic responsiveness.

A further example of this recognition-lack of recognition paradox in human filariasis can be seen in data describing the eosinophilic responses of these patients during infection and treatment. Recently, Beeson and then others (14-16) have shown unequivocally that in helminth infections the ability to generate eosinophilic responses is strongly dependent on intact T-cell immunologic mechanisms. Thus, eosinophil levels provide an additional immunologic parameter of importance in assessing the host responses to parasitic worm infections. Interestingly, however, when the levels of peripheral blood eosinophilia in patients with filariasis were examined (17), it was clear that the degree of blood eosinophilia in no way correlated with the intensity of infection or parasite worm burden, as gauged by the number of circulating microfilariae. (This, incidentally, is also the experience with other parasitic helminth infections.) On the other hand, if the steady-state situation of chronic infection was interrupted by chemotherapy with diethylcarbamazine (DEC), a posttreatment eosinophilic response developed within 7-14 days, and the magnitude of this response was clearly proportional to the host's microfilarial worm burden (or parasite antigenic load). While the functional importance of this response and its underlying mechanisms are both intriguing problems in themselves, the observations are noted here only to emphasize the host's simultaneous state of recognition and nonrecognition with respect to these parasites. In the steady-state situation of chronic infection, patients are immunologically aware enough of the parasites' presence to manifest eosinophilic responses in the blood and tissues, but presumably there exist modulating mechanisms responsible for keeping these responses at relatively modest levels regardless of the antigen load of parasite material within the host. On the other hand, when such mechanisms can be temporarily overcome, as following diethylcarbamazine (DEC) treatment, the magnitude of the response is clearly a direct function of the amount of parasite antigen available to the host.

Finally, the dissociation found among the various parameters of the immune response in patients with chronic filariasis may provide further evidence for a state of simultaneous host response and nonresponse, which presumably involves specific modulating mechanisms. For example, we have seen above that lymphocytes from infected individuals do not proliferate in response to filarial antigens *in vitro*; yet these same individuals often manifest delayed hypersensitivity skin test responses after challenge with filarial antigens (18). Such dissociations among the various correlates of cell-mediated immunity have been described in normal individuals (19) but it has been suggested that they are more common in patients

with chronic disease (20), and similar findings have been reported in patients with chronic schistosomiasis (12).

Pathology

   No one would deny that there is significant pathology associated with the human lymphatic-dwelling filariae. An important unanswered question, however, is how much of this pathology is immunopathology and how much develops independent of
the immune system. In the bancroftian and brugian filariases
there are two major sites of pathologic involvement. The more
common is that associated with lymph nodes and the lymphatic
drainage system. Acute episodes of filarial fever may occur
with a frequency of up to several times per year and be marked
by active lymphadenitis, lymphangitis, fever, and transient
edema. The local inflammation occurring during these episodes leaves residual scarring, and in time the lymphatics
become distorted and obstructed. Finally, the late sequelae
of filariasis develop--lymphedema, elephantiasis, hydrocele,
and chyluria. The role of the immune system in this pathogenetic sequence is entirely unknown. One can certainly speculate that the stimuli initiating episodes of filarial fever
are either entirely immunologic or at least work through the
immune system, but unfortunately as yet there is really no
compelling evidence for or against this hypothesis. The importance of the question is great, for these recurrent acute
episodes are in all likelihood responsible for the most significant pathology associated with chronic filarial disease.
Our own attempts at defining relevant immunologic differences
between those individuals with pathology and those with
filarial infection but without disease have included both
lymphocyte studies and extensive immunoglobulin and antibody
assessments. None of our studies, however, has as yet suc-
ceeded in defining these critical differences.
   The second major site of pathologic involvement in bancroftian and brugian filariasis is the lung--not through any
relationship of the parasites to pulmonary lymphatic system
but rather in a syndrome of immunologic hyperresponsiveness
involving the lung with what has been termed tropical pulmonary eosinophilia (TPE). This syndrome is characterized clinically by chronic lung disease with episodes of severe parox-
ysmal nocturnal asthma accompanied by high-grade blood eosinophilia (generally greater than $3000/mm^3$), markedly elevated
IgE levels, and very high filarial antibody titers. Patients
respond rapidly and dramatically to treatment with DEC, and
while details of the pathogenesis of the condition are still
obscure, it is reasonable to assume that individuals exhibit-

ing this syndrome have become "allergically" sensitized to
filaria (primarily microfilaria) or filarial products. As a
result of this sensitization, microfilaria in affected individuals are not free to circulate in the blood but instead
are trapped and cleared by the lung and sometimes other elements of the reticuloendothelial system. The price paid
clinically for this effective clearance of organisms, however,
is a state of severe asthmatic pulmonary disease that may
progress, if untreated, to chronic fibrosis of the lungs (21).

We have recently initiated studies on individuals with the
TPE syndrome to define in more detail the immunologic responses that distinguish this group of patients from those with
more "classic" lymphatic filarial disease (22). In these
studies, peripheral blood leukocytes from individuals with TPE
or with other manifestations of filariasis were incubated with
a variety of filarial antigens and the amount of histamine
released from their basophils *in vitro* was determined in a
highly sensitive radioenzymatic assay (23). A total of 29
individuals have been studied thus far--24 residents of the
endemic region (South India) and five North American unexposed
controls. The filarial antigens employed in this study were
derived from *Brugia* and *Dirofilaria* adult worms and from *Brugia, Dirofilaria,* and *Wuchereria* microfilariae. Both somatic
extracts and metabolic products from *in vitro* tissue cultures
were used as crude antigens. It was interesting, though perhaps quite predictable, that with all antigens tested patients with tropical pulmonary eosinophilia gave histamine release responses more vigorous than those of any other group
studied. Individuals with patent microfilaremia were least
responsive, and patients with chronic lymphatic pathology
were intermediate in responsiveness. Microfilarial antigens
(both metabolic and somatic) appeared especially effective in
discriminating between the responses of patients with TPE and
those with other types of filarial disease. And curiously
enough, the responses of the normal control population of
indigenous Indians did not differ significantly from those of
patients with elephantiasis--a situation fully in keeping with
the serologic findings in the Polynesian population described
above.

Such observations have put on a quantitative basis the
features of TPE already described clinically in more qualitative terms. The fact that histamine and other inflammatory
mediators are released from the basophils of these patients
with appropriate antigenic stimuli does take one somewhat
closer to the immunopathogenesis of this syndrome, but clearly
a great deal of work is still required to define precisely
the steps involved both in leading to and then modulating medi-

ator release *in vivo* and in determining the effects of these
mediators on the target tissues themselves.

SPECULATIONS

    The observations described above suggest that there may be
a number of stages in the development of the host response
during chronic filariasis, and our view of these has been
summarized in a hypothetical fashion in Fig. 2. Based on the
findings of vigorous cellular, antibody, and immunoglobulin
E responses in the exposed-but-not-infected individuals of
filarial endemic regions, we would speculate that when either
children from an endemic area or adults who come from outside
such an area are first exposed to infection, they initially
develop both cellular and humoral immune responses to filarial
organisms. This situation does not remain static, as reexposure to infecting organisms (and thus, parasite antigen) occurs
repeatedly in the environment on a many-times-per-day basis.
With the passage of time individuals appear to respond to
these repeated doses of infective "antigenic material" in at
least three distinct fashions. Most individuals seem to interpret the continual exposure to parasite material as "booster
immunizations," which keep antifilarial antibody titers and
perhaps even cellular immune responses at relatively high
levels. These are the people who remain free of infection,
and one is tempted to speculate that their heightened immune
responsiveness may play a role in determining this infection-
free state.
    Other individuals appear to respond differently. Many
become (or at least are found to be) relatively hyporesponsive
to filarial antigens, and these are the individuals who present
clinically with the various manifestations of lymphatic-related
filarial disease (i.e., microfilaremia, filarial fevers,
elephantiasis, hydrocele, or chyluria). In these patients both
serum and cellular inhibitory elements can be defined, and it
is quite likely that modulatory or suppressive mechanisms involving these elements play an important role in maintaining
the host's response to filaria at relatively low levels.
Whether these relatively low levels of responsiveness are the
cause or effect of chronic filarial infection remains to be
conclusively determined, but it is clear that it is in the
setting of such levels of responsiveness that filarial disease
of the lymphatic type is found.
    The third type of reaction, in our hypothetical schema,
which follows repeated exposure to infective filaria, is characterized by a hyperresponsiveness to parasite antigens. This

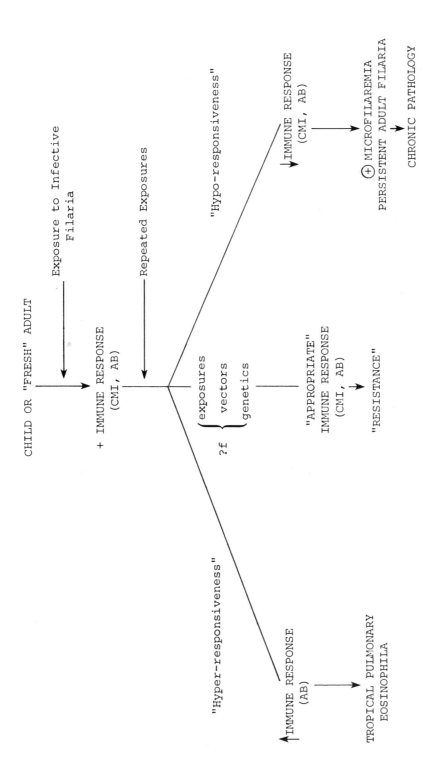

FIGURE 2. Hypothetical schema of the progression of clinical and immunologic responses of individuals living in an area endemic for W. bancrofti filariasis.

hyperresponsiveness is restricted almost exclusively to humoral immune responses and results clinically in the syndrome of tropical pulmonary eosinophilia described above.

What it is that determines just how an individual will respond immunologically to filarial infection and just who will develop clinical disease is still unknown. Clearly a number of nonimmunologic factors related to intensity of exposure, vector differences, and parasite strains may be important in this regard, and most of these still remain to be defined. Also, there may, of course, be genetic influences on the host that play a role in determining disease susceptibility. In this regard and in collaboration with others (24) during our study of the Cook Islands population, we attempted to correlate HLA markers with clinical and immunologic parameters in 225 individuals with or without bancroftian filariasis. Though analysis of the data is still incomplete, we have as yet been unable to find significant linkages between individual HLA specificities and clinical or immunologic responses. On the other hand, there did appear to be some evidence of a familial predisposition to filarial disease among these individuals. Children in families where one or both parents had filariasis were far more likely to have filarial infection than were children from families where neither parent had the disease (24). These results are still preliminary, and even though the differences were quite impressive, their interpretation is not entirely clear. One would like to think that they indicate an important genetic familial predisposition to developing disease, but it is also possible that these data reflect only a "familial predisposition" resulting from shared, common, nonimmunologic environmental influences.

In summary, the observations described above have only barely scratched the surface of the issues of penetration, persistence, and pathology in human filarial infections. Perhaps the most intriguing of these observations has been the paradoxical finding that in endemic areas it is *not* the patients with filariasis who have the most vigorous antifilarial immune responses but rather those *exposed but not infected* individuals of the "control population." This finding has been documented for the antigen-induced lymphocyte proliferation response, for specific antibody formation, and for immunoglobulin E responses. It suggests that chronic filariasis may be a disease state characterized by the presence of immunologic modulating mechanisms, and indeed there is some direct, though limited, evidence for the presence of both cellular and humoral inhibitory factors in these patients. Furthermore, from the data available at least some of these modulating mechanisms appear to have as one of their characteristics an important element of parasite antigen specificity. It is still unclear whether the relatively diminished responsiveness of infected individuals is a cause or an effect of chronic infection, but studies of an animal model suggest that the ability to generate early antibody responses is associated with protection from infection. In man, there is clear evidence for a familial predisposition to the development of filariasis, but the data do not allow one to decide with certainty whether this predisposition is genetically or environmentally determined. Finally, except for the syndrome of tropical pulmonary eosinophila, which is characterized by humoral immune hyperresponsiveness and clinical allergic-type disease, the correlation between the immunologic parameters and clinical features of individuals with filariasis has been poor.

References

1. World Health Org. Expert Committee on Filariasis. Third Rept. WHO Tech. Rep. Ser. #542, pp. 54, 1974.
2. Weller, P. F., Ottesen, E. A., and Heck, L. Manuscript in preparation.
3. Ottesen, E. A., Weller, R. F., and Heck, L. *Immunology 33*, 413, 1977.
4. Kagan, I. G. *J. Parasitol. 49*, 773, 1963.
5. Desowitz, R. S., Saave, J. J., and Sawada, T. *Ann. Trop. Med. Parasitol. 60*, 257, 1966.
6. Smith, D. H., Wilson, T., Berezoncev, J. A., *et al. Bull. Wld. Health Org. 44*, 771, 1971.
7. Ottesen, E. A., Weller, P. F., and Heck, L. Manuscript in preparation.
8. Gusmao, R. A., and Ottesen, E. A. Manuscript submitted for publication.
9. Portaro, J. K., Britton, S., and Ash, L. R. *Exp. Parasitol. 40*, 438, 1976.
10. Colley, D. G., Cook, J. A., Freeman, G. L., *et al. Int. Arch. Allergy Appl. Immunol. 53*, 420, 1977.
11. Chen, P., and Dean, D. A. *Am. J. Trop. Med. Hyg. 26*, 963, 1977.
12. Ottesen, E. A., Hiatt, R. A., Cheever, A. W., *et al. Clin. Exp. Immunol. 33*, 38, 1978.
13. Smithers, S. R., and Terry, R. J. *Adv. Parasitol. 7*, 41, 1969.
14. Basten, A., Boyer, M. H., and Beeson, P. B. *J. Exp. Med. 131*, 1271, 1970.
15. Fine, D. P., Buchanan, R. D., and Colley, D. G. *Am. J. Pathol. 71*, 193, 1973.

16. Larsh, J. E., Race, G. J., Martin, J. H., *et al.* *J. Parasitol.* *60*, 99, 1974.
17. Ottesen, E. A., and Weller, P. F. *J. Infect. Dis.* (in press), 1979.
18. Weller, P. F., Ottesen, E. A., and Heck, L. Manuscript submitted for publication.
19. Holt, P. G., Fimmel, P. J., Bartholomaeus, W. N., *et al.* *Int. Arch. Allergy Appl. Immunol.* *51*, 560, 1976.
20. Rocklin, R. E., Reardon, G., Sheffer, A., *et al.* *Proc. Fifth Leukocyte Culture Conference* (J. E. Harris, ed.), p. 639. Academic Press, New York, 1970.
21. Udwadia, F. E. "Pulmonary Eosinophilia," p. 270. Karger, Basel, 1975.
22. Ottesen, E. A., Tripathy, S. K., Thiruvengadam, K. V., *et al.* Manuscript submitted for publication.
23. Beaven, M. A. *In* "Jandbook of Psychopharmacology," Vol. 1 (L. L. Iversen and S. H. Snyder, eds.), p. 253. Plenum Press, New York, 1975.
24. Ottesen, E. A., Ward, F., MacQueen, M. M., *et al.* Manuscript in preparation.

DISCUSSION

DR. AMOS: I'm interested in your observation that only 70% of your Lewis rats became infected. Can you speculate on possible responsible mechanisms? Also, have you had any experience with gnotobiotic rats? If not, should this be considered?

DR. OTTESEN: Obviously, I haven't had any experience with gnotobiotics. I have no reason to expect that, although the Lewis rats are inbred, they would all respond identically to a given antigen.

DR. AMOS: I feel that you can assume that these inbred rats would be comparable in responsiveness to inbred mouse strains. I was hoping that you might speculate in the influence of environmental factors, including intercurrent infections.

DR. OTTESEN: I don't have any information at all on this. If there were intercurrent infections, they were subclinical; we did not detect gross body weight changes or unusual mortality. Your question certainly raises an interesting point, however, and is one well worth looking into.

DR. SHER: Have you tried to reinfect the rats that did not take the infection the first time around?

DR. OTTESEN: In our second group, where multiple small infections were being given as part of the experimental protocol, the answer is yes. However, we have not yet taken a group of uninfected but previously exposed rats and attempted to start a second infection. Thus the question of protective immunity in these animals is still unresolved.

DR. MUSHER: I would like to comment. Dr. Ottesen is interested in determining why some individuals become infected and others do not. Most of the data he presented compared already infected individuals with uninfected controls. If the attack rate is high enough it is important to examine the immunologic profile of the normal population prospectively and then determine who does and who does not become infected, as well as to measure the immunologic effects of the infection. It may be useful to return to the uninfected controls in Dr. Ottesen's series and see which of them will have become infected at some future point in time.

DR. OTTESEN: I agree; longitudinal studies of this type just haven't been done. The relative isolation and closed nature of our study population makes this group as close to the experimental laboratory situation as practical. A 5-year follow-up study of our group could provide some very interesting information.

DR. SISKIND: Is there a change in immune parameters in

filarial-infected subjects who are treated with drugs to reduce worm burden (antigen load)? If their immune response to
filarial antigens increases, does this not raise a question as
to whether the reduction is secondary to the antigen load
rather than the reason for these subjects acquiring infection?

DR. OTTESEN: This question has not been looked at in
filariasis but our studies in patients with schistosomiasis
where similar patterns of antigen unresponsiveness have been
seen in chronic infection *have* included such a follow-up. In
these individuals, antigen-responsiveness was detected (? re-
gained) beginning 3-4 weeks after treatment of the infection
with niridazole. Your suggested interpretation of these data
is a good one, and, in fact, we view our lymphocyte data in
both diseases as bearing more on mechanisms involved in the
persistence of the parasite within the host than on the
susceptibility of the host to acquiring the infection.

DR. SELL: What is the role of IgE in parasitic infections?
Postulate the mechanisms involved.

DR. OTTESEN: Clearly this is a difficult question, which
does not as yet have a defined answer. Presumably IgE has a
role in protective immunity in parasitic helminth infections
and because of its very low concentrations in the blood and
body fluids, it is likely that it works through amplifying
mechanisms provided by the multiple inflammatory mediators
found within mast cells and basophils to which it fixes. By
virtue of its association with mast cells, IgE is localized
along the body's surface barriers--the skin, mucosal surfaces,
and perivascular tissue. It is thus in an ideal position to
play a role in protective immunity at the penetration phase
of these helminth infections. In trichinosis and certain
other intestinal nematode infections, inflammation of the
gastrointestinal tract has been found to be a critical feature
of the "protective immunity" acquired by previously infected
animals and IgE antibodies may well play a role in the pathogenesis of this inflammatory response. Similarly, protective
immunity in some models of schistosomiasis has been shown to
involve eosinophils in regions (skin and lung) rich in mast
cells. It may well be that IgE-triggered release of mediators from these mast cells is involved in attracting cytotoxic
eosinophils to the sites of parasitic involvement and perhaps
even in direct toxic effects on the parasites themselves. A
great deal of work remains to clarify these and other potential roles for IgE antibodies in the host response to helminth
infections.

DR. SHER: I'd like to mention two other mechanisms by
which IgE could mediate parasite rejection. Dr. Andre Capron
at Lille has demonstrated a reaction in which schistosomula
are destroyed *in vitro* by an IgE-dependent reaction involving

macrophages; second, IgE might be acting as a "gatekeeper" controlling extravasation of other effector elements, such as antibodies and/or cells, at cutaneous infection sites.

DR. YUNIS: Did you consider the circadian variation in eosinophil levels in both your human and animal studies?

DR. OTTESEN: We certainly are aware of these circadian variations but did not study them directly. They were "taken into account" only by our performing all studies at fixed times of the day.

DR. EDELMAN: The discussion of filariasis today has centered about immune events and susceptibility and disease. You have not mentioned much about the microbiology of the parasite. Could two or more variants of the parasite exist in one locality, one being inherently more virulent than the other and at the same time less antigenic? Could it be that the weaker immune response seen in the infected person is not related at all to the reason for his being infected but rather to the virulence of the parasite that attacks him?

DR. OTTESEN: This is possible, but we have no way to test it. There are no animal models for human bancroftian filariasis.

IMMUNITY AND IMMUNE EVASION IN SCHISTOSOMIASIS

Alan Sher

Department of Pathology
Harvard Medical School
and
Department of Medicine
Robert B. Brigham Hospital
Boston, Massachusetts

Perhaps the most sophisticated evaders of the immune response are the metazoan parasites. In order to survive and perpetuate their species, these complex creatures require long periods of undisturbed development within the mammalian host. Therefore, they must be prepared for an extended onslaught from the immune system. Not only are the metazoan parasites highly successful defenders in this struggle, but many appear to actually utilize the immune response to regulate their own numbers, thus ensuring host survival. This remarkable adaptation is perhaps best illustrated by the schistosomes, a family of trematode worms responsible for the human and veterinary disease known as schistosomiasis.

Schistosome infections are initiated by water-borne infective larvae (cercariae) released from the snail intermediate host. The cercariae penetrate the skin of the mammalian host and undergo a rapid transformation into physiologically adapted parasites called schistosomula. The schistosomula then enter a four-week-long period of migration and maturation, which brings them first via the venous system to the lungs (where they can be recovered in large numbers) and later to the hepatic portal vessels where the larvae complete their development into adult worms. In the portal system, the male and female worms mate and proceed to their final habitat, which in the case of *Schistosoma mansoni*, the species of the parasite used in most laboratory work, lies within mesenteric veins of the lower intestine. The female worms then begin to produce large numbers of eggs. Although some are excreted enabling the para-

Portions reproduced from
*J. Exp. Med. 148:*46, 1978
by copyright permission of the Rockefeller University Press.

site to reinitiate its cycle by the infection of new snails, the majority of the eggs remain in the tissues where they induce the principal pathologic lesions of the disease. It should be emphasized that unlike most other infectious agents, schistosome worms do not multiply inside the vertebrate host.

Once established in the bloodstream, schistosomes produce long-lasting chronic infections, which in man may extend to decades in duration. During this period, the parasites are clearly evoking an immune response. A wide variety of different humoral and cell-mediated reactions against schistosomal antigens have been demonstrated in chronically infected human and experimental hosts (1). That the schistosomiasis-induced immune response is potentially effective against the parasite is evident in the fact that laboratory animals bearing adult schistosome worms acquire a partial or total resistance against subsequent challenge infections (1). This intriguing situation of a protective response induced by a parasite that itself is not damaged by the response has been termed "concomitant immunity" by analogy with a similar phenomenon described many years ago by Gershon *et al.* (2) in tumor-bearing animals. Concomitant immunity may well have evolved as a homeostatic mechanism ensuring parasite survival by protecting the host against the potentially lethal effects of superinfection. It can be thought of as a form of lysogeny operating at the level of the whole animal.

The phenomenon of concomitant immunity in schistosomiasis raises several important questions: (1) What is the target and effector mechanism of the protective immune response? (2) What is the nature of the adaptation enabling the established parasite to evade this response?

In studying the above problem we have used as our experimental model the *S. mansoni* infected inbred mouse. Aside from its obvious advantages as a tool for immunologic and immunogenetic investigation, the mouse is a host that is fully susceptible to chronic schistosomiasis (3) and is, in fact, the model most widely used for studies of the pathology induced by the parasite.

When mice are given a sublethal primary infection they can be shown to acquire a significant resistance against subsequent challenge infection with cercariae (4-7). This immunity develops gradually. It is first detectable at 6 weeks and reaches plateau levels at 12-16 weeks after primary exposure. At its peak, acquired resistance results in a 74-92% reduction in the number of challenge parasites reaching maturity. Although mice develop the capacity to reject challenge infections, the same immune processes fail to affect the survival of worms from the initial infection. Thus, acquired resistance to schistosomiasis in the mouse clearly represents a form of concomitant immunity.

Because immunity to challenge appears late in the primary infection and has been shown to persist 6 weeks following drug-induced elimination of primary infection worms (8) it is assumed that the adult schistosome must be the major stimulus of the protective response. However, there is also recent evidence suggesting that eggs produced by the adult females also are an important stimulus of immunity (9).

Although the immature developmental stages of the parasite do not appear to contribute significantly to the induction of acquired resistance, they appear to be the major target of the protective response. Thus, in immune animals challenged with cercariae the recovery of schistosomula from the lungs is significantly reduced with respect to the recovery from control animals (6). This reduction in challenge recovery appears to result from events initiated in the skin. For example, although schistosomula elicit significant tissue responses in the epidermis and dermis of the immune animals, they fail to do so during their transit through the lungs (10). Moreover, immunity against cercariae can neither be passively transferred into recipients (7) nor depleted (11) at time points after the exist of the challenge infection from the skin.

Based on the hypothesis that the early schistosomulum is the principal target of the effector mechanism of acquired resistance, von Lichtenberg and colleagues developed a model in which mice are challenged by the intravenous injection of *in vitro* prepared larvae (12). This experimental system provides several important advantages over the traditional technique of cutaneous cercarial challenge. After intravenous injection, schistosomula are carried immediately into the lungs, where their presence can be monitored both by histology and parasite recovery methods. Upon injection into immune animals, challenge schistosomula elicit eosinophil-enriched pulmonary tissue reactions in which the organisms appear to be rapidly damaged and phagocytosed. Although a similar process of reaction and destruction is observed in the lungs of nonimmune animals, this nonspecific response is slower and affects fewer parasites than the response occurring in immune mice. Moreover, fewer eosinophils appear to be present in the reactions elicited in normal lung tissue. That the events observed histologically reflect the actual elimination of parasites has been confirmed by demonstrating highly significant reductions in the numbers of viable schistosomula recoverable from the lungs of immune animals (Fig. 1) as well as corresponding reductions in the number of challenge larvae maturing into adult worms. In summary, by providing a method in which

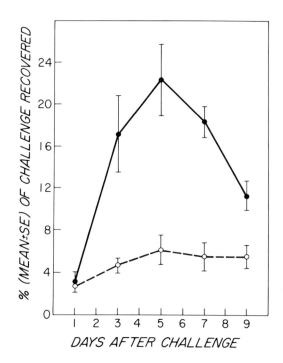

FIGURE 1. Recovery of schistosomula from the lungs of normal (◯) vs. immune (●) mice following intravenous challenge. The animals employed were C57BL/6 female mice infected for 10 weeks with 30 cercariae each and age-matched uninfected controls. The mice were challenged intravenously with 450 schistosomula each and the recovery of the larvae from chopped lung fragments determined as previously described (6,12).

the destruction of a defined stage of the parasite's development can be followed and quantitated in a defined tissue location, the intravenous larval injection model provides an excellent system in which to analyze effector mechanisms of schistosomulum rejection. As will be discussed later, the model also permits one to analyze the processes by which more mature parasites evade the immune response.

The mechanism by which injected schistosomula are destroyed in the lungs of previously infected mice is clearly immunologic. Thus, we have shown that athymic nude mice fail to react against challenge larvae despite appropriate sensitization (13). The inability of nude mice to reject challenge infections appears to result from the absence of a humoral factor rather than from a deficiency in effector T lymphocytes. This conclusion   .

is based on two observations (13):   (1) That significant immunity can be passively transferred to normal recipients from
heterozygote (nu/+) but not nude (nu/nu) infected donors.
(2) That nude and heterozygote recipients of immune serum displayed equivalent levels of immunity to larval challenge.

The nature of the thymus-dependent humoral component was
explored in a series of passive transfer experiments (13).
The results showed (1) that significant immunity against intravenous challenge can be passively transferred by the injection of as little as 50 µl of chronic immune serum per
recipient, and (2) that the factor responsible for transfer
of immunity has the molecular weight and chromatographic properties of an IgG molecule. Thus, it would appear that the
thymus-controlled humoral factor involved in the rejection of
schistosomulum challenges is antibody of the IgG class.

The observation of inflammatory reactions directed against
schistosomula dying in immune mouse lung (12) suggested that
parasite rejection was a cell-mediated process. In order to
confirm the requirement for effector cells in larval killing,
we examined the effects of whole-body irradiation on the rejection of schistosomulum challenges. We were able to show
that a 650R dose of gamma radiation completely ablated both
active and passive immunity to injected schistosomula when
administered 5 days before challenge (13). That the effect of
irradiation on challenge rejection was due to the depletion of
cells was confirmed in an experiment in which the injection of
syngeneic bone marrow was shown to restore the ability of irradiated, passively immunized mice to destroy challenge infections (13).

The passive transfer and cell depletion experiments summarized above suggest that the effector mechanism of schistosomulum rejection in the mouse is a form of antibody-dependent
cell-mediated immunity. A similar conclusion has been drawn
from the results of animal and human *in vitro* studies (14).
In this work from a number of different laboratories, schistosomula have been shown to be susceptible to damage by the
combined effects of antibody and cells (eosinophils, neutrophils, or macrophages) (14). It should be stressed that although the parasite appears to be vulnerable both *in vivo* and
in vitro to antibody-dependent cell-mediated mechanisms, to
date no evidence exists for a direct role of sensitized T
lymphocytes in larval killing (11,13,14).

If challenge infections in the mouse are susceptible to
the effector mechanism just described, how is it that older
worms are able to evade the effects of the protective immune
response? In studying this question we have focused on the
transition in susceptibility undergone by developing schistosomula. As discussed above, although in the natural percutan-

eous route of infection, challenge larvae elicit an inflammatory response in the skin of immune mice, they fail to do
so in the lungs (10). Nevertheless, intravenously injected
in vitro prepared schistosomula clearly evoke tissue reactions
and are killed after being introduced into the lungs (12).
Why then are injected newly transformed larvae so readily destroyed while older schistosomula arriving in the lungs via
the percutaneous route of challenge appear to be refractory to
the same immune mechanisms?

Our studies on this question have revealed that as schistosomula develop in the host they become progressively less
susceptible to attack by antibody (13). Thus, as summarized
in Fig. 2, injected schistosomula can be rejected in the
lungs by passively transferred immune serum only when the lat-

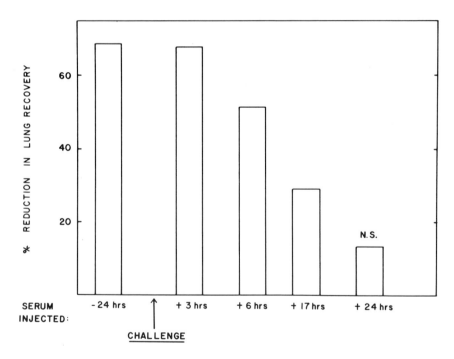

FIGURE 2. Effect of the injection schedule on the passive transfer of immunity to injected schistosomula. Immune
serum from a single pool was administered intravenously to
normal C57BL/6 mice at the times indicated. Immunity was
measured 5 days after the challenge by the lung assay. The reductions in recovery (with respect to recoveries from control
recipients of normal serum) were significant at all but the
last of the injection times indicated (13).

ter is administered before or within the first 17 hours after the challenge. It is clear from this experiment that developing schistosomula rapidly become resistant to the toxic effects of antibody *in vivo*. What then is the change in the parasite that accounts for the acquisition of resistance?

Unfortunately, the answer to this question is complex. We and other groups have discovered that maturing schistosomula undergo a number of different changes that could account for their loss of susceptibility to immune damage. Thus, within 48 hours the larvae lose their ability to activate complement via the alternate pathway (Sher, A., unpublished data) and acquire increased motility ("wriggle power") (15). Also occurring within the same period are complex changes in the structure of the surface of the parasite: the development of a double unit membrane (16) and the redistribution of intra-membraneous particles in that membrane (17). However, the most intriguing change occurring in the parasite during this period is the surface acquisition of host molecules.

The "host antigen" phenomenon in schistosomiasis was first described 8 years ago by Smithers *et al.* at Mill Hill (18). By means of an elegant series of worm transfer experiments in rhesus monkeys, these workers demonstrated that adult schistosomes living in a given host acquire surface antigens specific to that host. It was later demonstrated that the acquisition of these host determinants begins shortly after cercarial penetration and that the density of determinants reaches peak levels during the transit of the schistosomula through the lungs (19,20). It was also observed that as schistosomula acquire host molecules, they become progressively less reactive with antibodies directed against their own surface antigens, such that when they reach the lung stage no binding of antibody can be detected (19,20). Given these findings, it seems reasonable to propose that the process limiting the susceptibility of developing injected larvae to antibody attack in immune mouse lung is the acquisition of host molecules.

In attempting to test the latter hypothesis we used the following approach (13). Schistosomula were cultured in media containing red cells as a source of host molecules. By means of indirect immunofluorescence it was possible to demonstrate that worms cultured in this fashion acquire a thin coating of erythrocyte determinants. The red cell cultured larvae were then injected intravenously into immune mice and their survival assessed by the lung recovery assay. As shown in Fig. 3, worms cultured in a medium containing mouse RBC are rejected less efficiently than uncultured ("fresh") worms or worms cultured for the same period in a medium not containing the RBC host molecule source. It was also shown (Fig. 3) that RBC lysates could be substituted for intact cells as a source

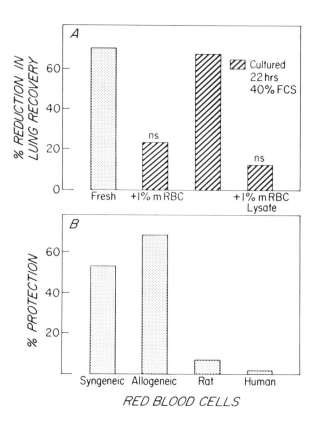

FIGURE 3. Effect of in vitro cultivation in red cells on
the survival of schistosomula after injection into immune
mouse lung. (A) Schistosomula obtained by the skin penetration method (35) ("fresh" worms) were cultured in media consisting of Earles' lactalbumin plus the ingredients listed on
the graph. The worms were then used to challenge immune and
normal C57BL/6 animals. Lung recoveries were performed on all
the animals on the same day (i.e., 5 days after the injection
of the fresh worms, 4 days after the injection of the cultured
worms). The erythrocyte lysate was prepared by subjecting
mouse red blood cells (mRBC) to five cycles of freezing and
thawing (13). (B) Comparison of the effects of syngeneic
(C57BL/6), allogeneic (DBA/2), and xenogeneic (rat and human) red
cells in promoting schistosomulum survival in immune mouse lung.
Percent protection refers to the percentage reduction in lung
recovery observed after challenge with worms cultured in fetal
calf serum (FCS) alone minus the percentage reduction obtained
with RBC (1%) cultured larvae divided by the percentage
reduction observed with FCS cultured worms, i.e.,

$$\frac{[\%R(FCS)]-[\%R(FCS+RBC)]}{[\%R \ FCS]}$$

of the *in vitro* protecting activity. Since it could be argued
that the added red cells were providing, in addition to surface binding hose molecules, nutrients necessary for the development of antibody-resistant worms, the effect of xenogeneic
RBC on the acquisition of protection was examined. As shown
in Fig. 3, neither human nor rat RBC cause a decrease in susceptibility to killing when added during the culture phase
of the experiment. On the other hand, allogeneic mouse RBC
are just as efficient as syngeneic cells in providing protection against immune attack. At present the explanation of
this unusual requirement for host molecules of the homologous
species in the acquisition of insusceptibility is unclear.
Finally, I should stress that the effects observed in the experiments described above were measured using a lung recovery
assay performed at a single time point. Additional work in
which recoveries of injected schistosomula were measured at
the adult stage has indicated that the numbers of worms protected against immune attack by preincubation in RBC may be
lower than the data shown here suggest. Nevertheless, it is
clear from these experiments that preculture in RBC has a
significant though partial effect in promoting the survival
of schistosomula in the immune animal (13).

Because of the probable importance of host molecule acquisition in protecting parasites against immune attack, we
have begun to examine the immunochemical identity of the substances that bind to developing schistosomula during murine
infection. In previous work, Clegg *et al.* (21) and Goldring
et al. (22) established that schistosomula cultured in the
presence of human red blood cells acquire A, B, H, and Lewis-
type blood group substances. Since these antigens were shown
to be acquired as glycolipids, whereas other blood group determinants that are glycoprotein in nature could not be detected on cultured worms (22), the Mill Hill group hypothesized
that the host substances absorbed by schistosomes are glyco-
lipid molecules.

Our approach to analyzing the chemical specificity of
mouse host antigens has been to examine lung stage schistosomula for the presence of known murine alloantigens. We began this study (Sher, A., Hall, B. F., and Vadas, M. A., *J. Exp.
Med. 148*, 46, 1978) by asking whether or not genetically
defined host determinants could be detected on the surface of
the worms. Alloantisera were prepared by cross immunization
of C57BL/6 and C3H/HE mice with spleen and lymph node cells
from donors of each strain. When tested by indirect immunofluorescence for its reaction with lung stage schistosomula,
each antiserum was found to give positive staining only with
worms recovered from the donors of the homologous strain, i.e.,
the anti-C57 serum reacted with C57 larvae but not with C3H

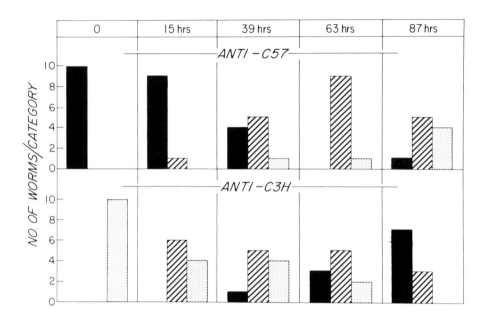

FIGURE 4. *Exchange of alloantigens after transfer of lung schistosomula into allogeneic recipients. Worms recovered from the lungs of C57BL/6 mice 5 days after the injection of newly transformed schistosomula were reinjected intravenously into C3H-HE mice. At the times indicated groups of animals were sacrificed and the transferred worms recovered from the lungs. The schistosomula were then reacted (see Table I) with either C3H anti-C57BL antiserum, C57BL anti-C3H antiserum, or normal mouse serum and after washing treated with fluorescein conjugated rabbit anti-mouse Ig. The larvae were then examined by fluorescence microscopy and scored either as negative (stipled bars), weakly positive (striped bars), or strongly positive (solid bars). Worms tested with normal mouse serum were negative at each of the time points examined.*

larvae, the anti-C3H serum reacted with C3H but not with C57 larvae. The allodeterminants detected in this manner on the larval surface appear to be tightly bound to the tegument. Thus, they can still be demonstrated on lung worms after 24 hours incubation *in vitro* and after 87 hours following transfer into allogeneic recipients (Fig. 4). As shown in the same experiment (Fig. 4), alloantigen acquisition occurs rapidly, new determinants being detected on the worms as early as 15 hours after allogeneic transfer.

TABLE I. *Acquisition of K- and I-Coded Determinants by Lung Stage Schistosomula*

Worm donor[b]	Antisera[a]			
	(1) anti-(K^k+I^k)	(2) anti-K^k	(3) anti-I^k	(4) anti-I^s
CBA (K^k-I^k)	10/10[c]	10/10	10/10	0/10
BIO/SN (K^b-I^b)	0/10	n.t.	n.t.	n.t.
BIO.BR (K^k-I^k)	10/10	n.t.	n.t.	n.t.
A.TL (K^s-I^k)	7/10	0/10	9/10	0/10
A.TH (K^s-I^s)	0/10	0/10	0/10	10/10

[a] The antisera employed were (1) BIO × LP.RIII anti-BIO.A (2R); (2) antiserum (#1) absorbed with A.TL spleen cells; (3) A.TH anti-A.TL; (4) A.TL anti-A.TH.

[b] Worms were recovered from the lungs of mice 5-6 days after the intravenous injection of in vitro prepared schistosomula. They were washed three times by centrifugation before testing.

[c] Number of larvae with positive tegumental fluorescence. The presence of surface alloantigens was assayed by incubating the worms in a 1/10 dilution of alloantisera for 1 hour at 37°C. After washing three times, the schistosomula were reexposed to a 1/10 dilution of fluorescein conjugated antimouse Ig (Cappel Laboratories) for 30 minutes at 23°C. They were then washed an additional three times and examined by fluorescence microscopy.

The identity of the mouse alloantigens acquired by schistosomula was examined by the use of monospecific antisera. With this approach, we were able to demonstrate that determinants coded for by the mouse major histocompatibility complex (MHC) are present as constituents of the parasite's coat of host material. Thus, an antiserum directed against antigens (K^k,I^k) within the K end of the locus was found to react with worms from $H-2^k$ strain animals (CBA and B10.BR), but not with worms recovered from $H-2^b$ (B10/SN) mice (Table I). Absorption of this antiserum with K^s-I^k (A.TL) spleen cells produced a reagent specific for K^k (i.e., the antiserum no longer reacted with larvae obtained from A.TL mice). The absorbed serum maintained its reactivity with $H-2^k$ (CBA) worms indicating that K-coded determinants are acquired by the parasites. The presence of I in addition to K-coded molecules on lung stage larvae was confirmed by showing reactions between anti-I^k sera (A.TH anti-A.TL) and worms from I^k (CBA and A.TL) but not I^s (A.TH) donors.

Although K and Ia antigens are clearly acquired by developing schistomula, other mouse alloantigens are not. Thus, in experiments of similar design to that summarized in Table I, we have been unable to detect Thy-1, Ly-1, or H-Y determinants on the surface of lung stage larvae. Similarly, we have also been unable to detect mouse IgG or C3, two examples of serum glycoproteins, on the larval tegument. Although these findings argue that the acquisition of K and I determinants by schistosomula is selective, other evidence suggests that K and I are not the *only* mouse molecules present on the worms. Thus, our antiserum prepared in C3H ($H-2^k$) mice against C57 ($H-2^b$) cells reacts with parasites recovered from B10.BR and AKR/J mice despite the fact that both strains are $H-2^k$. The identity of these non-MHC-coded host alloantigens remains to be determined.

The association of K and I antigens with immunologically insusceptible schistosomula is of interest for several reasons. First of all, the presence of these substances on schistosomes suggests that molecules other than glycolipids can be acquired by the parasite. Previous studies have indicated that K gene products are glycoproteins (23) and that Ia antigens are glycoproteins (24) or low molecular weight carbohydrates (25). Therefore, when taken together with the previous findings of the Mill Hill group, our observations suggest that the common chemical feature shared by schistosome-acquired host molecules (i.e., glycolipids, glycoproteins, and/or carbohydrates) is the presence of a carbohydrate moiety. One prediction of this hypothesis is that the schistosomulum surface bears receptorlike structures with affinity for certain oligosaccharide configurations and that these receptors determine the uptake of host molecules.

Of perhaps greater significance is the question of why schistosomes evolved a surface that binds substances such as the H-2K and Ia antigens--molecules thought to play an important role in immune recognition and cell cooperation (26). For example, by analogy with evidence from stusies on virus-infected (27) and chemically modified cell targets (28), one might suspect that the presence of H-2K antigens on schistosomula would facilitate rather than hinder their recognition and attack by the immune system. Yet, as I have stressed throughout this report, lung stage schistosomula appear to be insusceptible to immune damage by antibody-dependent as well as T-cell-mediated killing mechanisms. Therefore, it would seem that the acquisition of MHC-coded antigens by the larvae is not detrimental to their survival. On the contrary, it is more reasonable to assume that as "self"-determinants host MHC products *promote* survival by disguising accessible foreign determinants on the surface of the organisms. Although for the moment these considerations must remain speculative, they imply that schistosomes (and perhaps other parasites) have evolved mechanisms for utilizing the host MHC recognitory system to their own advantage!

In closing, I should stress that the evidence discussed above deals with only one of the many possible mechanisms of immune evasion that schistosomes might deploy during their extended lifespan in the susceptible host. Mechanisms other than host molecule addition have been proposed. These include the induction of tolerance or suppression (29), the production of blocking antibodies (30), parasite surface membrane turnover and repair (31), and "molecular mimicry" of host self-components (32). As has been demonstrated in the case of another helminth *Taenia taeniaeformis* (33,34), it is also possible that schistosomes produce inactivators or antagonists of inflammatory molecules (complement components, anaphylactic mediators, or lymphokines). Indeed, given its biologic sophistication and long evolutionary experience, the schistosome may have dozens of devices with which to thwart the immune system. Much of the fascination and challenge of the immunologic approach to controlling schistosomiasis lies in the unraveling of this parasitologic trickery.

Acknowledgments

I am grateful to Drs. J. R. David, A. E. Butterworth, and M. Vadas for their helpful discussions. I also thank Drs. Ulrich Hammerling and Gloria Koo for their generosity in supplying reagents used in our experiments. This work was supported by grants from the Edna McConnell Clark Foundation and the U.S.-Japan Program of the NIAID.

References

1. Smithers, S. R., and Terry, R. J. *Adv. Parasitol. 14*, 399, 1976.
2. Gershon, R. K., Carter, R. L., and Kondo, K. *Nature 213*, 674, 1967.
3. Warren, K. S., and Peters, P. A. *Am. J. Trop. Med. Hyg. 16*, 718, 1967.
4. Oliver, L., and Schneidermann, M. *Am. J. Trop. Med. Hyg. 2*, 298, 1953.
5. Hunter, G. W., *et al.* *Am. J. Trop. Med. Hyg. 11*, 17, 1962.
6. Sher, A., MacKenzie, P., and Smithers, S. R. *J. Infect. Dis. 130*, 626, 1974.
7. Sher, A., Smithers, S. R., and MacKenzie, P. *Parasitology 70*, 347, 1975.
8. Warren, K. S., Pelley, R. P., and Mahmoud, A. A. F. *Am. J. Trop. Med. Hyg. 26*, 957, 1977.
9. Dean, D. A., Minard, P., Murrell, K. D., and Vannier, W. E. *Am. J. Trop. Med. Hyg. 27*, 957, 1978.
10. von Lichtenberg, F., *et al.* *Am. J. Pathol. 84*, 479, 1976.
11. Mahmoud, A. A. F., Warren, K. S., and Peters, P. A. *J. Exp. Med. 142*, 805, 1975.
12. von Lichtenberg, F., Sher, A., and McIntyre, S. *Am. J. Pathol. 87*, 105, 1977.
13. Sher, A. *Am. J. Trop. Med. Hyg. 26*, 20, 1977.
14. Butterworth, A. E. *Am. J. Trop. Med. Hyg. 26*, 29, 1977.
15. Imohiosen, E. A. E., Sher, A., and von Lichtenberg, F. *Parasitology 76*, 317, 1978.
16. Hockley, D. J., and McClaren, D. J. *Int. J. Parasitol. 3*, 13, 1973.
17. McClaren, D. J., Jockley, D. J., Goldring, O. L., and Hammond, B. J. *Parasitology 76*, 327, 1978.
18. Smithers, S. R., Terry, R. J., and Hockley, D. J. *Proc. Roy. Soc. Ser. B 171*, 483, 1969.
19. McClaren, D. J., Clegg, J. A., and Smithers, S. R. *Parasitology 70*, 67, 1975.
20. Goldring, O. L., Sher, A., Smithers, S. R., and McClaren, D. J. *Trans. Roy. Soc. Trop. Med. Hyg. 71*, 144, 1977.
21. Clegg, J. A., Smithers, S. R., and Terry, R. J. *Nature 232*, 653, 1971.
22. Goldring, O. L., Clegg, J. A., and Smithers, S. R. *Clin. Exp. Immunol. 26*, 181, 1976.
23. Schwartz, B., *et al.* *Biochemistry 12*, 2157, 1973.
24. Cullen, S. E., *et al.* *Proc. Nat. Acad. Sci. USA 71*, 648, 1974.
25. Parish, C. R., Jackson, D. C., and McKenzie, I. F. C. *Immunogenetics 3*, 455, 1976.
26. Paul, W. E., and Benacerraf, B. *Science 195*, 1293, 1977.

27. Doherty, P. C., Blanden, R. V., and Zinkernagel, R. M. *Transplant. Rev. 29*, 89, 1976.
28. Shearer, G. M., Rehn, G. R., and Garbarino, C. A. *J. Exp. Med. 141*, 1348, 1975.
29. Weigle, W. O. *In* "Immunology of Schistosomiasis," *Bull. World Health Org. 51*, 578, 1974.
30. Sogandares-Bernal, F. *J. Parasitol. 62*, 222, 1976.
31. Perez, H., and Terry, R. J. *Int. J. Parasitol. 3*, 499, 1973.
32. Damian, R. T. *Am. Nat. 98*, 129, 1964.
33. Hammerberg, B., *et al. In* "Pathophysiology of Parasitic Infections" (E. J. L. Soulsby, ed.), p. 233. Academic Press, New York, 1976.
34. Leid, R. W. *Am. J. Trop. Med. Hyg. 26*, 54, 1977.
35. Clegg, J. A., and Smithers, S. R. *Int. J. Parasitol. 2*, 79, 1972.

DISCUSSION

DR. VAN ROOD: A Dutch group has recently shown that antibody titer and recovery of worms in mouse strains coisogenic
for H-2 differ significantly. Back-cross studies have not
been done but other data would be compatible with an H-2-linked
parasite-induced immune response.

DR. SHER: At present, we have no clear-cut data on the
influence of H-2 genotype on the response to schistosome antigens.

DR. DOHERTY: Could a cytotoxic T cell ever kill a schistosomula? For instance, can T cells dispose of parasites
grown in the relevant allogeneic environment?

DR. SHER: We are now attempting to kill lung stage schistosomula with T cells immunized against host alloantigen. As
your question implies, it is possible that T cells may not be
able to act against the parasite for the simple reason that
they lack the appropriate biochemical machinery for doing so.
Clearly, it is not because the targets lack the appropriate
MHC product required for recognition by these cells!

DR. BLOOM: Can you now ask the critical question whether
acquisition of "self"-MHC antigens is protective. One experiment would be the compare dose curves for infectivity of
schistosomulas cultured with self-antigens of a mouse strain
to organisms cultured in antigens of other strains or cultured in media lacking any mouse cellular antigen. Would that
be a feasible experiment?

DR. SHER: Yes, I think so if technical problems can be
resolved. You alluded to one in your presentation; that is
the problem of finding an appropriate host-antigen free medium
in which to do these experiments. In the experiment I described, we were looking at a very early time, 22 hours of culture, probably before an appreciable amount of fetal calf serum itself is adsorbed to the parasites and acts as the "host"
antigen. It's a very, very difficult problem.

DR. PREHN: Is there rigorous evidence that the new surface antigens are indeed supplied by the host rather than
generated by the parasite?

DR. SHER: No. However, such a process would require that
the parasite be able to recognize its host environment and
respond by synthesizing the appropriate alloantigen. This is
an incredibly sophisticated mechanism to explain a rather
simple phenomenon. Moreover, David Dean showed several years
ago that killed schistosomula express host antigens after incubation in host tissue. Therefore, I feel that it is extremely unlikely that worms actually synthesize the alloantigens that we have been studying.

DR. SACHS: Your evidence for selectivity of expression of MHC antigens depended on failure to detect a few other markers. Is it possible that this is a question of sensitivity of detection systems rather than selective uptake? Also, your C3H anti-B6 antiserum did react with B10-BR parasites. Have you looked at a backcross [(B10·BR × C3H)F1 × C3H] to determine how many different gene products were detected? I would imagine the number would be quite large.

DR. SHER: All of the alloantisera that failed to react with lung worms were found to react with lymphoid cells from the donor animals. We have not examined worms recovered from back-crossed mice. I agree with you that an experiment of this type would probably tell us that there are at least several alloantigens, other than H-2 and Ia, that are acquired by the parasites.

DR. PLATE: Do the lung stage parasites that you mix in culture with allogenic lymphocytes stimulate proliferation and the generation of killer cells to host antigenic targets?

DR. SHER: I don't know; we have planned experiments to answer this question.

DR. WYLER: Have you ever observed capping of host antigens on schistosomules?

DR. SHER: No, I have learned (L. Brink, personal communication), however, that "capping" or polarization of determinants on the surface of the parasite can be demonstrated using antibodies directed against schistosome antigens.

DR. LEVY: Why do you conclude that the determining molecule for attachment to the parasite is carbohydrate and not lipid?

DR. SHER: We hypothesize this because our results indicate that, in addition to glycolipids such as A, B, H, Le, and Forsmann substances, schistosomes can also acquire glycoproteins, that is, K and I gene products that are not known to contain lipids. However, as I mentioned, worms will not pick up all carbohydrate-containing molecules; immunoglobulins and C_3 are examples of glycoproteins not acquired by lung stage schistosomula. I should mention here, however, that Dr. Rosen has informed me that C_3 contains only a small amount of carbohydrate and, therefore, it may not be a relevant control substance.

CELL-CELL INTERACTION IN INFECTIOUS MONONUCLEOSIS*

Fred S. Kantor

Department of Medicine
Yale University School of Medicine
New Haven, Connecticut

Depression of delayed hypersensitivity has been observed
in a wide variety of viral infections (1-4). This depression
is usually quite transient lasting only a few days, but it may
be profound and prolonged. In this circumstance the virus may
act as an infectious, noxious agent, which destroys cells crucial to the development or the expression of delayed sensitivity. On the other hand, virus may act as a potent replicating
antigen, leading to regulatory immune responses that incidentally affect the host capacity to respond to other antigens in
a delayed hypersensitive fashion.

The present report explores the relationship of virus to
host in two infectious processes. The first involves canine
distemper virus infection of gnotobiotic puppies. This model
was selected because canine distemper so closely resembles
human measles infection and the anergy of measles virus infections, described earlier this century by Von Pirquet (5), is
the paradigm of viral induced anergy. The second model to be
explored is that of infectious mononucleosis, a disease associated with the Epstein-Barr virus (EBV), which is also incrim-
inated in nasopharyngeal carcinoma and Burkitt's lymphoma.
Finally, I wish to describe a system for the study of the interaction of virus and host *in vitro*, which may serve to elucidate important features of this relationship such as the
antigenic determinant recognized by the host and the mechan-
ism(s) whereby host immune responses are impaired.

*Supported by research grant AI-06706 from the National
Institutes of Health.*

MATERIALS AND METHODS

Patients

The population studied has been previously described (6) and consists of Yale University students with mononucleosis. The criteria for diagnosis included atypical lymphocytes in the blood smear, elevated heterophile antibody titers (>1:40 after guinea pig absorption), and the presence of antibodies to the Epstein-Barr virus as measured by the indirect immunofluorescence technique using the EB3 cell line as antigen.

The methods and antigens used for intradermal testing for delayed hypersensitivity has been previously described (6). Lymphocyte stimulation was undertaken using a micromethod (6); in brief, whole blood (20 units heparin/ml) was obtained by venipuncture. Lymphocytes were purified by centrifugation on Ficoll-Hypaque gradients and washed three times with Roswell Park Memorial Institute (RPMI) medium 1640. Leukocyte concentration was adjusted to 2×10^6/ml with RPMI medium 1640 containing 20% pooled human plasma, 50 units of penicillin, 300 µg glutamine/ml, and 50 µg streptomycin/ml. Cells (0.1 ml) were pipetted into quadruplicate microtiter wekks (Linbro Scientific, New Haven, Connecticut). Lymphocytes were stimulated with 0.1 ml of 1:500 dilution of phytohemagglutinin, 100 µg of pokeweed mitogen, 1:50 dilution of Candida albicans (Hollister-Stier Labs, Veadon, Pennsylvania) and 4×10^5 allogeneic lymphocytes (unless otherwise noted), which were obtained from four normal donors. These lymphocytes were irradiated with 3000 rads and pooled. Cultures were incubated in a 5% carbon dioxide and 95% air, humid atmosphere at 37°C. Tritiated thymidine was added to cultured containing phytohemagglutinin and pokeweed after 3 days and to cultures containing *Candida albicans* and allogeneic cells after 7 days of culture. After a 5-hour pulse cells were aspirated onto fiberglass filter paper with an automatic cell harvester and individual samples were placed in 3 ml of scintillation fluid and counted.

Enumeration of T and B Lymphocytes

Rosettes formed by lymphocytes with sheep erythrocytes were used as a marker for T cells as previously described (6). Two hundred lymphocytes were counted and all cells binding more than three sheep erythrocytes were considered to be T cells. B lymphocytes were enumerated by the presence on their surface of immunoglobulins. Lymphocyte suspensions containing 1×10^6

cells were incubated with 0.1 ml of fluoresceinated polyvalent antihuman immunoglobulin serum. The cells were washed three times and the final pellet resuspended in two drops of fetal calf serum. A smear of this preparation was evaluated in a dark-field microscope with an ultraviolet illuminator. Four hundred cells were examined and the percentage of fluorescent cells noted. The percentage of monocytes present was calculated using a myelo-peroxidase stained dry smear of cells.

Animals

Gnotobiotic mongrel puppies susceptible to canine distemper virus (CDV) were immunized with KLH in complete Freund's adjuvant and infected with CDV strain R252 as previously described (7).

Preparation of B Lymphocytes

Suspensions of mononuclear cells separated on Ficoll-Hypaque gradients were purified by exposure to neuraminadase-treated sheep red cells and centrifuging the resulting T rosettes at 300 g (8). Lymphocyte suspensions thus prepared retained fewer than 6% rosetting cells. Cell suspensions (4 × 10^6/ml) prepared in RPMI 1640 medium with 15% human AB+ serum and 10% DMSO (dimethylsulfoxide) were frozen at a rate of 1°C/ minute in a specially designed apparatus (Cryo-Med, Mt. Clemens, Michigan). After freezing, cells were stored in the vapor phase of liquid nitrogen and were rapidly thawed by immersion in a 37°C water bath and immediately diluted by 15% human serum and then washed free of DMSO.

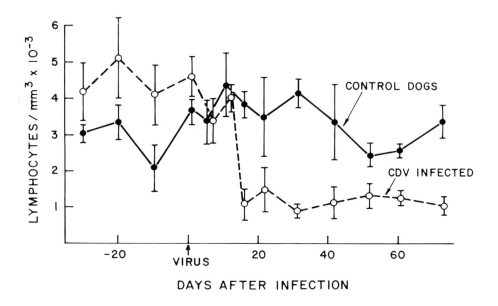

Figure 1. Lymphocyte counts in puppies infected with canine distemper virus.

RESULTS

Infection of gnotobiotic puppies with canine distemper virus related in a profound reduction in skin test reactivity and lymphocyte stimulation by antigen or mitogen. Stimulation was reduced even when numbers of lymphocytes were adjusted for the marked leukopenia which occurred. As shown in Fig. 1, the lymphocyte count dropped in the second week after infection to 25% of its usual value. Canine distemper virus shares with measles certain antigenic similarities, including affinity for T cell receptors (9,10). In this instance canine distemper virus directly infected T cells, and by destroying them rendered the animal immunodeficient.

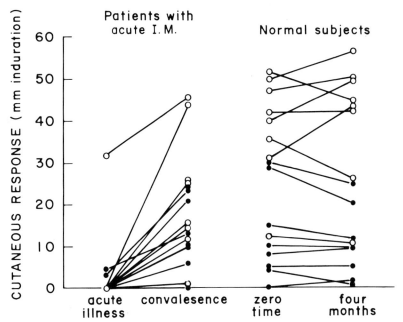

FIGURE 2. *Skin tests with SKSD and Candida antigens in normals and in patients with infectious mononucleosis.*

The immunological events in infectious mononucleosis are quite different; human "T" cells do not have receptors for EB virus (11). At the first visit, patients with infectious mononucleosis already had evidence of marked impairment of delayed skin reactions as well as depressed lymphocyte function. As shown in Fig. 2 the skin reactions with strepokinase-streptodornase and with Candida revealed markedly depressed reactions during the acute phase of the illness. When each individual was retested 4 months later an increase in skin reactivity to the same antigens was observed; retesting normal subjects with the same antigens did not enhance skin reactivity.

Several important alterations in tests of cell-mediated immunity *in vitro* in cells from patients during the acute phase of infectious mononucleosis were observed (Fig. 3). Cells obtained during the acute phase of the illness and cultured *in vitro* incorporated more tritiated thymidine in the

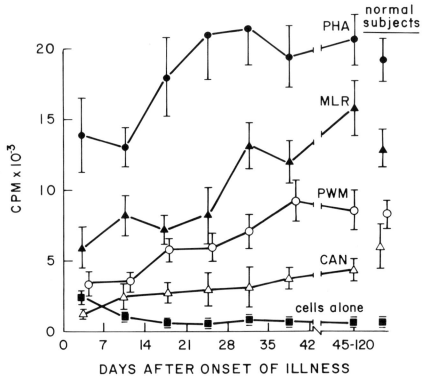

FIGURE 3.   *Responses of lymphocytes during acute I.M.*

absence of any stimulants such as mitogens or antigens.   This
was not surprising since at the time of diagnosis there were
already many atypical (stimulated) cells in the circulation.
Stimulation with phytohemagglutinin, pokeweed mitogen, Candida
antigen, and in a mixed lymphocyte reaction universally resulted in reduced reactivity during the acute illness as seen
in Fig. 3.   However, the time required for return of these
functions varied considerably; return to normal stimulation
indices after cells were exposed to Candida antigen was delayed for at least 6 weeks after the onset of acute illness.
In contrast, the deficiency seen with mitogen stimulation and
in mixed lymphocyte reactions returned to normal within the
third to fourth week.   Numbers of peripheral B and T cells
were increased absolutely and relatively during the early
weeks of illness.   It is important to note, however, that maximum elevation of B lymphocytes (Fig. 4) was seen in the first
week of illness with a gradual decline to normal values with-

in 3 or 4 weeks. In contrast, T cells usually reached peak numbers at the end of the second week of illness and declined to normal in 2 to 4 weeks as shown in Fig. 5.

These changes are significant for several reasons. The nuclear antigen of Epstein-Barr virus (EBNA) has been estimated to occur in a frequency of about 10^{-3} or 10^{-4} in cells of patients with infectious mononucleosis (12). This is inconsistent with the observation that 20-50% of peripheral blood mononuclear cells are transformed atypical cells. In the first week of illness approximately half of them are B cells. There is thus a disparity in the number of transformed B cells and the number of cells bearing EBNA antigen. Several workers have suggested that atypical B cells represent cells induced to transform by virus (13-15). The surface of these transformed cells is thought to contain a neoantigen induced by virus, which is recognized by host T cells causing a proliferative response. The disparity in numbers of EBNA positive cells and transformed B cells may reflect ability of EB virus to initiate transformation by interaction with cell surface receptors without going through all the steps of cellular infection. Whether the putative neoantigen is host or viral in origin is not clear, but lymphoblastoid cell lines containing EBV have been shown to stimulate T cells from patients convalescing from infectious mononucleosis (IM) while concentrated virus did not (14).

To study this system further we separated peripheral B cells from two patients acutely ill with IM by forming T cell rosettes and centrifuging them away. We then stored the resultant B cell suspension by cryopreservation. Approximately 4 weeks after obtaining the cells and 6 weeks after the onset of illness, cells were thawed, irradiated with 3000 rad so that they would not take up tritiated thymidine, and exposed to autologous fresh lymphocytes. Freezing whole lymphocyte suspensions (Table I) for 56 days did not significantly reduce cell numbers, viability, or the distribution of T and B markers. We exposed stored B cells obtained during the acute phase of the illness to convalescent whole lymphocyte suspensions from the same person in a mixed lymphocyte culture and the results are shown in Table II. It is evident that when normal control cells are treated in this way there is no stimulation when fresh and stored cells are cocultured. However, in the case of both of our patients with infectious mononucleosis, a distinct stimulation of convalescent T cells was obtained with acute phase B cells indicating that a surface antigen had appeared on B cells that was recognized by the individual's own T cells.

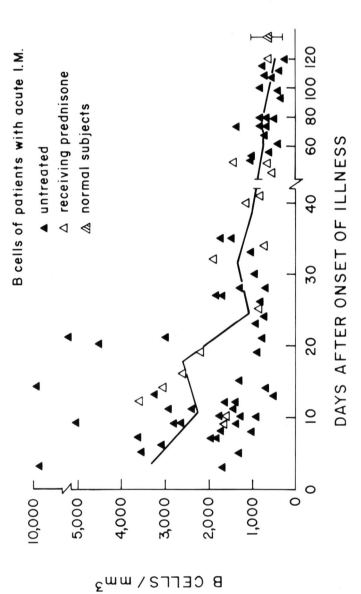

FIGURE 4. B cells of patients with acute I.M.

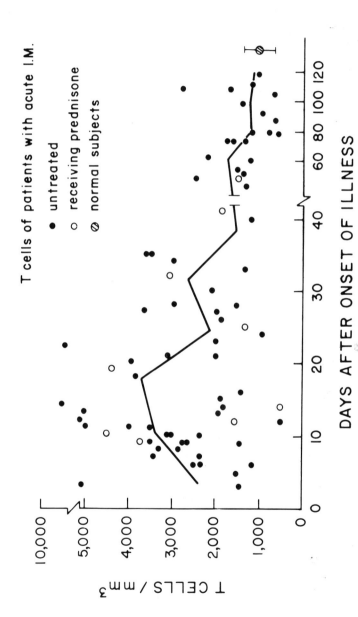

FIGURE 5.   T cells of patients with acute I.M.

261

TABLE I. *Recovery and Viability of Frozen Human Lymphocytes*

Time (days)	No. of cells frozen (×10⁶)	No. of cells removed (×10⁶)	%Viable	T cell	B cell
0	16	14.6	91	61	14
14	12	11.9	93	61	13
28	11	10.2	80	63	14
56	16	12.5	71	56	17

TABLE II. Coculture of Lymphocytes from Patients with Infectious Mononucleosis Obtained during Acute Illness and 4-5 Weeks Later

	Responder		Target			
Source	Type	No. ($\times 10^5$)	Type	No. ($\times 10^6$)	Condition	CPM
C	Lymph	2	–	–	–	454
C	–	–	B	2	Froz 28 d	340
C	Lymph	2	B	2	Froz 28 d	686
IM_1	Lymph	2	–	–	–	630
IM_1	–	–	B	2	Froz 28 d	1111
IM_1	Lymph	2	B	2	Froz 28 d	6434
IM_2	Lymph	2	–	–	–	760
IM_2	–	–	B	2	Froz 31 d	1222
IM_2	Lymph	2	B	2	Froz 31 d	9324

DISCUSSION

Infection of naive puppies with canine distemper virus led
to a profound leukopenia and a concomitant loss of delayed
skin reactivity and *in vitro* cell mediated immune reactions.
This finding is highly consistent with the known receptor on
T cells (11) for the measles-distemper-rinderpest group of
viruses and the presumption of viral infection and destruction
of functional T cells. In contrast, studies of children immunized with measles-mumps-rubella vaccine have indicated that
impairment of delayed hypersensitivity occurs in this circumstance without reduction of total or T lymphocyte numbers (16).
We have not excluded the possibility that a specific clone of
reactive T cells was infected and destroyed, but the rapid return of function suggests a temporary suppression rather than
destruction of a selected population.

The situation in infectious mononucleosis is clearly different and is diagrammactically shown in Fig. 6. Interaction
of virus and specific B cell viral receptors leads to stimulation of the cell and induction of a surface antigen that is
recognized by autologous T cells. The sequence of events
suggested above is associated with depression of cutaneous
skin reactions to unrelated antigens and to depressed T cell
responsiveness to mitogens, recall antigens, and allogeneic
lymphocytes *in vitro* (6). Augmentation of antibody production
may be seen in these circumstances and is represented in the
right portion of the diagram. Royston *et al.* (14) have shown
that T lymphocyte proliferative responses to mitomycin-treated
lymphoblastic cell lines containing EB virus antigen are present during the acute episode of mononucleosis, even though
they confirmed that cell-mediated immunity to other unrelated
antigens was depressed. In Fig. 6 this is reflected by a putative stimulation of suppressor T cells by virus-cultured B
cells.

Preliminary data obtained from two patients with infectious mononucleosis were presented above; convalescent peripheral lymphocytes were stimulated by acute phase B lymphocytes taken from the same patient and stored frozen during the
intervening period. Stimulatory indices of 6 and 9 times were
obtained. Considerably more data will be required to confirm
these findings and to determine optimal multiplicities of responder to target cells and the duration of responsiveness of
convalescent T cells. Previous studies have suggested that
the number of lymphocytes containing EB antigens during the
acute phase of the disease is relatively small. These estimates may be of antigens quite unrelated to the present stimulatory system. Indeed, one of the exciting aspects of having

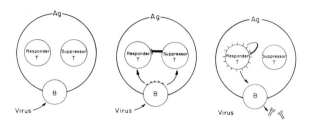

FIGURE 6. *Schematic representation of EBV infection. Virus infects and/or induces neoantigen on B cell surface which stimulates responder and suppressor T cells leading to anergy and increased antibody production.*

altered B cells and normal B cells from the same patient concurrently is the opportunity to investigate the nature of the antigen on the altered cell to determine if it is of viral or host origin.

Several previous workers have demonstrated proliferative or cytotoxic responses of lymphocytes obtained from patients with IM directed against lymphoblastoid cell lines derived from autologous cells (13-15). Junge et al. have previously stimulated cells from convalescent IM donors with frozen acute-phase whole lymphocyte suspensions and the present work confirms and extends their findings (17). Several possibilities are consistent with the ability of preserved acute-phase B cells to stimulate convalescent lymphocytes. Production or release of a blastogenic factor from previously frozen acute-phase B cells even after irradiation is not excluded by the present findings but seem unlikely in view of experiments (not reported here) in which supernates of irradiated, stored acute-phase B cells failed to stimulate normal allogeneic lymphocytes.

Secondly, stimulated B cells (blasts) may be able to trigger resting T cells by exposure of a new nonspecific blast antigen on their surfaces. This is easily approached experimentally and needs to be ruled out. EBV may induce a new specific host antigen on the surface of stimulated cells, but this is likely to require infection of the B cell and the small number of EBNA positive cells reported in acute IM makes this possibility unattractive. Virus itself may induce a T cell response, but in one study this was not successful. I

would like to suggest a possibility that is consistent with
the available data. EBV stimulates (not "transforms") B cells
by interacting with the receptor for virus and producing the
necessary surface perturbation to trigger the cell. The stimulus to the T cells may be the conjugate of EBV and receptor
in a fashion analogous to induction of delayed hypersensitivity
to haptens coupled to autologous serum protein. Thus, neither
the cell alone, nor the virus alone, would be sufficient.

In any case, the capacity of storing cells capable of stimulating autologous T cells should permit a detailed investigation of the mechanism of anergy induced during the acute
disease. Specifically, the question of whether stimulation
of convalescent cells includes a population of suppressor
cells is amenable to experimental investigation.

SUMMARY

Two examples of host-virus interaction producing impairment of cell-mediated immunity have been presented. In naive
animals canine distemper virus infects and destroys T lymphocytes, while EBV alters B lymphocytes causing them to stimulate autologous T cells. A system of cryopreservation of
acute-phase B lymphocytes is presented that permits study of
the interaction of such cells with convalescent T cells and
may help elucidate the regulatory mechanisms involved.

References

1. Mellman, W. J., and Wetton, R. *J. Lab. Clin. Med. 61*,
   453, 1963.
2. Starr, S., and Berkovich, S. *N. Engl. J. Med. 270*, 386,
   1964.
3. Mims, C. A., and Wainwright, S. *J. Immunol. 101*, 717, 1968.
4. Penhale, W. J., and Pow, I. A. *Clin. Exp. Immunol. 6*,
   627, 1970.
5. Von Pirquet, C. *Dtsch. Med. Wochenschr. 34*, 1297, 1908.
6. Mangi, R. J., Niederman, J. C., Kelleher, J. E., Dwyer,
   J. M., Evans, A. S., and Kantor, F. S. *N. Engl. J. Med.
   291*, 1149, 1974.
7. Mangi, R. J., Munyer, T. P., Krakowka, S., Jacoby, R. O.,
   and Kantor, F. S. *J. Infect. Dis. 133*, 556, 1976.
8. Galili, U., and Schlesinger, M. *J. Immunol. 112*, 1628,
   1974.
9. Imagawa, D. T., Goret, P., and Adams, J. M. *Proc. Nat.
   Acad. Sci. U.S.A. 46*, 1119, 1960.

10. Valdimarsson, H., Agnarsdottir, G., and Lachmann, P. *Nature 255*, 554, 1975.
11. Greaves, M. F., and Brown, G. *Clin. Immunol. Immunopathol. 3*, 514, 1975.
12. Rocchi, G., deFelici, A., Ragona, G., and Heinz, A. *N. Engl. J. Med. 296*, 132, 1977.
13. Svedmyr, E., and Jondal, M. *Proc. Nat. Acad. Sci. U.S.A. 72*, 1622, 1975.
14. Royston, I., Sullivan, J. L., Periman, P. O., *et al. N. Engl. J. Med. 293*, 1159, 1975.
15. Hutt, L. M., Huang, Y. T., Dascomb, H. E., *et al. J. Immunol. 115*, 243, 1975.
16. Munyer, T. P., Mangi, R. J., Dolan, T., and Kantor, F. S. *J. Infect. Dis. 132*, 75, 1975.
17. Junge, U., Hoekstra, J., and Deinhardt, F. *J. Immunol. 106*, 1306, 1971.

DISCUSSION

DR. HUTT: I agree that the non-B cell lines used by
Svedmyr and Jondal are not good controls. I believe you and
others have used non-EBV cell lines and found cytotoxicity of
convalescent IM cells.

DR. KANTOR: Yes, we have seen increased cytotoxicity in
mononucleosis patients for both EBV-positive and -negative
cells. Also, the increased cytotoxicity is seen in patients
with CMV- as well as EBV-associated mononucleosis.

DR. AMOS: It would be very convenient to use EBV-transformed HLA homozygous cells for HLA-D typing, but in many instances background stimulation of cells sharing the HLA-D
type is inconveniently high. Do you think this is due to
prior sensitization of the responder, and do you have information about the duration of immunity?

DR. KANTOR: We have examined only two patients for about
1 month each. I should have an answer for you within the
next 4-6 months. Previous reports have noted that cytotoxicity of host T cells for autologous transformed cell lines
diminishes with time so that the level of cytotoxicity is
near normal in 6 months but we do not yet know about proliferative responses.

DR. ROSEN: Why don't we encounter a lot more cases of
fatal EBV infection in the immunocompromised patient? It appears to be a rare occurrence. How do you explain that?

DR. AMOS: As a supplementary question, I'd like to ask
Dr. Kantor about a suggestion made by Dr. Simmons of The University of Minnesota. He believed that some of the host
transplant lymphomas are due to uncontrolled proliferation of
IM cells in the compromised host.

DR. KANTOR: Dr. Simmons' report, as yet unpublished, supports the view that host T cell responses to the EBV-infected
cells (B lymphocytes, salivary gland, or whatever) is a necessary condition for control of the proliferative phase of
infection. His patient died with a lymphoproliferative disease, which I hear was polyclonal. Whether cell transplant
patients' monoclonal B cell lymphomas went through a polyclonal lymphoproliferative phase is not known but possible
and should be investigated as a possibly treatable phase of
disease.

DR. GOOD: I have a comment concerning the observation
that Dr. Amos cited. I do not know the case mentioned, but
it may be that this malignancy, like EBV-associated Burkitt
lymphoma, has an initial precancerous proliferation or transformation and that a second stage is the change to a true
malignancy. The crucial issue is whether this proliferation

was invasive, disturbed architecture, invaded capsule, etc. If so, like Burkitt lymphoma, this may be another malignancy associated with EBV.

DR. J. SANFORD: Patients who are EBV negative are frequently immunosuppressed by the administration of live, attenuated, viral vaccines such as rubella, which is associated with immunosuppression. Is infectious mononucleosis more severe under these circumstances or is the immunosuppression not sufficient?

DR. KANTOR: This is an important question about which we have no hard data. I suspect that both of the circumstances you mention may be seen in different individuals. In those with mild, transient viral infections with attendent mild, transient anergy, little influence on the course of infectious mononucleosis would be expected; in those circumstances where prolonged and profound anergy is produced by viral infection or vaccination a real possibility for modification of infectious mononucleosis exists and should be studied. It is fortunate that the immunologic experience of the adult population with this virus is rather widespread, which lessens the probability that a patient who is susceptible becomes immunologically vulnerable because of unrelated disease or immunosuppressive drugs and *then* is exposed and infected with the virus. The likelihood of being aware of all these events in time to study them is small indeed.

DR. GOOD: It is of great interest that another malignancy that occurs with great frequency in patients who have been transplanted is Kaposi's sarcoma. This is a tumor that has also been linked to a herpes virus, namely, cytomegalovirus. Geraldo and his co-workers have shown that, in Africa and in America, seroepidemiological evidence associates this malignancy with cytomegalovirus. It would be interesting to know if this association holds in the transplantation patients.

DR. KANTOR: There are some interesting data from certain families who have been studied at the Children's Hospital, Boston. They exhibit an X-linked susceptibility to one of three outcomes of EBV infection: fatal mononucleosis, agammaglobulinemia, or B cell lymphoma.

DR. GOOD: There is another situation where a herpes virus produced polyclonal, clinically malignant, proliferation. This is the H tumor infection that F. Deinhardt has studied, in the marmoset I believe. I have argued whether this is a "true" malignancy, but it surely is a malignant hematopoietic polyclonal proliferation. Malignancy often, if not always, comes in two major steps: premalignant proliferation, not necessarily associated with monoclonality, and monoclonal malignant proliferation.

DR. SCHWARTZ: In Simmons' case, the "tumor" cells were polyclonal, and not the monoclonal type expected in the case of a true neoplasm.

DR. ESSEX: It has been mentioned elsewhere that EBNA positive cells taken from infectious mononucleosis patients, as well as those "cord blood cells" altered *in vitro* by EBV, lack certain characteristics (i.e., the ability to grow as tumors in nude mice) that are exhibited by malignant lymphoid cells taken from monoclonal Burkitt tumors. Do these two populations differ on the basis of any cell surface antigen? What is the role of the LYDMA antigen in the immune responses?

DR. KANTOR: I don't know of a comparison of cell surface antigens such as you desire. Certainly cells obtained from patients with infectious mononucleosis are distinguishable from those from patients with Burkitt's with respect to motility, cloning efficiency, and other characteristics, which suggest that their surfaces are different.

DR. BLOOM: If I remember correctly, these experiments were done by K. Nilsson and G. Klein and are of profound importance. Fresh IM cells and *in vitro* EBV-transformed lymphocytes are pseudodiploid in karyotype and fail to grow in nude mice. Biopsies from Burkitt's lymphoma are aneuploid, often with an 8/14 translocation, I think, or trisomy, and do grow in nude mice. When *in vitro* EBV-transformed cells were carried for long periods of time *in vitro*, many grew in nude mice, and, interestingly, all had chromosomal changes. These results suggest strongly that there is a real dichotomy between *in vitro* transformation or immortalization and malignant potential, at least in the nude mice. If EBV is involved at all in malignant transformation, it must be regarded as a necessary but not sufficient condition. In the terminology of an earlier generation, it serves as a "promoter" of carcinogenesis. The possibility that chromosomal changes are requisite for neoplastic potential was suggested in the 1940s by Foley, and generally dismissed.

DR. ESSEX: I'd like to add to that. Ruscetti and Gallo have recently obtained evidence that certain primate C type viruses have the capacity to take these EBV-altered lymphoid cells one step further to allow them to grow as tumors in nude mice.

DR. ROSEN: Hasn't George Miller induced metastatic disease in subhuman primates with EBV transformed cells?

DR. KANTOR: I believe he has.

DR. LEVY: Experiments have been performed in which peripheral lymphocytes from patients with acute infectious mononucleosis have been cloned in culture and only about 1% of these cells will become established into continuous lines. I don't know if karyology was performed but this observation has been used to explain Burkitt's lymphoma in some EBV-infected individuals. One could say that, in patients who cannot immunologically attack these cells capable of continuous growth, a lymphoma would develop. An interesting observation would be whether the antibodies against EBV are made only by cells infected with the virus. Perhaps these infected cells are needed to maintain the resistant state in the EBV-infected individual.

DR. KANTOR: I don't know.

DR. GOOD: I am not sure that the nude mouse is as good a model as we can have for transplantation of lymphoid malignancy. Perhaps the LASAT mouse, lacking spleen and thymus, or another nude and immunosuppressed model might be more revealing.

DR. PREHN: To expand Dr. Good's comment, growth in the nude mouse is indeed a poor criterion of neoplasia. Even MCA-induced sarcomas that grow well in the strain of origin may grow poorly in nude mice. Liisa Prehn and Tony Oatzen were able to show that X-irradiated nude mice were better hosts for immunogenic sarcomas, so perhaps growth in irradiated nudes would be the best presently available criterion of neoplasia.

UPS AND DOWNS OF IMMUNE RESPONSIVENESS
DURING PRIMARY EB VIRUS INFECTION

Sven Britton

Department of Infectious Diseases
Danderyd Hospital
Danderyd, Sweden

Immune responsiveness is characteristically affected during the infectious mononucleosis (IM) syndrome or, as it should be called, primary EB virus infections. These effects include a transient rise of serum immunoglobulins mostly comprising IgM, a transient depression of *in vivo* delayed hypersensitivity reactions to recall antigens and a much decreased *in vitro* proliferative response of blood lymphocytes from IM patients to primarily lectins but also allogeneic cells (1).

The polyclonal rise of serum immunoglobulins--the so-called nonsense antibodies, which include various autoantibodies--during primary EB virus infection has been difficult to explain, but we have recently shown (2) that the effect of EB virus infection on resting B cells is one of derepressing the cell and thus allowing it to functionally mature into an antibody secreting cell. Below I shall somewhat elaborate on these experiments. The second phenomenon, i.e., the depression of T cell responsiveness *in vivo* and *in vitro* has mostly been explained by a mechanism akin to antigenic competition, where nonspecific active suppression (T suppressor cells) has been implied. An alternative less-favored hypothesis for *in vivo* anergy has been brought forward (3) i.e., that the monocytes, which are instrumental cells in DH reactions, cannot orient themselves to the site of application of the recall antigen because their receptors for monocyte chemotaxins are already blocked by chemotaxins released from *in vivo* activated T and B lymphocytes, which are abundantly present during this syndrome. I have previously (3) presented data to support this hypothesis and in this communication I include experiments that suggest a rather trivial explanation for why lymphocytes during primary EB virus infection do not respond to lectins.

METHODOLOGY

This has been explained in previous publications and thus I shall dwell on it only very shortly. Polyclonal activation of B lymphocytes by EB virus lymphocytes was obtained after Ficoll-Hypaque separation of human blood (2). As target cells for the polyclonal activation of EB virus in *in vitro* normal donors were used regardless of immune status vis-a-vis EB virus, although they most likely were immune as are most adults. The source of EB virus were supernatants of B 95-8, i.e., marmoset monkey cells infected with and releasing EB virus. One ml of a supernatant from such cultures was added to 10^7 lymphocytes for 1 hour, after which the cells were washed and cultivated further for 5 days. The detection of single cells making IgM immunoglobulins after *in vitro* exposure to EB virus was done in a single cell plaque assay, utilizing various heterologous red cells as targets (2).

Lectin-Dependent Lymphocytotoxicity

Lymphocytes from acutely ill IM patients were isolated as above and exposed for 2 hours to ^{51}Cr-labeled heterologous target cells (mouse lymphoma cells) in the presence of lectins as described before (4). In addition, the same cells were exposed under identical conditions to labeled lymphoma cells coated with rabbit IgG antibody so as to measure K cell-mediated cytotoxicity (4). In this system control lymphocytes from (a) convalescent IM patients (>8 weeks after onset of symptoms) (b) patients suffering from other acute phase diseases such as streptococcal pharyngitis and normal controls were also tested. Direct autocytotoxicity data were obtained by studying uptake of vital dye (trypan blue) of lymphocytes exposed to lectins for short time periods as above.

RESULTS

Mechanism of Polyclonal Activation of B-Lymphocytes by EB Virus

When blood lymphocytes were exposed to EB virus *in vitro*, polyclonal antibody formation could be detected after 5 days'

TABLE I. *Polyclonal Activation of Human Blood Lymphocytes in Vitro[a] by EB Virus*

Pretreatment of cells	Number of PFC/10^6 against	
	SRBC	HRBC
Live virus[b]	210	170
Killed virus[c]	5	0
Killed + live virus[d]	40	60
PWM[e]	290	165
Killed virus + PWM	300	160
None	0	0

[a] *After pretreatment the lymphocytes were cultivated 5 days in 10% FBS before tested for polyclonal antibody formation.*

[b] *1 ml of supernatant from B 95-8 culture cells was added to 10^7 lymphocytes for 1 hour at 37°. Thereafter the cells were washed twice and recultivated.*

[c] *Supernatant from B 95-8 kept at 56° for 30 minutes.*

[d] *First 1 hour with killed virus then 2 hours with live virus with intermediate washings.*

[e] *20 µg pokeweed mitogen present for the whole culture period.*

culture as revealed by increased numbers of direct plaque-forming cells to horse and sheep red blood cells, respectively (Table I). These two blood cells cross-react to less than 2% at the antibody level. When heat-killed (56% for 30 minutes) virus was used in the same manner no polyclonal activation took place, but preexposure to killed virus could inhibit subsequent activation by live virus (Table I), which indicated that killed and live virus competed for the same receptor on the B cell. Killed virus did not negatively effect polyclonal activation by pokeweed mitogen (PWM), indicating both that such virus preparation did not have a mere toxic effect on the B cells and that EB virus and pokeweed mitogen used different receptors for activation of the B cells.

Further studies to characterize the surface receptors used by live EB virus to polyclonally activate the B cells were done by preexposing the test lymphocytes to sheep red blood cells (E), sheep red blood cells coated with rabbit IgG (Fc), and sheep red blood cells coated with rabbit IgM and activated mouse C5 deficient complement (EAC) before they were exposed

TABLE II.   Receptor Blockade of Polyclonal Activation by EB Virus

Treatment of cells	Number of PFC/10^6 against	
	SRBC	HRBC
Virus[a]	200	160
SRBC (E)[b]	10	0
SRBC-IgG (EA)[c]	0	0
SRBC-IgM-C' (EAC)[d]	0	0
Virus + E	245	170
Virus + EA	260	155
Virus + EAC	15	0
None	0	0

[a] 1 ml supernatant of B 95-8 added to 10^7 cells and present throughout culture period of 5 days.

[b] Sheep red blood cell (SRBC) at ratio 100:1 added to test lymphocytes for 5 days.

[c] SRBC coated with rabbit IgG added at ratio 100:1 to test lymphocytes for 5 days.

[d] SRBC treated with specific rabbit IgM plus C5 deficient mouse serum added to test lymphocytes at ratio 100:1 for 5 days.

to live virus (Table II). These experiments showed that only red cells coated with activated complement could block subsequent activation by live EB virus indicating that the virus uses structures similar or close to the complement receptor to polyclonally activate the B cell. The experiment also shows (Table II) that this *in vitro* system under these conditions does not allow specific antibody formation to sheep red blood cells as lymphocytes cultivated in the presence of these cells do not display more antibody-forming cells to sheep red cells than to horse red cells.

Lectin-Dependent Cytotoxicity during Primary EB Virus Infection

It is well known that blood lymphocytes from acutely ill IM patients proliferate very poorly in response to lectins (1). This has been confirmed by us and in an attempt to explore the cellular background of the lack of such prolifera-

TABLE III. Specific Cytotoxicity[a] of Various Effector Lymphocytes on a ^{51}Cr-Labeled Lymphoma Target Cell in the Presence of Phytohemagglutinin (LDCC) and Rabbit Antibody to the Target Cell (ADCC)

Source of effector cells[b]	Specific ^{51}Cr release (%)	
	LDCC	ADCC
Acute IM (26)	29.6 ± 1.4	44.5 ± 2.6
Convalescent IM (20)	7.2 ± 0.4	46.0 ± 1.5
Streptococcal pharyngitis (16)	5.8 ± 1.6	44.8 ± 1.1
Normal controls (42)	5.4 ± 0.4	46.6 ± 0.4

[a] Details of assay and calculations to be found in reference 4.

[b] Blood lymphocytes from indicated sources. Numbers in parentheses are numbers of individuals tested.

tive response we have studied lectin-dependent cytotoxicity of lymphocytes from acutely ill IM patients and compared it to various controls (Table III). The nature of the effector cell in lectin-dependent lymphocytotoxicity is not well known (6) but it is important to stress that this cytotoxicity is mechan-istically different from lectin-induced cytotoxicity (7), which requires long-term exposure to lectins in order to be expressed. The lectin-dependent cytotoxicity (LDCC) des-cribed here as well as elsewhere merely requires short-term exposure (2 hours) to lectins. At any rate it can be seen that blood lymphocytes from patients with acute infectious mononucleosis display strong cytotoxicity to a ^{51}Cr-labeled heterologous lymphoma target cell as compared to various con-trol lymphocytes (Table III), whereas antibody-dependent cellular cytotoxicity (ADCC) to the same target cells is com-parable between these groups of cells. If viability of lym-phocytes from these various sources were tested before and af-ter 2 hours exposure to lectins *in vitro* it was evident (Table IV) that lymphocytes from acutely ill IM patients showed dras-tically decreased viability after exposure to lectins as com-pared to controls.

TABLE IV. *Viability*[a] *of Lymphocytes of Various Origins
after Varying Time* in Vitro *in the Presence or Absence of
Phytohemagglutinin*[b]

	Time in vitro		
	0 hours	2 hours	
Source of cells	Without PHA	With PHA[b]	Without PHA
Acute IM (11)	87.6 ± 4.5	24.0 ± 5.2	78.6 ± 9.1
Convalescent IM (12)	96.5 ± 2.2	94.0 ± 7.6	91.2 ± 6.0
Normal controls (16)	95.8 ± 2.6	92.7 ± 1.8	89.6 ± 4.3

[a]*Measured by uptake of trypan blue. Recovery of cells
after 2 hours was >95% except for the acute IM cases, where
it was ≥75%.*

[b]*1 μg PHA/ml. No agglutination was evident at this dose.*

DISCUSSION

The really puzzling thing about primary EB virus infection
as it is expressed during the infectious mononucleosis syndrome
is how the monumental changes that occur within the lymphoid
system at this instance are so efficiently regulated. Only
very rarely, such as in Duncan's syndrome and in occasional
fatal cases (8), do the surveillance mechanisms seem to fail.
The experiments described above have some bearing on this
regulation. They show that *in vitro* exposure of blood lymphocytes to EB virus results in rapid proliferation (2) and
maturation of B lymphocytes into antibody-secreting cells.
This is most likely the mechanism underlying the increased
serum levels of primarily IgM accompanying this infection. It
is not clear though whether the increased heterophile titers
can be explained exclusively by this mechanism. In addition,
the experiments indicate that the virus needs intracellular
access to the B cells in order to activate it to proliferation
and maturation because killed noninfectious virus cannot turn
on the B cell although it apparently binds to the same surface
receptor (Table I). Thus it seems quite clear that EB virus
activates B cells via a mechanism different from most B cell
mitogens such as LPS and the like, as these compounds appear
to act via cell surface events that do not require intracellular access of the activating molecule. From blocking experiments (Table II) it seems evident that the EB virus uses struc-

tures similar or close to the complement receptor on the B cell surface to gain intracellular access and start the activation process.

Incidently the proliferative response of convalescent lymphocytes when mixed with syngeneic acute phase B lymphocytes from IM patients reported by Kantor in this volume may well result from direct viral transformation of B lymphocytes in the convalescent mixture from EB virus released from the acutely infected B lymphocytes.

In addition to this direct activation and proliferation of B cells by EB virus there is apparently an intense generation of cytotoxic cells, which becomes expressed *in vitro* when mixed with target cells in the presence of lectins (Table III and IV). It is already known that there appear two sets of cytotoxic cells during primary EB virus infection *in vivo*, one with specificity against EB virus antigen expressing cells and one of unknown specificity (9). The specificity of the cytotoxic cell in the lectin-dependent cellular cytotoxicity (LDCC) described here is not known, but it is evident that it can kill autologous target cells in the presence of lectins and that it has gained an active cytotoxic potential *in vivo*. I therefore suggest that the poor proliferative response to lectins during acute infectious mononucleosis is due to lectin-dependent autocytotoxicity. Dead cells cannot proliferate. In addition I propose that the LDCC effector cell is the key regulator cell in infectious mononucleosis, i.e., the cell that guarantees that the lymphoid system reaccomplishes its normal size after primary EB virus infection.

References

1. Magni, R., Nicolerman, J., Kelleher, X., *et al.* *N. Engl. J. Med. 291*, 1149, 1974.
2. Rosén, A., Gergerly, P., Klein, G., and Britton, S. *Nature 267*, 1977.
3. Britton, S. *J. Infect. Dis. 134*, 395, 1976.
4. Elhilali, M., Britton, S., Brosman, S., *et al.* *Cancer Res. 36*, 132, 1976.
5. Britton, S., and Rosenblatt, J. *J. Infect. Dis.*, in press, 1978.
6. Bonavida, B., and Bradley, T. *Transplantation 21*, 94, 1976.
7. Holm, G., and Perlmann, P. *Nature 207*, 818, 1965.
8. Britton, S., Andersson-Anvret, M., Gergely, P., *et al.* *N. Engl. J. Med.*, in press, 1978.
9. Svedmyr, E., and Jondal, M. *Proc. Nat. Acad. Sci. 72*, 1622, 1975.

DISCUSSION

DR. VAN ROOD: It might be of interest to see whether IM virus induction of PFC can be blocked by HLA antibodies.   It would be of special interest to test antibodies against not only the so-called short antigens but also antibodies against the long antigens, Bw 4 and Bw 6, because of their possible correlations with the C_3 receptor (see Villanez and Ferreuireir, *Nature*, 1976).

DR. BRITTON: I quite agree, especially since Dr. Rosen seems to have evidence for nonidentity between the C3b receptor and the EBV receptor on B cells.   Such an experiment would also answer the question whether addition of anti-Bw sera per se could activate human B lymphocytes to antibody secretion.

DR. WYLER: Will blocking C3d receptor on B cell actually prevent infection of the cell by EBV if you look for EBV antigen in the cells?

DR. BRITTON: Blockade of the C3b receptor by activated complement prevents superinfection and thus intracellular expression of EBV, as shown by Jondal and Klein.

DR. ROSEN: I have a comment for Dr. Britton.   You are looking at the C3b receptor.   It is not identical to the EBV receptor.   We had studied several patients with common variable agammaglobulinemia who have B cells with normal C3b receptors but few or no EBV receptors.   We have sent these cells to George Klein and he has confirmed these observations.   At any rate the C3b and EBV receptors appear to be adjacent but not identical.

DR. LEVY: What is the level of cross reactivity between the antibodies produced against sheep RBC and horse RBC? Could the same antibody be involved?

DR. BRITTON: On the order of less than 1% at the antibody level.

DR. LEVY: To explain the reaction against horse RBC, you may be dealing with antiheterophile antigen.   A forthcoming publication shows that cells grown in fetal calf serum pick up heterophile antigen.   The virus might then activate the cell to respond to the heterophile antigen picked up in the virus preparation since the virus was obtained from cells cultured in fetal calf serum-containing medium.

DR. BRITTON: In that case killed virus would yield the same polyclonal response, which it does not.   Furthermore, you also see an increase of antihapten (FITC) antibody forming cells which cannot be explained by your pick-up suggestion.

DR. HUTT: We find that live, but not inactivated, EB virus induces increased levels of cAMP in B lymphocytes.   Do you have any direct evidence as to whether inactivation of EBV inhibits binding to lymphocytes or inhibits capping of the virus?

DR. BRITTON: We have evidence to the contrary; killed virus can inhibit binding of live virus and killed and live virus bind to and compete for the same receptor of the B cells. Also, killed virus has been shown by Gerber to bind to specific T cells, as revealed by DNA proliferative assay of immune blood cells.

DR. HUTT: We have seen several patients with reactivation of EBV infection but no heterophile antibody.   Could you comment on this?

DR. BRITTON: If my data are correct, this would suggest that, in the case of reactivation of EBV infection, you have no *de novo* infection of immunocompetent B lymphocytes because in such instances you would see an increase in heterophile antibody as well as IgM antibodies of other specificities. I would assume then that the major lymphocyte mediated response in reactivation syndromes is specific, that is, mediated by specific anti-EBV lymphocytes in the B and T population.   Incidently, I believe that the lack of heterophile antibody in EBV infection in the very young is due to lack of stimuli (beef and sheep alimentary products) for expansions of those clones.

DR. HUTT: Since the K562 cell does not express normal histocompatibility antigens, do you think it is a valid target cell to use as a control for EBV containing B cell lines?

DR. BRITTON: I did not know that it did not carry HLA antigens.   Considering Zinkernagel's data I then agree that cytotoxicity should be tested on an EBV-negative, HLA-positive, target.

DR. YUNIS: Is it possible that T lymphocytes may bind EB virus or antigens?   Have you demonstrated B lymphocytes in the thymus of your patients with positive EBV?   Binding alone could alter T cell function without infection or transformation.

DR. BRITTON: The demonstration of B lymphocytes in the thymus of these patients rests on the presence of EBNA positive cells, which have invariably been known to be B cells.   I believe T cells can bind EB virus but that would have to be specific (with antigen-specific receptor for EB virus) T cells. It would only be a surface binding, not intracellular infection, which is revealed by EBNA positively.

DR. THEIS: Do you have evidence of EBV replication in thymic epithelium?

DR. BRITTON: No, I do not.   That is an interesting question because nobody knows what happens to the virus between the time of infection and the appearance of lymphoproliferative disease.   The incubation time is thought to be between 60 and 90 days; many people think that the virus is actually replicating, perhaps in the salivary gland, during this period.

IS SUSCEPTIBILITY TO TUBERCULOID LEPROSY
DUE TO A RECESSIVE HLA-LINKED GENE?*

R. R. P. de Vries
J. J. van Rood

Department of Immunohematology
University Hospital
Leiden, The Netherlands

R. F. M. Lai A Fat

Dermatological Service
Paramaribo, Surinam

N. K. Mehra
M. C. Vaidya

Cellular Immunology Laboratory
A.I.I.M.S.
New Delhi, India

INTRODUCTION

The demonstration by Lilly *et al.* that resistance of mice
to Gross leukemia virus is controlled by the H-2 system (1),
and the observation by McDevitt and co-workers that the anti-

*Supported in part by a grant from De Nederlandse Stichting
voor Leprabestrijding, NIH contract (NO1-A1-4-2508), the Dutch
Foundation for Medical Research (FUNGO), which is subsidized
by the Dutch Organization for the Advancement of Pure Research
(ZWO) and the Dutch Organization for Health Research (TNO), and
the J.A. Cohen Institute for Radiopathology and Radiation Protection (IRS).*

283

TABLE I. Disease Predisposition and HLA

	HLA antigen
Rheumatology	
Ankylosing spondylitis	B27
Rheumatoid arthritis	Dw4
Dermatology	
Psoriasis vulgaris	Bw17/B13
Dermatitis herpetiformis	B8/Dw3
Gastroenterology	
Gluten-sensitive enteropathy	Dw3
Autoimmunity, endocrinology	
Myasthenia gravis	B8
Addison's disease	B8
Juvenile diabetes mellitus	B8/Bw15
Neurology	
Multiple sclerosis	B7/Dw2
Psychiatry	
Manic depression	Bw16
Schizophrenia	Cw4

body response to synthetic polypeptides is controlled by H-2 linked Ir (immune response) genes (2,3), have caused an avalanche of immunogenetic research in experimental animals and in man. Amiel's finding that patients suffering from Morbus Hodgkin carried the cross-reactive antigen R twice as frequently as healthy controls led to a study of other malignancies (4). The assumption was that the HLA system might have a role in the control of malignant mutation. Such studies proved largely to be unproductive but led to studies of diseases of allergic, immunopathologic, and even psychiatric origin. Significant associations were found with many (Table I) (5). It seems reasonable to assume that these disease associations are due at least in part to Ir genes, which are either hyporeactive (e.g., multiple sclerosis?) or hyperreactive (e.g., gluten enteropathy?).

The impact of these findings can hardly be overestimated. They have led to new diagnostic criteria and broadened our insight in the genetics and pathogenesis of these diseases. Nevertheless because they occur to a large extent in advanced life, i.e., after offspring have been born, it is difficult to see how the associations of HLA with those diseases could have exerted selection pressure. It seemed a priori more likely that resistance or susceptibility against infectious diseases, if influenced by HLA, could be responsible for the selection pressure that caused the enormous complexicity of the HLA system and the large variations of its gene frequencies in different parts of the world.

To analyze this problem further it was decided to study the importance of the HLA system for the immune response against a number of bacterial and viral antigens (6,7). Table II summarizes the positive findings of our group and those of others (8). It can be concluded from these studies that HLA-linked genes influence cellular immunity (streptococcus and vaccinia) and antibody response (rubella) but genes not linked to HLA do so as well (diphtheria). These studies strongly suggest that the HLA system might play an important role in the control of endemic or epidemic infections. Individuals with low- or nonresponder genes might more easily become victim to such infections. If the findings in the mouse would hold true in man, one would expect such low-responder genes to be recessive to the dominant responder genes. Although suggestive, the data in Table II provide no evidence for this assumption, because they are based for the greater part on vaccination studies and not on the study of epidemic or endemic infections. To test this assumption further it was decided to study the segregation of HLA in leprosy patients. There were several reasons why we choose to study leprosy.

One is that it seems reasonable to assume that genetic host factors could play a considerable role in which type of leprosy occurs. We know of two extreme types: (1) the lepromatous form with an almost absent cellular immunity. In biopsies, one finds an abundance of *Mycobacterium leprae*. This form is infectious. (2) The tuberculoid form; cellular immunity is still present, but is apparently inappropriate. In the biopsy one finds only a small number of mycobacteria or none at all. Nerve damage occurs here very early. The patients are generally not infectious. It is not definitively proven what is cause and effect, i.e., whether infection with *M. leprae* causes a diminution of cellular immunity or vice versa. In the second place, insight in genetic factors that influence the host response to *M. leprae* may have important implications for control and therapy of leprosy:

1. If genetic markers for susceptibility were available, one might be able to delineate in a population those individuals most prone to develop (a particular type of) leprosy. Preventive measures could then be directed to those at highest risk, a small fraction of the population, and would be less expensive and more effective.

TABLE II. Example of Possible Immune Response Genes in Man[a]

Antigen	Exposure	Measurement	Genetics	Population
Au antigen	endemic	presence of antigen	Bw35 assoc.	Australian aborigines
Streptococcal antigens	ubiquitous	LTT	B5 assoc.	Caucasians?
Vaccinia	vaccination	LTT	Cw3 assoc.	Caucasians
Rubella virus	vaccination	antibody titers	Bw17 + A28 association[b]	Caucasians
Influenza virus (Alice strain)	vaccination (nasal spray)	antibody titers	Bw16 association[b]	Caucasians
Measles virus	ubiquitous	antibody titer	twin study; HLA linked?[c]	Caucasians
Diphtheria toxoid	vaccination	antibody titer	twin study non-HLA linked[c]	Caucasians

[a] See reference 8 for further references.

[b] With low response.

[c] Mean difference in titer of monozygotic and dizygotic twins compared.

2. Identification of the products of susceptibility genes might enable us to study possible mechanisms of interaction between these products and *M. leprae*. This could give more insight in the immunopathology of leprosy and might have implications for immunotherapy of individual patients.

We shall present data from family studies, which indicate that susceptibility to at least tuberculoid leprosy is controlled by possibly recessive genes linked to the HLA system. First the genetics of the HLA system will be briefly discussed.

THE HLA SYSTEM*

The HLA system, the major histocompatibility complex (MHC) of man, is an extremely polymorphic genetic system, which contains information for the major histocompatibility or strongest transplantation antigens. It is situated on chromosome 6. At least four loci may be distinguished, A, B, C, and D, each with a large number of alleles (see Fig. 1). Only one allele of each locus will be present on each chromosome. A set of combination of alleles on the same chromosome is called a haplotype.

On the A, B, and C loci, genes that code for transplantation or histocompatibility antigens are localized. These antigens are present on the surface of all nucleated cells and can be recognized by antisera. The products of the D locus are mainly present on B lymphocytes and monocytes. Because of their probable close relationship to the Ir genes, recognition of these determinants is of prime importance for the studies to be undertaken. The HLA-D determinants were originally de-

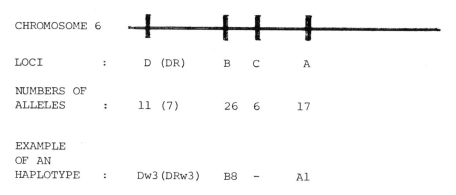

CHROMOSOME 6					
LOCI	:	D (DR)	B	C	A
NUMBERS OF ALLELES	:	11 (7)	26	6	17
EXAMPLE OF AN HAPLOTYPE	:	Dw3 (DRw3)	B8	–	A1

FIGURE 1. *The HLA system.*

*For references see ref. g

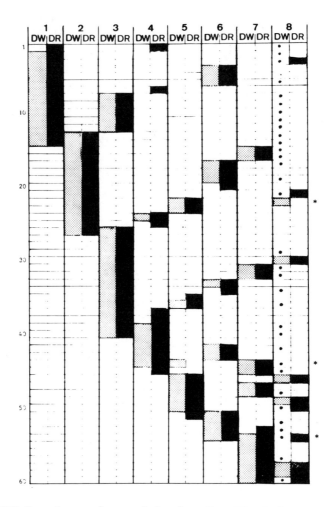

FIGURE 2. Comparison of typing for HLA-D by HTC and/or
PLT and for HLA-DR by serology. Dw, HLA-D determinants recognized by HTC and/or PLT; DR, B cell determinants recognized
by anti-DRw sera. *, Possibility of triplets not formally
excluded. ●, Not done.

fined by means of mixed lymphocyte cultures. Because this procedure does not lend itself to field testing, serological techniques have been developed for the detection of antigens present on B lymphocytes, which are identical or closely related
to the products of HLA-D (10-12). The antigens recognized by
serology were called HLA-DR (for D-related) antigens (13).

HLA-DR is the human equivalent of the mouse H-2-Ia antigens. The HLA-D and -DR products are also histocompatibility antigens, but biologically, chemically, and functionally different from HLA-A, -B, and -C products. Figure 2 illustrates how remarkably good the agreement is between the results obtained by cellular typing techniques (MLC) and by serology (14). Although DR typing can substitute for HLA-D typing by HTC for several determinants it is still unclear whether the two approaches recognize the same determinant, different determinants on the same molecule, or two determinants carried by two different closely linked structures. It should be noted that these data are from Dutch Caucasians and that it is uncertain whether they would hold true in other races. Available data suggest but do not yet prove that the HLA-D and -DR genes are alleles of one locus. The gene frequency of the null gene (i.e., determinants for which no reagents are yet available) is less than 0.05.

The HLA system also contains less precisely mapped genetic information for the complement factors Bf, C2, and C4, and for the bloodgroups Chido and Rodgers. However, it should be noted that there is still "room" for perhaps as much as 100 or more as yet not identified loci.

HLA AND LEPROSY

Several groups have searched for an association between leprosy and HLA antigens (for references see reference 15). A summary of the results is shown in Table III. The most important conclusion from this table is that not one of the HLA antigens showing a deviating frequency in one population is the same in another population. Some investigators have concluded because of this irreproducibility that the observed differences were due to chance. On the other hand these findings could be compatible with the assumption that the observed differences between the leprosy patients as compared with controls are due to genes linked with but not identical to the HLA-A and -B alleles. The "irreproducibility" is then simply caused by the fact that we are as yet unable to type for the products of these susceptibility genes directly. Therefore, if leprosy susceptibility genes are closely linked to HLA, we should observe that in studies of families in which two or more siblings suffer from leprosy, affected siblings would share one (or two?) parental HLA haplotypes more often than expected on the basis of the Mendelian segregation rules. It was therefore decided to study such families.

TABLE III. Leprosy and HLA: Population Studies[a]

Population	HLA antigen[b]	Antigen frequency[b]			
				Leprosy	
		Control	Total	Lepromatous	"Nonlepromatous"
(1) Ethiopia	Bw21	0(26)	26(39)	0(19)	33(20)
(2) Spain	B14	4(149)	23(30)	35(17)	8(13)
(3) India	A9	27(40)	10(70)	18(40)	0(30)
(4) Philippines	B5	4(50)	9(82)	0(38)	16(44)

[a]For references, see reference 15: (1) Thorsby et al. (1973), (2) Kreisler et al. (1974), (3) Dasgupta et al. (1975), (4) Smith et al. (1975).

[b]Only typing for HLA-A and -B antigens was performed, and only deviating frequencies (percentages) are given in this table. The number of controls, respectively patients studied are given in parentheses.

METHODS

Typing for HLA-A, -B, and -C antigens was performed using a set of 180 highly selected sera in the two-stage cytotoxicity test (16). Typing for the HLA-DR antigens was done by the two-color fluorescence assay (12) using 60 highly selected platelet absorbed sera. The statistical analysis has been described (15).

RESULTS

The Surinam Study (15)

From the out-patient files of the Leprosy Service in Surinam (a South-American country where leprosy is hyperendemic) we selected 16 families on the following criteria: (1) at least two siblings affected with leprosy; (2) at least two healthy siblings older than the youngest affected sib and living in the same environment; (3) both parents available for study.

Patients were classified on the basis of clinical and histological criteria and assigned to one of three groups: tuberculoid (TT and TT/BT), borderline (BT, BB and BL), or lepromatous (LI and LL). Both parents and affected siblings were typed for HLA-A, -B, and -C antigens. We deduced the four parenteral HLA-haplotypes from the phenotypes and tested whether a parenteral HLA-haplotype was seen more or less often in affected siblings than expected in the case of Mendelian segregation. Table IV summarizes the most important results:

(1) Siblings affected with the same type of leprosy shared significantly more often than expected a parenteral haplotype. It should be noted that in all cases the leprosy type was tuberculoid (TT or TT/BT). These findings indicated that susceptibility to tuberculoid leprosy is controlled by HLA-linked genes.

(2) In a few families with siblings affected with the two different types of leprosy the segregation was random. This could either indicate that only susceptibility to tuberculoid leprosy is controlled by HLA-linked genes, or that different types of HLA-linked susceptibility genes predispose to different types of leprosy.

We did not observe an association between a particular HLA-A, -B, or -C antigen or haplotype and leprosy or leprosy

TABLE IV.   HLA-Haplotype Sharing in Siblings in Leprosy[a]

Country	Leprosy classification	Obs.	Exp.	p
Surinam	tuberculoid	36	24	<0.01
	lepromatous	–	–	–
	different types	8	12	n.s.
India	tuberculoid	23	14.5	<0.05
	lepromatous	10	8	n.s.
	different types	20	15.5	n.s.

[a] "Tuberculoid" or "lepromatous" indicates that the affected sibs suffered from the same form of leprosy, i.e., either tuberculoid or lepromatous. "Different types" implies that the siblings suffered from different forms of leprosy. Sibling pairs sharing an HLA-haplotype are given in the column observed.

type, which implies that the susceptibility gene(s) for leprosy cannot be identical to these antigens.

In conclusion, these data indicate that susceptibility to tuberculoid leprosy is linked to HLA, but not associated with a particular HLA-A, -B, or -C antigen. Typing for the HLA-DR determinants was not yet possible at the time this study was done.

The Wardha Study (17)

To confirm the HLA-linked susceptibility to tuberculoid leprosy in another population living in another environment a study was performed in the Ghandi Memorial Leprosy Foundation in Wardha (India), where the same type of family was studied as in the Surinam study. This was done with the help of Dr. Gupte (director) and his staff and personnel; V. Periaswami performed the biopsies. In this study we typed not only for the HLA-A, -B, and -C antigens, but also for the HLA-DR or B cell antigens.

Table IV shows the result of the segregation analysis for the Wardha families. It appeared very difficult to find complete families containing two or more siblings affected with the lepromatous type, because in most cases the patients did not have contact with their family at all, or only with some family members.

An excess of identical haplotypes was observed again in siblings affected with tuberculoid leprosy but not in the (few) siblings with lepromatous leprosy nor in those affected with the two different types of leprosy. Thus, these studies confirm that susceptibility to tuberculoid leprosy is controlled by HLA-linked genes, whereas such an influence is not detectable in lepromatous leprosy. A total of 71 patients was studied in Surinam and India; the majority (47) was of tuberculoid type.

Again we observed no striking differences in frequencies of HLA-A, -B, and -C antigens between children affected with tuberculoid and/or lepromatous leprosy and healthy parents. However, healthy parents and children with tuberculoid leprosy both showed a very high frequency of HLA-DRw2 (over 75 and 90%, respectively). Preliminary studies indicate that the frequency of DRw2 in healthy controls in this population is about 50%. In contrast to the parents as one group of unrelated individuals who were mainly heterozygous for DRw2, the majority of the oldest sibs with tuberculoid leprosy were homozygous for DRw2 (Table V). Whether this is due to recessitivity of the predisposing gene or simply to twice as great a chance for the disease predisposing gene to be present in DRw2 homozygous individuals cannot be ascertained at this moment. That the gene predisposing to tuberculoid leprosy is linked to DRw2 finds further support if we analyze the segregation of DRw2 in healthy parents heterozygous for DRw2 (Table VI). If DRw2 were not associated with the leprosy-predisposing gene, an average of 50% of these children should receive DRw2, which is the case in children with lepromatous leprosy. However, children affected with tuberculoid leprosy inherited DRw2 significantly more often than expected.

Finally Table VII shows that whereas all but one of the unrelated patients suffering from tuberculoid leprosy were DRw2

TABLE V. DRw2 Phenotypes in Four Groups of Unrelated Individuals

	w2,w2 N	w2,non-w2 N	w2 neg. N
Healthy parents	3	10	3
Children with tuberculoid leprosy	8	5	1
Children with lepromatous leprosy	4	6	5
Healthy controls	4	16	18

TABLE VI.   Segregation of HLA-DRw2 from Heterozygous Healthy Parents to Children Affected with Tuberculoid or Lepromatous Leprosy

	Segregation	
	+	−
Children with tuberculoid leprosy	9	2 (p = 0.03)
Children with lepromatous leprosy	9	8 (p = 0.50)

positive all but one were DRw6 negative. These data could indicate that whereas the gene that predisposes to tuberculoid
leprosy, possibly because it can only lead to inadequate immunity, is linked to HLA-DRw2, the gene that can protect a-
gainst tuberculoid leprosy is linked to HLA-DRw6. This raises,
of course, the question whether the predisposing and protecting gene are alleles. The distribution of the other DR antigens was normal.

SUMMARY

   The conclusions that may be drawn from these two studies
are

   (1) Susceptibility to tuberculoid leprosy is controlled
by (an) HLA-linked gene(s);
   (2) Such (a) gene(s) might be situated to the D-side of
HLA, which is known to be involved in the regulation of immune
response (18,8). At least in the Wardha families DRw2 seems
to be a genetic marker for susceptibility, while DRw2 might
be a marker for resistance.

TABLE VII.   DR Antigens in Tuberculoid Leprosy

	DRw2		DRw6	
	pos.	neg.	pos.	neg.
Patients	13	1	1	13
Controls	20	18	22	16
p	0.01		0.001	

The Indian data could be compatible with a recessive inheritance, which was not the case in Surinam families, but these were not typed for HLA-DR. It cannot be exluded that different susceptibility genes exist in different populations, or that complementation of two HLA-linked genes situated more or less often on the same chromosome in different populations confers susceptibility.

It is clear that these studies are only a beginning in the unraveling of the disease predisposition for leprosy. One of the first questions that can and should now be answered is whether the positive association with HLA-DRw2 and a negative with DRw6 can be reproduced in a larger Indian series and whether it can be found in the Surinam population. Further it should be determined if these findings are of importance for the *in vitro* study of the lymphocyte response to *M. leprae* and whether it will be possible to identify individuals carrying high responder genes in this manner. It should be pointed out that although association with DRw2 is almost complete, there is one exception indicating that not DRw2 but a closely linked gene predisposes to tuberculoid leprosy. Whether this gene is an Ir gene is completely speculative at this moment: it could equally well be a gene that controls monocyte function or the access of the *M. leprae* to the nervous tissues. So far the data have been only significant for the tuberculoid form of leprosy. It is, however, not impossible that the susceptibility to the lepromatous form of leprosy is also influenced by HLA. Larger numbers of patients may have to be studied before this becomes clear.

Although much experimental work remains to be done, it is clear that if these findings can be reproduced in a larger patient sample even in the Wardha region alone, DR typing could be an useful adjunct in identifying those maximally at risk and those minimally at risk for tuberculoid leprosy. This in itself might be of importance in areas where 1% of the population suffers from leprosy.

References

1. Lilly, F., Boyse, E. A., and Old, L. J. *Lancet II*, 1207, 1964.
2. McDevitt, H. O., and Sela, M. *J. Exp. Med. 122*, 517, 1965.
3. McDevitt, H. O., and Benacerraf, B. B. *Adv. Immunol. 11*, 31, 1969.
4. Amiel, J. L. "Histocompatibility Testing 1967," p. 79. Munksgaard, Copenhagen, 1967.
5. Dausset, J., and Svejgaard, A. (eds.). "HLA and Disease." Munksgaard, Copenhagen, 1977.

6. Haverkorn, M. J., Hofman, B., Masurel, N., and van Rood, J. J. *Transplant. Rev. 22*, 120, 1975.
7. De Vries, R. R. P., Kreeftenberg, H. G., Loggen, H. G., and van Rood, J. J. *N. Engl. J. Med. 297*, 692, 1977.
8. Van Rood, J. J., de Vries, R. R. P., and Munro, A. J. *Proc. 3rd Int. Congr. Immunol., Sydney 1977*, Progress in Immunology III, T. E. Mandel *et al.* (eds.), p. 338. *Austr. Acad. Sci. Canberra 1977.*
9. Bach, F. H., and van Rood, J. J. *N. Engl. J. Med. 295*, 806, 872, 927, 1976.
10. Van Leeuwen, A., Schuit, H. R. E., and van Rood, J. J. *Transplant. Proc. 5*, 1539, 1973.
11. Van Rood, J. J., van Leeuwen, A., Keuning, J. J., and Blussé van Oud Alblas, A. *Tissue Antigens 5*, 73, 1975.
12. Van Rood, J. J., van Leeuwen, A., and Ploem, J. S. *Nature 262*, 795, 1976.
13. Bodmer, W. F., *et al.* (eds.). "Histocompatibility Testing 1977." Munksgaard, Copenhagen, 1977.
14. Van Rood, J. J., van Leeuwen, A., Termijtelen, A., and Bradley, B. A. *Tissue Antigens 10*, 125, 1977.
15. De Vries, R. R. P., Lai A Fat, R. F. M., Nijenhuis, L. E., and van Rood, J. J. *The Lancet II*, 1328, 1976.
16. Van Rood, J. J. *In* "Manual of Tissue Typing Techniques" (J. G. Ray *et al.*, eds.), p. 75. Bethesda, Maryland, 1974.
17. De Vries, R. R. P., Mehra, N. K., Vaidya, M. C., Gupte, M. D., and van Rood, J. J. *N. Engl. J. Med.* in press.
18. Munro, A., and Bright, S. *Nature 264*, 145, 1976.

DISCUSSION

DR. BLOOM: In my opinion, your most interesting finding is that DRw6 correlated negatively with tuberculoid leprosy. I wonder if it would have correlated well with the anergic, immunologically nonresponsive form of the disease, lepromatous leprosy.

DR. VAN ROOD: You're absolutely right; we plan to pursue this question as we continue our study.

DR. MOLLER: A recessive Ir gene is certainly possible, if the gene determines lack of recognition of the bacillus. However, if this is so, there would not be any difference between the two forms of the disease?

DR. VAN ROOD: Not necessarily if you assume that tuberculoid leprosy is mainly due to one gene linked to DRw2 and that lepromatous leprosy is due to several factors, for example, a DRw2-linked gene and a non-HLA-linked gene, or a nongenetically determined factor such as protein starvation. In this case, the clear-cut association with DRw2 found in tuberculoid leprosy could be far less clear in the lepromatous form.

DR. DOHERTY: I'd like to comment in reference to Dr. Moller's point. I don't think that it is a particular problem that there are two forms of the disease, the nature of which may be related to immune response. For instance, mouse-adapted influenza virus may cause disseminated neurological disease in nu/nu mice, whereas nu/t mice tend rather to develop severe pneumonia.

DR. BLOOM: It should be emphasized that leprosy does not have only two forms, but an infinite number of forms ranging across a wide spectrum. Immunologists tend to be most interested in the extremes, but these are relatively small portions of the spectrum.

DR. VAN ROOD: I agree.

DR. SACHS: Was the frequency of DRw2/DRw6 heterozygotes in your populations consistent with the frequency predicted by individual gene frequencies or could there be some other reason for an inverse correlation between these two genes and the disease?

DR. VAN ROOD: The individuals studied were in Hardy-Weinberg equilibrium but the number of persons studied is too small to form a definitive conclusion on this important issue.

DR. JANICKI: I encourage you to follow up on your plans to examine your patient's immune responses, including various *in vitro* tests and skin testing. My co-workers and I (Goldstein, R. A., *et al.*, Veteran's Administration Hospital, Washington, D.C.) have found an association between increased morbidity (reactivation, extrapulmonary manifestations) in black tuberculosis patients and the presence of Bw 15. However, we found no striking differences in *in vitro* reactivity. Do you yet have any such indications in your population of tuberculoid leprosy patients?

DR. VAN ROOD: We plan to start these studies soon.

DR. NOWINSKI: I have difficulty understanding this disease. You can have two different forms of influenza in compromised and competent hosts. But if you look at the immune response genes to that virus, they're still involved. I have the impression that different response genes are involved in leprosy. Is this correct?

DR. VAN ROOD: It would appear to be so. It should be emphasized, however, that the mycobacteria present a variety of antigens, so it also is possible that we're dealing with multiple immune response genes.

DR. DOHERTY: Perhaps I can clarify a point for Dr. Nowinski with respect to the influenza model. An Ir gene associated with strong T cell responsiveness might tend toward an immunopathological consequence, as in the severe pneumonia in nu/t or t/t animals. On the other hand, an Ir gene determining defective T cell responsiveness could lead to failure of virus clearance and dissemination, as occurs in the nu/nu.

DR. STANLEY COHEN: Desensitization to soluble proteins is nonspecific; desensitization using tubercle bacilli is specific. This could be analogous to the specific anergy that Dr. Bloom mentioned as occurring in leprosy. Regarding the disease spectrum, could this be related to infecting dose? Stated another way, do they escape from anergy following chemotherapy? Finally, are there associations between leprosy susceptibility and minor blood groups? For example, anti-Lewis antibodies could react with putative lymphokine receptors and induce partial anergy.

DR. VAN ROOD: This is a very important question because preliminary evidence from French workers has shown the Lewis system to be a transplantation antigen system. That is, lele patients reject kidney grafts more significantly more often than Lele and LeLe patients.

DR. BLOOM: I have information relevant to the first part of Dr. Cohen's remarks. In general, lepromatous patients who are considered "cured" after prolonged chemotherapy can react or retain their reactivity to a battery of antigens, but remain anergic to the antigens of the lepra bacillus.

DR. KIRKPATRICK: I'd like to comment on a question raised by Dr. Stanley Cohen. Certain patients with chronic mucocutaneous candidiasis recover immune responses spontaneously after treatment. These patients were normal during infancy and childhood and then, during the early teens, developed candidiasis, often after antibiotic therapy for relatively innocent

infections.   They usually are unresponsive by skin testing and
MIF production to candida but will respond to other common antigens.   After therapy with adequate doses of amphotericin B,
they will spontaneously recover both *in vivo* and *in vitro*
responses to candida.

DR. VAN ROOD: Your anergic patients thus have a different
response pattern from that which Dr. Bloom described for leprosy patients.

DR. PREHN: Is the armadillo subject to both forms of
leprosy and, if so, would this not be a good model for the
study of some of these questions?

DR. VAN ROOD: I don't know; perhaps Dr. Bloom can answer
this question.

DR. BLOOM: Approximately 50 to 70% of a group of arma-
dillos injected intravenously with *M. leprae* will develop a
lepramatous type of disease.   Interestingly, the remaining
animals do not exhibit any clinical disease although granu-
lomas are detectable.

Session V
Therapeutic Manipulation

OVERVIEW: THERAPEUTIC MANIPULATION

Thomas A. Waldmann

Metabolism Branch
National Cancer Institute
National Institutes of Health
Bethesda, Maryland

Over the past few years there has been a dramatic increase
in our knowledge of immunological mechanisms. There have been
new insights into the mechanisms of genetic control of the immune response, into the pathways of antigen processing and recognition, and into the events of cellular maturation, cellular interaction, and biosynthesis of the effectors of the
immune response. The discovery that immune responses are controlled by a series of negative as well as positive regulatory factors has been especially critical in our understanding
of immune surveillance. More recently it has been recognized
that many infectious, parasitic, autoimmune, allergic, and
malignant diseases are associated with immunological deficiency
characterized in some cases by abnormalities in the differentiation of effector cells of the immune system or in the positive interactions of these cells and in other cases by disorders of the negative regulatory or suppressor cell systems.
    An understanding of the normal events of immune regulation
as well as the abnormalities of these processes that occur in
disease is absolutely critical in developing new effective
therapeutic approaches. A number of recent examples emphasize
the point that the mere immunization with antigenic infectious
agents or the use of certain procedures to augment immune
responses nonspecifically may, on occasion, lead to accentuation rather than prevention or elimination of disease. The
problem of accentuation of disease on reexposure to an infectious agent after an initial immunization with an inactivated
microbial vaccine has recently been reviewed (1). Vaccination
with formaldyhyde-inactivated rubeola vaccine led to an accen-
tuated disease following reexposure to the virus, characterized
by inordinate fever, pneumonia, pleural effusion, and an atypi-

ISBN 0-12-055850-5

cal distribution of a severe rash. Accentuation of disease was also an unexpected complication of immunization with Trachoma, respiratory synicitial virus, and *Mycoplasma pneumoniae* vaccines when such vaccination procedures were performed with vaccines that did not produce prolonged long lasting immunity. It was concluded that in some cases, the production of circulating antibody or induction of cellular immunity may be hazardous if the local immune mechanisms of the mucosa are not operative (1). Augmentation of unwanted pathological processes has also been observed in tumor immunization schemes. In these systems these undesirable responses reflect the activation of suppressor rather than cytotoxic or killer systems. For example, Ilfeld and co-workers (2) demonstrated that lymphocytes sensitized *in vitro* with syngeneic tumor cells enhanced tumor growth when the lymphocytes were inoculated with the tumor cells into syngeneic mice. In a number of other studies, there has been a paradoxial reduction in the host resistance to tumor by treatments that superficially resembled immunization or by procedures such as the injection of *Corynebacterium parvum* into tumor cells, a procedure that had been performed to augment nonspecific immune responses (3). It is clear from these examples that therapeutic manipulation of human disease must be based on a broad understanding of normal immune regulation, on the disorders that occur in disease, and on the effect of the proposed therapeutic maneuvers on the immunological system.

A major approach directed toward augmenting immune responses has been the replacement of effector cells of the immune system or their humoral products. This approach has been especially widely utilized in primary immunodeficiency diseases, where failure of the development of these immune effectors is commonly the primary defect. Dr. Good has reviewed many of these approaches in his introduction to the immunopathology section of this conference. As our understanding of the primary immunodeficiency diseases has increased, our ability to reconstitute immunodeficient patients has progressed. Certain patients with severe combined immunodeficiency disease have been reconstituted by the transplantation of bone marrow from HLA-D matched siblings. In addition, some but not all of the patients with the autosomal recessive form of severe combined immunodeficiency associated with adenosine deaminase deficiency have been reconstituted immunologically by transfusions of irradiated red blood cells from individuals with normal quantities of this enzyme. Patients with the DiGeorge syndrome have a failure of the development of the organs derived from the third and fourth brancheal pouch and have a consequent failure of development of the thymus and abnormalities of cell-mediated immunity. Such patients have been reconstituted by the administration of a fetal thymus, cultured adult thymic epithelial cells, or by the administration of thymic humoral factors. Although each of these

approaches has been of value, they are not entirely satisfac-
tory. Thymic humoral factors may act predominantly on postthy-
mic cells and do not fully reconstitute the defective immune
response in these patients. In addition, on the basis of studies in mice it has been suggested recently (4) that transplantation of a thymus from an HLA-D, -A, -B incompatible source may
not reconstitute thymus-deficient patients entirely but may lead
to an individual who is still T-cell immunoincompetent, except
for allograft rejection or mitogen-induced T-cell reactivities.
The bone marrow stem cells might differentiate under the influence of the donor thymus to express the surface specificities of
the transplanted thymus rather than those expressed on the B
lymphocytes and macrophages of the recipient. As a consequence
the T cells might not participate normally in the multiple lymphocyte interactions required for such responses as antivirus
specific responses and T-cell-dependent antibody responses. It
was suggested (4) that for functional reconstitution certain HLA
matching rules for fetal grafts should be observed. It was proposed that the recipient and the fetal thymic graft should share
at least one HLA-D haplotype and at least one of the HLA-A or
-B antigens. Other approaches directed toward replacing or augmenting immune effector function that have applicability to other
diseases include the administration of immunoglobulins and antibody molecules and the stimulation of the production of humoral
products such as interferon by host lymphocytes. We shall hear
more about this latter approach in Dr. Merigan's discussion of
antiviral therapy.

A second type of potential immune intervention is suggested
by the observation that excessive numbers of activated suppressor T cells may be involved in the abnormalities of the
immune response observed in certain patients with primary immunodeficiency disorders, in patients with widespread fungal
infections, or in patients with malignancy. An abnormal number or an abnormal state of activation of suppressor T cells
has been demonstrated in a subset of patients with common variable hypogammaglobulinemia and in some patients with selective
IgA deficiency (5). Suppressor T cells inhibiting delayed
hypersensitivity responses have also been demonstrated in the
circulation of patients with anergy associated with widespread
fungal infections (6). Suppressor T cell have also been implicated in the immunological enhancement of tumor growth.
Fujimoto and co-workers (7) and others (8,9) have demonstrated
that tumor-specific suppressor T cells may prevent the effective elimination of tumor cells and thus enhance tumor growth.
With these disorders our goal should be the reduction of suppressor T-cell activity. For that small subset of patients
with primary immunodeficiency disease who have a disorder of
suppressor cell activity as the primary causative event in
the immunodeficiency, the use of drugs such as corticosteroids

or cyclophosphamide that inhibit suppressor T-cell activity may be of significant value in reversing the immunodeficiency. Even for those patients who have the development of suppressor cells as a secondary event, the elimination of suppressor cells may be required before other therapies are effective. Another approach to the elimination of suppressor T cells is the administration of antisera that recognize and eliminate these cells. In mice, suppressor T cells and certain specific soluble suppressor factors derived from such cells contain antigens coded by the *I-J* subregion of the H-2 complex (10). Therefore, antibodies directed against such *I-J* determinants would be expected to nullify the suppressor activity *in vivo*. Recent studies have in fact, shown that alloantisera directed against the appropriate *I-J* antigen caused significant enhancement of IgM and IgG immune responses to sheep erythrocytes (11). Based on these observations Greene and co-workers (12) tested the hypothesis that the *in vivo* administration of antisera directed against *I-J* coded determinants would eliminate suppressor T cells from tumor-bearing mice and cause an inhibition of syngeneic tumor growth. Spleens of tumor-bearing mice treated with anti *I-J* antiserum no longer contained specific suppressor cells. In addition there was a highly significant retardation of tumor growth in mice after daily intravenous treatment with microliter quantities of anti-*I-J* antiserum. These experiments provide a model for the removal of suppressor T-cell activity and a new approach to the therapeutic manipulation of the immune response.

Activated monocytes and other non-T-cell suppressor cells have also been implicated in immunodeficiency states including the polyclonal immunoglobulin deficiency associated with multiple myeloma (13), the anergy associated with Hodgkin's disease (14), and the depressed cell-mediated immunity in certain patients and animals with advanced solid tumors and with widespread fungal or parasitic infestations. Therapeutic manipulations directed against such non-T-cell suppressor effectors might take a number of forms. One approach would be to prevent the activation of these monocyte suppressors. An initial T-cell recognition step appears to play a role in the events leading to activation of monocyte suppressors such as that observed associated with antigen competition. Presumably the activated T cells in turn activate monocytes by a mechanism analogous to that described for immunity against certain microorganisms. The activated monocytes then cause a nonspecific inhibition of lymphocyte cellular proliferation and antibody production. Thus, one could approach the disorder of monocyte suppressors at the initial T-cell activation step. Alternatively one could attack the steps whereby the macrophage inhibits the immune system. It has recently been suggested that the *in vitro* hyporesponsiveness found in certain patients with Hodgkin's disease may be due to the excessive production of protaglandin E2 by glass-adherent mononuclear suppressor cells (15). Following this, lead indomethacin, a prostaglandin synthetase inhibitor, was shown to restore *in vitro* blastogenic responses to lymphocytes from certain patients with Hodgkin's disease (15). These observations may eventually have clinical relevance by providing a relatively safe pharmacological basis for manipulating non-T-cell suppressor cell activity in certain disease states.

The suppressor system will also have to be considered in immunotherapeutic manipulation, including desensitization procedures directed toward abrogating unwanted immune reactions. The administration of anti-Rh antisera immediately postpartum to inhibit sensitization of an Rh-negative mother by her Rh-positive offspring is a classic example of the rational use of a known specific physiological negative immunoregulator in the prevention of an undesired immune response. Loss of suppressor T-cell function has been demonstrated in the NZB/W animal model of autoimmunity and in patients with certain autoimmune disorders, including systemic lupus erythematosus (16). Even if loss of suppressor cells in patients with autoimmunity is not the primary event but only one link in the chain of causation, therapy directed toward augmenting suppressor mechanisms may be of value in reducing the manifestations of autoimmunity. The studies demonstrating that the administration of humoral immunosuppressive products of activated suppressor T cells can prevent the autoimmunity observed in NZB/W mice suggest that the use of physiological products of suppressor T cells might also be of value in the therapy of such autoimmune diseases of man as systemic lupus erythematosus (17). A more ideal approach would be to activate specific suppressor T cells. The studies of Eichmann (18) and Binz and Wigzell (19) suggest that the activation of such specific suppressor T cells by the administration of anti-idiotype antibodies might be possible.

The use of techniques to augment antigen-specific suppressor T cell function may also be a critically important maneuver for the management of various allergic diseases since IgE antibody responses are particularly susceptible to suppression (20). The demonstration by Ishizaka and co-workers (21) that the structure of ragweed antigen can be modified so that it stimulates T cells but does not stimulate antibody production suggests that the activation of antigen-specific suppressor T cells may be an effective approach to hyposensitization.

In summary, there have been major advances in our understanding of the systems regulating immunological processes. More recently, disorders in these regulatory systems have been

demonstrated in association with a number of infectious,
parasitic, immunodeficiency, autoimmune, allergic, and malignant diseases. There is hope that in the near future these
insights into the physiological role played by regulatory
cells and into the role played by disorders of these regulatory systems in the pathogenesis of various diseases may lead
to more rational therapeutic strategies for the prevention and
therapy of these human diseases with disorders of immunological surveillance.

References

1. Craighead, J. E. *Infect. Dis. 131*, 749, 1975.
2. Ilfeld, D., Carnaud, C., Cohen, I. R., *et al*. *Int. J. Cancer 12*, 213, 1973.
3. Broder, S., Muul, L., and Waldmann, T. A. *J. Nat. Cancer Inst. 61*, 5, 1978.
4. Zinkernagle, R. F. *N. Engl. J. Med. 298*, 222, 1978.
5. Waldmann, T. A., Broder, S., Krakauer, R., *et al*. *Fed. Proc. 35*, 2067, 1976.
6. Stobo, J. D., Paul, S., Van Scoy, R. E., *et al*. *J. Clin. Invest. 56*, 467, 1975.
7. Fujimoto, S., Greene, M. I., and Sehon, A. H. *J. Immunol. 116*, 791, 1976.
8. Umiel, T., and Tranin, N. *Transplantation 18*, 244, 1974.
9. Kirkwood, J. M., and Gershon, R. K. *Progr. Exp. Tumor Res. Immunol. Cancer 19*, 157, 1974.
10. Tada, T., Taniguchi, M., and David, C. S. *J. Exp. Med. 144*, 713, 1976.
11. Pierres, M., German, R. N., Dorf, M. E., *et al*. *Proc. Nat. Acad. Sci. (USA) 74*, 3975, 1977.
12. Greene, M. I., Dorf, M. E., Pierres, M., *et al*. *Proc. Nat. Acad. Sci. (USA) 74*, 5118, 1977.
13. Broder, S., Humphrey, R., Durm, M., *et al*. *N. Engl. J. Med. 293*, 887, 1978.
14. Twomey, J. J., Laughter, A. H., Farrow, S., *et al*. *J. Clin. Invest. 56*, 467, 1975.
15. Goodwin, J. S., Messner, R. P., Bankhurst, A. D., *et al*. *N. Engl. J. Med. 297*, 963, 1977.
16. Waldmann, T. A., and Broder, S. *Progr. Clin. Immunol. 3*, 155, 1977.
17. Krakauer, R. S., STrober, W., Rippeon, D. L., *et al*. *Science 196*, 56, 1977.

18. Eichmann, K. *Eur. J. Immunol. 4*, 296, 1974.
19. Binz, H. and Wigzell, H.. *Cold Spring Harbor Symp. Quant. Biol. 41 (1) 275*, 1977.
20. Tada, T. *Progr. Allergy 19*, 122, 1975.
21. Ishizaka, K., Kishimoto, T., Delepesse, G., *et al.* *J. Immunol. 113*, 70, 1974.

SUCCESSFUL ANTIVIRAL THERAPY REQUIRES
THE COOPERATION OF IMMUNE RESPONSES*

Thomas C. Merigan

Division of Infectious Diseases
Stanford University School of Medicine
Stanford, California

Because of the close relationship between the replication
of animal viruses and host cell functions, successful antiviral therapy has demanded agents specifically directed a-
gainst virus-infected cells. In addition, the spread of virus within an infected individual involves a wide variety of
cells in which antiviral drugs may or may not act with similar efficacy. Recent studies (1) have demonstrated that host
defense to viral infection involves a multitiered series of
interrelated, but independent responses, which act on virus-
infected cells as well as on extracellular virus to diminish
spread of the agent within the host. Various host defenses
act both at the portal of entry and in the target organs with
relative efficacy, which differs from one virus to another--
or even between strains. In addition to local actions of IgA
antibody and macrophages, systemic IgM and IgG antibodies and
antibody-dependent cellular cytotoxic mechanisms come into
play, together with thymus-derived lymphocyte cytotoxicity
and lymphokine production. Such host factors are clearly
critical in dictating the pathogenesis of infection of any
particular virus. The proper function of all of these events
obviously depends on a complex series of host biosynthetic and
differentiation steps.

*Supported by a grant from the United States Public Health
Service (AI 05629).*

IMMUNOSUPPRESSION AND CHEMOTHERAPY

The systemic use of antivirals in such a setting is hazardous if they do not have specificity for the virus-infected cell. A number of studies have demonstrated that the host may be relatively immunosuppressed in a variety of cellular and humoral immune responses during systemic virus infections (2). It is quite possible that the pathogenicity of certain agents depends upon their having evolved such immunosuppressive abilities. In the absence of certain host defenses, others may be called upon for more efficient function and thus spread somewhat more thinly, making those remaining functions quite vulnerable to the action of metabolic inhibitors. Thus, skillful use of antiviral agents that are specific is particularly important when they are to be used therapeutically in order to avoid adding to immunosuppression. It seems quite likely that if we could measure specific host defenses to tumors with accuracy in man we would find that they also must function in close concert with antitumor agents for their most efficient therapeutic action.

This situation with viruses should be contrasted with chemotherapeutics active against more complicated microorganisms such as bacteria and fungi. Here, the site of action of the antimicrobial can be so selected as to preclude any effect on the cells of the host. For example, penicillin and amphotericin B are directed against components of the parasite's cell wall that are not present in host cells (3) and immunosuppression is not reported with their use. With other agents the selectivity is based on an action on enzymes unique to the parasite. For example, the antifolates, pyrimethemine and trimethoprim, used against protozoa and bacteria, are much more active against the dihydrofolate reductase of the parasite than that of the host (4). In the case of the antifungal 5-fluorocytosine, its selective toxicity for the parasite depends upon the organism but not the host cell possessing cytosine deaminase, which will degrade the drug to the toxic metabolic 5-fluorouracil (5). On the other hand, chloramphenicol and rifamycin have been demonstrated under certain conditions to inhibit host humoral and cellular immune functions (6,7) as well as having potent antimicrobial properties. The antihelminthic niridazole also inhibits cell-mediated immune responses in man and animals (8). However, in neither the case of this agent nor that of the two previously mentioned antibiotics is there any direct evidence for the immunosuppressive capacity leading to increased susceptibility to infection.

However, it has been observed that prompt treatment of tularemia with tetracycline or streptomycin impaired the pa-

tient's production of precipitin antibody (9). An increased
frequency of relapse or susceptibility to reinfection was observed with the impaired antibody response produced by the
bacteriostatic and the bacteriocidal antibiotic, respectively.
Thus, treatment clearly compromised full development of immunity although the mechanism of immune suppression was not determined.

PRESENT STATUS OF ANTIVIRALS

Initially the focus for development of human antivirals
was either (a) on local therapy to sites, which could be exposed to high concentration of antiviral agents without systemic adsorption, or (b) on systemic prophylaxis. For example,
the initial success of iododeoxyuridine (10) and cytosine
arabinoside (11) in herpetic keratitis depended on their local
application to the cornea, a site where quite high concentrations could be built up without effects on lymphatic or bone
marrow cells, which would have been manifest if the agents
were given systemically. Furthermore, the use of amantadine
in influenze (12) and isatin in smallpox (13) prophylaxis
during the incubation period has prevented or diminished infection. As this action occurs quite early in the infectious
process, the need for cooperation with host defenses is mini-
mized. In fact, with the effective use of both these agents,
antibody responses are inhibited in contrast to untreated controls. This is most likely because the therapy prevents development of an antigenic mass sufficient for immune sensitization. The net result was that the drug-protected host not
only did not have symptomatic disease but did not develop immunity and was susceptible on rechallenge. In controlled
trials with volunteers, locally applied interferon has also
been effective in preventing respiratory tract infection (14)
as well as vaccinial skin lesions (15), and here again immunity did not develop--most likely because of the restricted
development of antigenic mass.
It is only in recent years that we have begun to under-
take antiviral therapy. The first systemically applied antiviral therapeutic agent, iododeoxyuridine, had already shown
efficacy in local treatment of acute herpetic keratitis before it was employed in the systemic treatment of herpes simplex encephalitis (16). Despite early enthusiasm, careful
studies (17) demonstrated that side effects and complications
of the therapy outweighed any possible benefit. Specifically,
severe thrombocytopenia and leukopenia was observed with little
evidence of significant concentrations of the drug in the cen-

tral nervous system and frequent isolation of the virus from
lesions after the full course of therapy. In addition, tissue and CSF levels of the drug in treated cases were found to
be so low as to not be expected to influence viral replication (18).

Cytosine arabinoside was utilized systemically for varicella or zoster in a number of patients with immunosuppressive
disease on the basis of single anecdotal cases. Carefully
controlled trials revealed no evidence that the course of
zoster was improved by this agent (19-22). In fact, in a
randomized placebo controlled double-blind trial (19) in
patients with lymphoma at Stanford, it was observed that parenteral cytosine arabinoside actually prolonged the course
of disseminated zoster concomitantly with its delay of host defenses. Specifically, it delayed the appearance of varicella-
zoster complement-fixing antibody in the serum and the local
vesicle fluid interferon responses in the treated patients who
had received recent chemotherapy and irradiation when their
responses were compared to similar placebo treated controls.

Amantadine has lately also been discovered to be effective therapeutically if given early in symptomatic influenza.
It produced a shortening of the duration of fever, both in
controlled trials in volunteers (23) as well as in field disease (12). This beneficial effect, like its prophylactic effect (24), was more marked in volunteers who carry some antibody to the infecting influenza virus prior to infection (12),
pointing to a cooperative effect of immunity with the antiviral agent.

In the last 2 years, beneficial results have been reported
with systemic administration of agents that seem to inhibit
virus replication when given after symptoms have appeared.
Specifically, we have found (25) intramuscular leukocyte interferon appears to shorten the course of zoster in immunosuppressed individuals as others have also observed in similar studies with intravenously administered adenine arabinoside (26). Adenine arabinoside also decreased mortality in
the encephalitis produced by type I herpes simplex (27). Both
these agents (28-30), as well as iododeoxyuridine (31) and
cytosine arabinoside (32), can decrease urinary excretion of
cytomegalovirus, although the response is somewhat variable
and only a transient suppression is observed in most treated
individuals. This latter result may be due to the lack of
specific antiviral host responses available to cooperate with
these antivirals in the neonates and transplant recipients
who were treated.

Optimal usage and demonstration of therapeutic efficacy
of interferon and adenine arabinoside has depended upon early
utilization of these antiviral agents. It has been important

to carefully follow the effect of these agents on the development of the immune response in the treated individuals because
they were given in the midst of critical events in host response to the antigens of the infecting agents. Although large
doses of mouse interferon have been demonstrated to suppress
antibody production (33) and cellular immunity (34), these are
greater than those required to limit acute viral infection.
Adenine arabinoside has been observed to be not as toxic *in
vivo* as cytosine arabinoside or iododeoxyuridine (35) and
actually was selected as an antiviral agent for widespread
trials because of its lack of immune suppression (36,37).
Furthermore, in contrast to iododeoxyuridine and cytosine arabinoside, it was able to produce a therapeutic effect, even
when given as late as 7 days after vaccinia or herpes simplex
infection of immunosuppressed mice (38,39). The leukocyte interferon trials in zoster were conducted primarily in lymphoma
patients. No impairment was observed in the antibody production of the interferon recipients as compared to that of the
placebo recipients, even at a level of 35 million reference
units per day. It is possible that this occurs because this
antibody response is an amnestic one to an agent with which
the host is persistently infected. In a smaller uncontrolled
and unconfirmed trial, it was suggested that lower doses, that
is, 3 million reference units daily, would terminate new lesion
formation in the primary dermatome in normal individuals with
zoster (40). Normal individuals may require less of this antiviral agent because of their intact immune responses.

   As most patients who have herpes simplex encephalitis
develop good antibody titers early in the disease, or have
preexisting titers, the disease is thought to be a recrudes-
cent infection in many cases, with immune responses present at
the time of recurrence. Whether host responses complement the
therapeutic action of adenine arabinoside in this infection is
not clear.

FUTURE PERSPECTIVES FOR ACUTE AND CHRONIC INFECTIONS

   There is now evidence that it takes one or more days for
antivirals to begin to act, and many herpesviral diseases in
which they are to be used only last a few days. Hence, there
is a strong rationale for the use of antiviral agents in such
infections as early as possible in the infection, if maximum
prevention of pathology in the treated individuals is to be
achieved. Yet it is also clear that in many this is one of
the most sensitive times for possible interference with the
immune response and thus immunological parameters should be

measured in all such trials to determine whether certain pa-
tients--rather than being helped--may be further immunocompromised by such agents. Assays of specific cellular immunity to viruses in man are being developed and will be particularly useful to monitor during trials considering the apparent importance of thymus-derived lymphocytes in recovery.

   The neonate is at special risk for persistent herpesviral
infections, and significant pathological sequelae are present
in children who have been born infected with HSV, CMV, rubella,
and varicella-zoster virus. Evidence is presently emerging
that specific deficiencies associated with the immunological
immaturity of the newborn (41) may be associated with the establishment of such neonatal disease, which is often quite
prolonged as compared to that in more mature individuals.
Numerically, chornic CMV infection is probably the most important of these four and the long-term neurological sequelae
of such infections are of significant economic importance in
our society. Yet, as mentioned previously, adenine arabinoside and interferon have only transiently suppressed CMV viru-
ria (28-30) and the effect of interferon on cells chronically
infected with rubella (42) suggests it also will be resistant
to such therapy. It is possible that some carefully planned
combination of chemo- and immunotherapy will be required to
clear such persistent infections. For example, prevention
of herpes simplex encephalitis in mice with adenine arabinoside was improved by the concomitant administration of specific immune globulin (43). The use of such combined therapy
was particularly beneficial in infections of newborn or immunodeficient nude mice (44). Whether such effects can be obtained with Cornynebacterium parvum, BCG, levamisole, or
other agents (45-49) requires further study.

   Recently our group has observed both leukocyte interferon
and adenine arabinoside will influence hepatitis B infection
(50,51). This persistent infection appears suppressible by
both treatment modalities. Utilizing a 50-fold range of interferon dosage, and a 6-fold range of adenine arabinoside,
we find some patients appear much more responsive to this
therapy than others, although all demonstrate a progressively
increasing effect with increased dosage. The most responsive
appear to have the most prolonged responses, and in two followed over a year the particles have not returned. If Dane
particles can be fully cleared from the blood by either agent,
the effect persists and Hb_SAg titers fall as well. So far,
even in patients who have become cleared of Hb_SAg, antibody
to this antigen has not been detectable. Yet it appears to
us that host factors condition the outcome of such therapy.
We are currently trying to determine the optimum dosing regimen for both agents alone and in combination, as well as to

determine the role of various host responses in the outcome
of our therapeutic effects. We are encouraged by present results that, by determining the extent of Dane particle suppression in the first weeks of therapy, we might be able to
predict the outcome of the several-month course of therapy
that is required to eradicate the infection.

It is apparent that greater sophistication in selecting
agents that are less likely to be immunosuppressive has been
crucial in producing a second generation of systemically administered antiviral agents, specifically adenine arabinoside and leukocyte interferon. Hopefully, better insights
into the natural history and the nature of the host defenses
will allow the development of more and better agents. Particularly interesting classes of agents at present fall into
two categories (52). The first, which appears to include adenine arabinoside, includes agents with greater affinity for
the viral DNA polymerase than for the host DNA polymerase.
Secondly, novel nucleotides have been found that are phosphor-
ylated by the virus pyrimidine kinase but not but the host
cell thymidine kinase. Hence, these nucleoside analogs can
only be incorporated inot the DNA of virus-infected cells but
not normal cells. Such agents as thymine arabinoside and
the halogenated pyrimidines fall into this latter category.
If such agents can be discovered that have appropriate pharmacologic distribution properties and lack of significant
side effects, it is anticipated their specificity will restrict their action to antiviral effects. Thus, one would
avoid significantly effecting lymphoid cells or bone marrow,
two of the most critical and easily compromised rapidly di-
viding cell populations in the whole animal.

Of course, there are other characteristics that are important in an ideal antiviral. In the long run, the fact that
interferon, like antibody, is part of normal host defenses,
also may be of special advantage in its potential lack of the
two most difficult to assess long range toxicities, that is,
mutagenicity and teratogenicity. Iododeoxyuridine and cytosine arabinoside have been observed to be teratogenic in rodents (53), and the latter also has been noted to increase
the number of chromosome breaks in herpes simplex infected
cells (54). The recently described mutagenic and teratogenic
effects of adenine arabinoside must be taken into consideration in its use (55). Finally, the long exposure of pathogens to interferon without development of resistance also
might be a special advantage in its clinical application.

The greatest challenge to antiviral chemotherapy is the
eradication of persistent infection in locations like the
sensory ganglia, where it is already known that potent antivirals such as adenine arabinoside and phosphonoacidic acid

(56,57) cannot inhibit or depress the extent of ganglia involvement in mice once the herpes simplex has reached that
site. It is possible that virus replication is not in a productive phase at that site and thus is even less susceptible
to selective chemotherapeutic action. On the other hand, it
is also possible that certain antigens may be expressed in
such persistently infected cells, which might make them susceptible to selective immunotherapy. Alternatively, if viral
enzymes are produced in the latently infected cell, then it
is possible they may provide the key to selective kill of
those cells as mentioned above. Obviously work will be continuing on such questions in years to come.

SUMMARY

This review has attempted to synthesize work on antiviral
chemotherapy, particularly pointing up the possibility of immunosuppression by drugs and the importance for antivirals of
cooperative effects with immune and nonspecific recovery mechanisms. With the current successes and crucial need for antiviral chemotherapy, it is likely present efforts will be
superseded by future work. A particularly attractive possibility that has only just begun to be investigated is the combination of chemo- and immunotherapy.

References

1. Notkins, A. L. (ed.). "Viral Immunology and Immunopathology." Academic Press, New York, 1975.
2. Woodruff, J. F., and Woodruff, J. J. *In* "Viral Immunology and Immunopathology" (A. L. Notkins, ed.), p. 393.
   Academic Press, New York, 1975.
3. Pratt, W. B. "Chemotherapy of Infection." Oxford Univ.
   Press, New York, 1977.
4. Burchall, J. J., and Hitchings, G. H. *Mol. Pharmacol. 1,*
   126, 1965.
5. Koechlin, B. A., Rubio, F., Palmer, S., et al. *Biochem.
   Pharmacol. 15,* 435, 1966.
6. Della Bella, D., Petrescu, D., Marca, G., et al. *Chemotherapy 18,* 99, 1973.
7. Sanders, Jr., W. E. *Ann. Intern. Med. 85,* 82, 1976.
8. Webster, L. T., Butterworth, A. E., Mahmoud, A. A. F., et
   al. *N. Engl. J. Med. 292,* 1144, 1975.
9. Vosti, K. L., Ward, M. K., and Tigertt, W. D. *J. Clin. Invest. 41,* 1436, 1962.

10. Kaufman, H. E., Martola, E.-L., and Dohlman, C. H. *Arch. Ophthalmol. 68*, 235, 1962.
11. Kaufman, H. E., and Maloney, E. D. *Arch. Ophthalmol. 69*, 626, 1963.
12. Jackson, G. G. *Hospital Practice,* Nov., 75, 1971.
13. Bauer, D. J., St. Vincent, L., Kempe, C. H., *et al.* *Am. J. Epidemiol. 90*, 130, 1969.
14. Merigan, T. C., Reed, S. E., Hall, T. S., *et al.* *The Lancet i*, 563, 1973.
15. Scientific Committee on Interferon. *Lancet i*, 872, 1962.
16. Nolan, D. C., Carruthers, M. M., and Lerner, A. M. *N. Engl. J. Med. 282*, 10, 1970.
17. Boston Interhospital Virus Study Group and the NIAID Sponsored Cooperative ANtiviral Clinical Study. *N. Engl. J. Med. 292*, 600, 1975.
18. Lauter, C. B., Bailey, E. J., and Lerner, A. M. *Proc. Soc. Exp. Biol. Med. 150*, 23, 1975.
19. Stevens, D. A., Jordan, G. W., Waddell, T. F., *et al.* *N. Engl. J. Med. 289*, 873, 1973.
20. Davis, C. M., VanDersarl, J. V., and Coltman, C. A. Jr. *JAMA 224*, 122, 1973.
21. Schimpff, S. C., Fortner, C. L., Greene, W. H., *et al.* *J. Infect. Dis. 130*, 673, 1974.
22. Betts, R. F., Zaky, D. A., Douglas, Jr., R. G., *et al.* *Ann. Int. Med. 82*, 778, 1975.
23. Wingfield, W. L., Pollack, D., and Grunert, R. R. *N. Engl. J. Med. 281*, 579, 1969.
24. O'Donoghue, J. M., Ray, C. G., Terry, Jr., D. W., *et al.* *Am. J. Epidemiol. 97*, 276, 1973.
25. Merigan, T. C., Rand, K. H., Pollard, R. B., *et al.* *N. Engl. J. Med. 298*, 981-987, 1978.
26. Whitley, R. J., Ch'ien, L. T., Dolin, R., *et al.* *N. Engl. J. Med. 294*, 1193, 1976.
27. Whitley, R. J., Soong, S.-J., Dolin, R., *et al.* *N. Engl. J. Med. 297*, 289, 1977.
28. Ch'ien, L. T., Whitley, R. J., Dismukes, W. E., *et al.* *J. Infect. Dis. 130*, 32, 1974.
29. Emödi, G., O'Reilly, R., Müller, A., *et al.* *In* "Antivirals with Clinical Potential" (T. C. Merigan, ed.), p. 199. Univ. of Chicago Press, Chicago, 1976.
30. Arvin, A. M., Yeager, A. S., and Merigan, T. C. *In* "Antivirals with Clinical Potential" (T. C. Merigan, ed.), p. 205. Univ. of Chicago Press, Chicago, 1976.
31. Barton, B. W., and Tobin, J. O. *Ann. N.Y. Acad. Sci. 173*, 90, 1970.
32. McCracken, G. H., and Luby, J. P. *J. Pediatr. 80*, 488, 1972.

33. Chester, T. J., Paucker, K., and Merigan, T. C. *Nature* *246*, 92, 1973.

34. De Maeyer-Guignard, J., Cachard, A., and De Maeyer, E. *Science 190*, 574, 1975.

35. Kurtz, S. M., Fisken, R. A., Kaump, D. H., et al. *Antimicrobiol. Agents Chemother. 1968*, 180, 1969.

36. Zam, Z. S., Centifanto, Y. M., and Kaufman, H. E. *Intersci. Conf. Antimicrobiol. Agents Chemother., Am. Soc. Microbiol. 4*, abstr. 139, 1974.

37. Steele, R. W., Keeney, R. E., Brown, J. III, et al. *J. Infect. Dis. 135*, 593, 1977.

38. Worthington, M., and Conliffe, M. *J. Gen. Virol. 36*, 329, 1977.

29. Worthington, M. G., Conliffe, M., and Williams, J. *Proc. Soc. Exp. Biol. Med. 156*, 168, 1977.

40. Emödi, G., Rufli, T., Just, M., et al. *Scand. J. Infect. Dis. 7*, 1, 1975.

41. Gehrz, R. C., Knorr, S. O., Marker, S. C., et al. *The Lancet*, 844, 1977.

42. Desmyter, J., Rawls, W. E., Melnick, J. J., et al. *J. Immunol. 99*, 771, 1967.

43. Cho, C. T., Feng, K. K., and Brahmacupta, N. *J. Infect. Dis. 133*, 157, 1976.

44. Cho, C. T., and Feng, K. K. *J. Infect. Dis. 135*, 168, 1977.

45. Starr, S. E., Visintine, A. M., Tomeh, M. O., et al. *Proc. Soc. Exp. Biol. Med. 152*, 57, 1976.

46. Kirchner, H., Hirt, H. M., and Munk, K. *Infect. Immun. 16*, 9, 1977.

47. McCord, R. S., Breinig, M. K., and Morahan, P. S. *Antimicrobiol. Agents Chemother. 10*, 28, 1976.

48. Glasgow, L. A., Fischbach, J., Bryant, S. M., et al. *Infect. Dis. 135*, 763, 1977.

49. Fischer, G. W., Podgore, J. K., Bass, J. W., et al. *J. Infect. Dis. 132*, 578, 1975.

50. Greenberg, H. B., Pollard, R.B., Lutwick, L. I., et al. *N. Engl. J. Med. 295*, 517, 1976.

51. Pollard, R. B., Smith, J. L., Neal, E. A., et al. *JAMA, 239*, 1648-1650, 1978.

52. Cohen, S. S. *Cancer 40*, 509, 1977.

53. Percy, D. H. *Teratology 11*, 103, 1975.

54. O'Neill, F. J., and Rapp, F. *J. Virol. 7*, 692, 1971.

55. Petrick, T. Discussion at Adenine Arabinoside Collaborative Study Group, Bethesda, Marlyland, Nov. 17, 1977.

56. Wohlenberg, C. R., Walz, M. A., and Notkins, A. L. *Infect. Immun. 13*, 1519, 1976.

57. Klein, R. J., and Friedman-Kien, A. E. *Antimicrobiol. Agents Chemother. 12*, 577, 1977.

DISCUSSION

DR. B. SANFORD: You mentioned effects of interferon on
specific viral infections in lymphoma but what about effects
on the lymphoma itself?   Do you have any evidence you can present at this time?   What is your personal level of optimism
at this time about treatment of lymphoma or leukemia with interferon?

DR. MERIGAN: We have had poor results in previously treated patients with advanced histocytic lymphoma.   Recently we
have had a dramatic improvement on administration of interferon to a patient with lymphocytic lymphoma who had not been
treated previously.   We shall try to confirm this observation
in other patients in the near future.

DR. VAN ROOD: Have you checked whether host factors such
as HLA determine the effect of interferon?

DR. MERIGAN: No, but it is an interesting idea and we
plan to do it.

DR. LEVY: While I find your treatment trials with interferon very encouraging for hepatitis B, I am a bit worried.
It looks as if you are blocking the replication of the virus,
but viral antigens continue to be made for a period of time
and perhaps virus remains locked in the liver.   In other virus systems, such as with herpes or C-type viruses, it has become evident that a block in the replication of a virus may
enhance its transforming properties.   I am worried that while
the infection hepatitis is arrested you might see development
of primary liver cancers.   The association of hepatitis B infection and liver cancer has been made in Africa.   Unfortunately the tissue culture studies that showed the damaging
effect of herpes and C-type viruses cannot yet be done with
hepatitis B virus to examine *in vitro* the possibility of the
transform capacity of hepatitis B virus.

DR. MERIGAN: We realize this concern but we feel that
tumor production is less likely if we can eradicate the infection completely.

DR. DVORAK: How confident are you that the therapeutic
effects you have observed are in fact attributable to interferon and not to another lymphokine present in your lymphocyte
supernatants?

DR. MERIGAN: We are not absolutely certain but it does
copurify with antiviral activity through a 100-fold purifica-
tion from our standard material.

DR. WALDMANN: In terms of your introductory remarks,
are the interferons immunosuppressive?

DR. MERIGAN: With mouse interferon, 10 to 100 times the
minimum *in vivo* antiviral dosage is required to suppress the

production of antibody.   Because we do not know the minimum
in vivo immunosuppressive dose, we are carefully monitoring
immune responses in our patients undergoing treatment with
interferon.

    DR. THEIS: Are there any adverse effects on the patients
undergoing treatment with the very large doses of interferon?

    DR. MERIGAN: Yes, we have noted two effects that need to
be followed carefully.   The first occurs early in treatment;
4 to 6 hours after intramuscular injection of the high doses
of interferon, some patients exhibit fever and weakness.
This effect tends to wear off after continued administration
of interferon.   The second type occurs 3 to 4 days after initiation of treatment; an effect on the hemopoietic system,
mainly involving platelets and leukocytes, is observed.
This effect has been reversible, disappearing shortly after
therapy is stopped, and has not led to any complications such
as bleeding or infection.   As the threshold for this effect is
variable, hematopoeitic function is carefully evaluated before
deciding on a long-term dosage regimen.

IMMUNE REACTIVITY IN MAREK'S DISEASE
DURING VIRAL ONCOGENESIS AND PROTECTIVE VACCINATION

Gail A. Theis [*]

Department of Microbiology
New York Medical College
Valhalla, New York

INTRODUCTION

Marek's disease (MD) is an avian lymphoproliferative disease caused by infection with a herpesvirus (1-4), which in nature is highly contagious and epizootic. Marek's disease virus (MDV) can be spread by contact infection. The virus, which
replicates to fully infectious form in feather follicle epithelial cells (3), is probably shed into the environment and
inhaled or ingested by contact birds. The established causative relationship between infection with this herpesvirus and
the development of visceral lymphomas and lymphoproliferative
lesions had focused attention on research problems associated
with MD. The lymphoproliferative nature of MD, the herpesvirus etiology, and the contagion of the virus suggests that
MD provides a model for the studies of lymphoproliferative disorders of man. In addition, MD can provide a system for
studies of the efficacy of vaccination against oncogenic herpesviruses, since vaccines suppressive of viral oncogenesis
in MD have been developed (5). The future importance of such
vaccines in treatment of other oncogenic viral diseases can
only be glimpsed at present. From an epidemiological point
of view, it is important to note that control of oncogenesis
in MD does not depend on elimination of this epizootic virus.
Rather, vaccination appears to prevent only the development of

*Recipient of Research Career Development Award #K04 CA70-
812 from the National Cancer Institute.*

the visceral and peripheral nerve lymphoproliferative lesions
that characterize acute diseases (4,5). The mechanisms of
acquired resistance to oncogenic transformation have been under investigation.

Infection of susceptible chickens with MDV results in any
of three expressions depending on virulence and tropism of the
virus strain: (a) lytic and productive; (b) abortive and non-
productive; (c) neoplastic. The lytic productive virus replication occurs almost exclusively in squamous cells of the
stratified epithelium in feather follicles (3). Cell-free en-
veloped infectious virions of MDV may be found among degenerated epithelial cells. At late stages of acute MD, fully en-
veloped virions have been demonstrated in cell-free form in
the thymus, bursa, or kidney, where tissue degeneration has occurred (4). However, it is not certain that the virus replicates completely in these tissues, although it is possible
that epithelial elements in these organs support lytic virus
development.

The persistence of infectious MDV *in vivo* is related to
the nature of virus association with monuclear cells in peripheral blood and cells of lymphoid tissues (6). MDV is disseminated *in vivo* via cells of peripheral blood, in which
virus undergoes nonlytic replication. Although the virus
extracted from peripheral blood leucocytes (PBL) shows loss
of infectivity (6), the infectivity of PBL for passage of virus both *in vivo* and *in vitro* has been established. MDV is
apparently transmitted from cell to cell by contact (7). It
may be an important long-term survival mechanism for this
herpesvirus that infectivity can be maintained in cell-associated form, protected against a hostile environment of humoral antibodies directed against viral antigens. Evidence
that MDV is present in infectious form in peripheral blood
leucocytes (PBL) and in cells of lymphoid organs has been established by: (a) the *in vivo* transmission of MD after injection of unexposed chickens with cells from MDV-infected
birds; (b) the formation of plaques in tissue culture monolayers exposed to such cells. In addition, the intracellular
presence of MDV has been demonstrated by detection of viral
antigens (8) and herpesvirus-like particles (9) in cells of
blood and organs of MD chickens with MD.

The major interest in MD for studies of tumor viruses
relates to its classification as a contagious herpesvirus
that can cause transformation and lymphoma development in certain infected cells. Major questions in MD involve the nature
of the specific target cell that ultimately becomes transformed, and the variety of potential interactions between MDV
and target cells; the nature of lymphoproliferative stimuli
resulting from MDV infection; and the immune reactivity that

accompanies infections with both nonpathogenic and pathogenic strains of MDV. With respect to lymphoma development, data suggest that the T lymphocyte is the major target for oncogenic transformation, since the majority of cells of the MD lymphomas exhibit antigens in common with T cells (10,11). Similar observations pertain to the MD lymphoblastoid cells maintained by continuous passage *in vitro* (12,13).

The availability of the lymphoblastoid cell lines (12-14) as well as an *in vivo* transplantable lymphoblastic leukemia (15) and a lymphoma (16) has facilitated studies of the association of the MDV genome with host cell genetic material. When the cells become transformants, neither virus-specified antigens nor virus particles are detectable under normal conditions (17). However, in a proportion of cells from both lymphoblastoid lines maintained *in vitro* (18) and virus-induced primary lymphomas obtained from MDV-infected chickens (19), portions of the MDV genome can be demonstrated by nucleic acid hybridization methods.

A recent development of considerable importance to the tumor immunology of MD has been the demonstration of a Marek's associated tumor-specific surface antigen (MATSA) shared by the transformed cell lines MSB-1, JMV, and HPRS (18). The MATSAs expressed by each transformed cell lines have both cross-reactive and specific determinants (20). MATSA appears to be specific for neoplastic cells in MD, since it cannot be demonstrated on cells of MDV-infected tissue culture monolayers in which the MD viral antigens are readily expressed (20). It is particularly relevant to observe that MATSA may be present on cells in lymphoproliferative lesions of peripheral nerves (21), as well as on MD lymphoma cells (22). The transformed nature of all lymphoproliferative lesions in MD is suggested. Thus, neoplastic transformation in MD appears to specify neoantigens distinctive and unrelated to those antigens associated with intracellular nonlytic replication, or with the virus particle *per se*. This is an important concept for studies of immunity and immunosuppression in MD. The effective immune responsiveness to the virus-associated antigens and to the tumor-specific antigens must have different significance in determining the outcome of MDV infection.

IMMUNOLOGY OF MAREK'S DISEASE

The duality of the central lymphoid organs (bursa and thymus) of the chickens allows for manipulation of humoral and cellular immunity. The effects of selective extirpation of the thymus and bursa have been investigated in relation to immune reactivity and oncogenic transformation in MD. Demon-

stration of avian T lymphocyte surface antigens on cells of
both MD lymphomas (10,11) and lymphoblastoid cell lines (12,
13) by inference supports the suggestion that T lymphocytes
are the target cells for MDV neoplastic transformation (13,
22). Whether a specific subset of T lymphocytes is sensitive
to oncogenesis is also an unresolved issue. The definitive
determination of target cell will await a method for oncogenic
transformation *in vitro*, with display of MATSA as indicator
of the transformation event. With respect to B cell-mediated
immunity, data are less convincing that antibody to virus or
MDV-specified cellular antigens has a critical role in containment of viral disease (23-25). Suppressed antibody responses in MDV-infected chickens probably result from the degeneration of lymphoid tissues in the wake of cellular infiltrations (4). Most significantly, bursectomy does not alter
the outcome of MD (26). However, anti-MDV antibody may play
some role in containment of virus upon initial exposure, as it
was noted that newly hatched chickens protected by maternal
anti-MDV antibody developed less severe symptoms after exposure to virulent MD (27). The specificities of the anti-MDV
antibodies in these studies were not established.

Accumulating experimental data indicate overwhelmingly
that the primary disequilibrium in immune reactivity occurs in
the T cell-mediated responses after infection of chickens with
oncogenic MDV. Observations support the early hypothesis of
Payne (28) that T cells act as both the targets for MDV-induced
oncogenic transformation and the reactive or effector immunocytes in immunosurveillance. T cells are also implicated as
targets of MDV oncogenesis by the studies of Sharma *et al.*
(29), who showed a decrease in incidence of lymphomas in T
cell-depleted chickens.

The role of T lymphocytes as both targets and effector
cells in MD have led to investigations in my laboratory of
the specific effects of MDV on T lymphocyte subpopulations.
At the beginning of these studies, we noted that in terminal
stages of acute MD, thymus tissues were degenerated or completely atrophic. The reason for the severity of these lesions
has not yet been established, but it has been noted by others
(4) that degenerative lesions in MD follow infiltration of
lymphoblastoid cells. Perhaps these infiltrations of lymphoblastoid MD cells, as observed commonly in lymphoid organs
and peripheral nerves, indicate an autoimmune response, a proliferation of cells activated by virus-associated cellular
antigens of infected cells in these sites. As for induction
of oncogenesis, it may be that the neoplastic transformation
event can occur on the substrate of activated cells in specific tissue sites. With respect to the thymus, tissues may degenerate from MDV replication in epithelial cells that produce

TABLE I. Effects of MDV Infection on Allograft Rejection and Immune Response to Sheep Erythrocytes (SE)

MDV inoculation[a]	No. of birds with surviving allografts[b]	Immune response to SE mean $\log_2$ hemagglutination titer			
		First response[c]		second response[d]	
		IgM	IgG	IgM	IgG
−	0/8	6.9	0.1	5.3	3.0
+	7/8	5.6	0.3	5.1	2.5

[a] MDV inoculated at 16 days after hatching.

[b] Ratios: number of birds with surviving allografts/total number of birds grafted.

[c] First response to SE determined on day 6 after first injection of SE.

[d] Second response to SE determined on day 6 after second injection of SE.

thymic differentiating factors or hormones (30,31). In addition, thymic tissue may be depleted of lymphocytes as cytotoxic cells arise in response to virus-associated cellular antigens of nonlytically infected or transformed cells. The detection of MATSA-specific cytotoxic cells (21,32) in chickens early after infection will be discussed further below. The immunological outcome on the thymus functions of these autoimmune and degenerative processes, associated with development of acute MD, would be pronounced immunosuppression of T cell reactivity as MD progressed. Suppression of T cell immune responses in MD has been observed repeatedly.

The immunosuppressive effects of MDV on T cell-mediated allograft reactivity was demonstrated in experiments summarized in Table I (33). The results presented show that selective virulent effects of MDV infection can suppress T cell reactivity of chickens, even when infected at 16 days after hatching. While allograft reactivity is obviously inhibited, humoral antibody response in the infected chickens remains similar to uninfected controls. Thus, as indicated above, the humoral immune responses are not affected in the initial stages of MD pathogenesis, and eventual depression of antibody responses is probably a secondary effect of destruction in thymus and bursa (4).

We have studied more intensively the effect of virulent MDV infection on T lymphocyte reactivity by using tissue culture systems (34-36). T cell mitogen responsiveness of lym-

TABLE II. Quantitative Comparison of Viable Cells Responsive to PHA in Spleen Cultures from Normal and MDV-Infected Chickens

Spleen cell donors (no. of chickens studied)	^{3}H-Tdr incorporation in spleen cell cultures		Mean stimulation index[b]
	Mean cpm/10^5 viable cells[a]		
	+PHA	−PHA	
MDV-infected chickens (10)	30.3	25.3	1.2
Uninfected normal chickens (7)	2727.1	28.1	97.1

[a] cpm/10^5 viable cells: mean counts per minute (cpm) triplicate cultures, calculated per 10^5 viable cells in cultures at time of termination.

[b] Stimulation index: cpm per 10^5 viable cells stimulated by PHA/cpm per 10^5 unstimulated viable cells.

phocytes cultured from MDV-infected and uninfected chickens of susceptible strains has been studied as the indicator of integral T cell function. Our results have shown that blastogenic responses to PHA and Con A in cultured spleen and thymus cells are increasingly inhibited as symptoms of MD exacerbate (34). In chickens with acute MD and visceral lymphomas, the loss of mitogen responsiveness might be predicted, if only on the basis of atrophy in the thymus, since no gross anatomic evidence of this tissue was detected. Thus, depleted mitogen reactivity could result from dilution or absence of differentiated T cells from peripheral lymphoid tissues. However, immunosuppression may also result from interactions with a variety of suppressor cells, which can be T, B, or M cells. The problem of distinguishing among the various forms of immunosuppression, which could be relevant to MD pathogenesis, has been under study in my laboratory. The favored premise has been that the depressed mitogen reactivity seen in lymphocytes cultured from MDV-infected chickens resulted from a depletion of responsive cells. Early data summarized in Table II show that fewer lymphocytes from MDV-infected birds underwent blastogenic transformation under conditions optimal for normal spleen lymphocytes (NS). It should be noted that in other studies we have not been able to determine any concentration of phytomitogens that was stimulatory for lymphocytes from chickens with acute MD. Thus we assume that mitogen responsiveness in cultures of spleens (MDS) from MDV-infected chickens is generally depressed or absent. Further evidence, derived from cell separation studies (36), has reinforced our working hypothesis that depletion of certain cell subpopulations provides the physical basis for immunosuppressed T cell reactivity *in vivo*. Some data from these studies are summarized in Figs. 1 and 2 and in Table III. The distribution profiles in Fig. 1 show that NS cells are predominantly in denser fractions 5-7 in both unimmunized (exp. 1) and 5-day primary sheep erythrocyte (SE)-sensitized (exp. 11) chickens. In contrast, data in Fig. 2 show the majority of cells in the more buoyant fractions 1-4 in spleens of (exps. IV, VI) chickens with acute lymphoblastoid leukemia JMV (JMV-S) and (exp. V) chickens with visceral MD lymphomas. Denser cells of fractions 5-7 are depleted in spleens of chickens with acute disease symptoms. When calculated in terms of cell number, we have shown that depletion in these fractions is absolute, that is, that there is an absence of denser cells in JMV-S. In contrast, cells from spleens of chickens with less acute symptoms of JMV leukemia (exp. VII, Fig. 2) distributed as NS (Fig. 1) among denser fractions 5-7. Cells cultured from different fractions of the NS and MDS were tested for blastogenic responses to T cell mitogens PHA and Con A. Results are shown

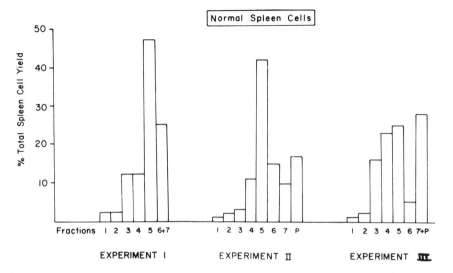

FIGURE 1. *Cell density profiles of normal chicken spleens (NS) after separation of cells on a discontinuous gradient of Ficoll. Exp. 1, unsensitized; exp. II, primary sensitization with SE; exp. III, secondary sensitization with SE.*

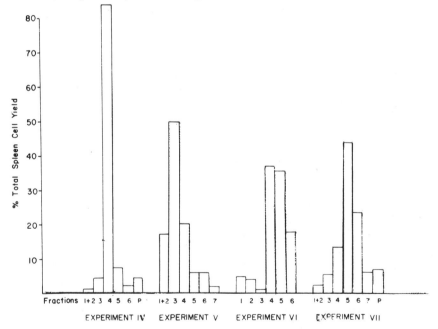

FIGURE 2. *Cell density profiles of spleens from JMV- and MDV-infected chickens after separation on a discontinuous Ficoll gradient. Exp. IV, JMV-S, acute symptoms; exp. V, MDS, acute symptoms; exp. VI, asymptomatic; exp. VII, asymptomatic, 5 days postinjection.*

in Table III. Among NS fractions tested, cultured cells that
were isolated in fraction 5 were most vigorous in blastogenic
responses to the mitogens. By contrast, the separated cells
cultured from JMV-S (exps. IV, VI) and MDS (exp. V) showed
either inhibited or depressed uptake of T cell mitogen reactivity in cell fractions. At this time, we cannot state definitively that depletion of immunoresponsive cells results
in the observed depressed reactivity of these fractionated cell
populations. However, the data support the view that gradual
tissue infiltration and disruption of thymic architecture (4)
in MD provide the anatomical rationale for the loss of differentiated T cells in the periphery. Depression of T cell-mediated immunity, as measured by mitogen-induced blastogenesis, may
be mediated by soluble factors. Such suppressive factors can
be produced in certain cultures of MDS, in response to exposure
to PHA (35). Are these factors produced by activated T lymphocytes? This question becomes particularly important in view of
a recent report that herpesviruses have mitogenic capacity *in
vitro* (37). Immunosuppression in MD might be the outcome of interaction of competent lymphocytes with soluble suppressive factors, produced by activated lymphocytes, which were stimulated
by herpesvirus in cell-associated or free form. In investiga-
ting mechanisms of immunosuppression in MD, it is possible
that specific cell depletion and soluble inhibitory factors
could act in synergy. With the use of enriched cell populations obtained by gradient separation of lymphoid tissues, we
feel that we may investigate more critically these and other
aspects of altered immunosurveillance in MD.

ACQUIRED IMMUNITY AND PROTECTIVE VACCINATION IN MD

Specific T cell reactivity can be induced against both
virus-associated antigens and MATSA of T lymphoblastoid cell
lines derived from MD lymphomas. Using a plaque-inhibition
assay, T cells from spleens of virus-immunized chickens were
shown to inhibit specifically the development of MDV plaques
in vitro (31). Thus, these studies demonstrated the capacity
of viral antigens to evoke virus-specific cellular immunity in
adult chickens. The *in vivo* significance of the containment
of infection afforded by this kind of T cell immune response
may be found in future studies of chickens resistant to severe
effects of MDV infection by virtue of age (39) or genotype
(40). Experiments have already shown that T cells are implicated in age resistance to MD, since neonatal thymectomy abro-

TABLE III. Comparison of Proliferative Responses to T Cell Mitogens in Spleen Cells Cultured from Normal (NS) and MD-Infected (MDS) Chickens[a], after Separation of Cells by Buoyant Density in Ficoll Gradients

Cells tested	T Cell mitogens[b]	^{3}H-Thymidine uptake in unseparated spleen and spleen cell fractions (E - C), cpm[c]					
		UnS	Fractions				
			3	4	5	6	7
NS	PHA	+18,862	−[d]	+9523	+8522	—	—
	Con A	+17,202	—	+24,416	+22,935	—	—
	Con A	+17,873	+1839	+4701	+11,518	+5170	+6734
	PHA	+4800	—	+2360	+3923	+1076	—
	Con A	+1920	—	757	+4292	+13,331	+21,662
MDS	PHA	−2296	−1229	−2915	−534	—	—
	Con A	−1957	−19	−1510	−590	—	—
	PHA	−5545	+1700	−478	−168	−435	—
	Con A	−9882	+1534	−1310	+38	−379	—
	PHA	—	—	−414	−8735	+3475	—
	Con A	—	—	+1363	−4584	+50	—
	PHA	+1468	+1778	+644	−186	+1136	—
	Con A	+2241	+839	−78	−388	+120	—
	PHA	−4893	+1324	−1932	−455	+936	—
	Con A	−6745	−2437	−2377	−566	+234	—

[a] 21-28-day-old FP chickens used in these studies.

[b] Maximum stimulatory doses of mitogens: PHA, 2 μg/0.25 ml culture; Con A, 2 μg/0.25 ml culture.

[c] (E−C): (Experimental ^{3}H-Tdr uptake) − (Control ^{3}H-Tdr uptake) in counts per minute per 10^6 cells in each of the replicate cultures.

[d] Fractions omitted when there were insufficient numbers of cells for studies.

gates this age resistance (41). Another kind of T cell immunity has been demonstrated in cytotoxic assays against MSB-1 lymphoblastoid targets (21). Cytotoxic T cells have been detected in spleens of MDV-infected birds 7 days after exposure to virus. The presence of cytotoxic cells specifically sensitized to tumor-associated antigens suggests that viral transformation is an early event after MD^S infection, although tumors may not be detected until later in the disease. However, further study is necessary to interpret the role of the cytotoxic cells at this early stage after infection. For example, the age of the chicken at the time of infection and its ultimate response to the virus must be evaluated. Would the neonatally infected bird respond in similar fashion with the appearance of these specific cytotoxic cells? Several other questions can be presented. Although the susceptibility of MATSA-bearing lymphoblastoid cells indicates specificity of the cytotoxic cells (21), it is not clear that MATSA is the only antigenic determinant against which the effector cells are reactive. The cluster of sensitizing antigens may also be related to viral antigens. Although these antigens are not expressed on transformant cells *in vitro*, IUDR treatment of lymphoblastoid cells will result in some viral antigen induction (42,43), showing the potential in these cells for such expression. The viral and tumor antigenic determinants could serve as immunogens for developing cellular immunity.

The interrelationship between immune responses to membrane-associated viral and tumor antigens in MD is enigmatic. Although these antigenic groups appear to be distinctive, immunity to either determinants can result in prevention of MD lymphoma development. Thus, vaccination of chicks with plasma membranes (44,45) from MDV-infected cells that exhibit MDV antigens but no MATSA or with glutaraldehyde-fixed lymphoblastoid cells (with MATSA but no MDV antigens) of tissue culture lines (46) will abort neoplastic transformation. These observations provoke speculation on a possible relationship between appearance of cell-associated viral antigens and tumor antigens in the MDV-infected cells. Perhaps all cells are potentially capable of expressing MATSA and viral antigens, or transformants may express viral antigens at different stages of the cell cycle *in vivo*. Also, different cells may be non-lytically infected and transformed, thus providing several separate populations for sensitization. A further point of interest relates to the time required for transformation and establishment of transformants *in vivo*. There is a rapid appearance of MATSA in cells after MDV infection. Sharma (21) detected significant levels of anti-MATSA cytotoxic T cells at 7 days after MDV. Thus, cellular immunity, presumably directed toward control of transformants, would appear concurrently

with anti-MDV immunity. The interrelationship between effective anti-MDV immunity and suppression of oncogenesis (44,45)
can be understood if it is assumed that control of virus
spread and replication will limit contact with cells potentially susceptible to transformation. The apparent rapid appearance of MATSA-bearing cells at high enough concentrations to
generate specific cytotoxic T cells raises basic questions related to the transformation event in vivo.

   Vaccination with either nonpathogenic MDV or cross-reactive herpesvirus from nervesvirus tumors (HVT) of turkeys has
been successful in protecting susceptible fowl from the acute
pathological symptoms of MD (5). While vaccination will abrogate the oncogenic process, the chickens can be infected
nevertheless with either virus. This concept is supported by
Witter (46) in studies of protective effects of nonreplicating
MDV isolates. Thus, the persistence of attenuated MDV or HVT
in cells of MDV-infected birds maintains a constantly available pool of virus and virus-associated cellular antigens.
In addition, the generation of MATSA-specific cytotoxic T cells
may be associated with sensitization by microscopic clones of
transformants or abortively infected cells, as seen in vaccine-
protected birds (21).

   Other stimuli of immune reactivity must be considered, in
view of the studies of Kaaden and co-workers (44,45), which
show protective vaccination with plasma membranes of virus-
infected tissue culture cells. Mechanisms of vaccine protection are not understood. However, protection may relate, at
least in part, to abortive transformation in a small number of
cells, which then act as immunogenic stimulus for the T lymphocytes in the control of the further emergence of transformed
clones. Sharma (21) suggested the transformation of cells in
HVT-vaccinated birds, and predicted that MATSA would be detected among these cells. However, the appearance of MATSA-
sensitized cytotoxic cells cannot be the only significant expression of vaccine protection, since cells of equivalent cytotoxicity have been detected in chickens that succumb to MD
(21). The need for transformation in eliciting vaccine protection implies that vaccine virus must replicate and cause the
expression of cross-reacting antigens (47,48). Cells expressing
immunity against these vaccine-virus-induced membrane antigens
could amplify the immune response and thus contain the cell-
associated viremia of MD. Cells susceptible to transformation
would be protected by lessening the concentration of virulent
virus.

   Whatever the complexity of cellular interactions operative
in vaccination against oncogenesis in MD, the integrity of the
immune system is pivotal to effectuation of the protection.
Depressed immunity, which follows injection of cyclophosphamide
(Cy), will abrogate HVT protection (49). Although originally

TABLE IV. Comparison of Proliferative Responses to PHA
in Spleen Cells Cultured from HVT-Vaccinated and Unvaccinated
Chickens 20-28 Days after Injection of MDV

Chickens injected with:	Ratio of visceral tumor development	Proliferative responses to PHA in spleen cell cultures, stimulation index[a] (±S.E.M.)
HVT[b] + MDV[c]	0/4	29.8 (±6.93)
MDV	5/5	2.7 (±1.08)
HVT	0/4	35.7 (±7.55)

[a] Stimulation index: ^{3}H-Tdr uptake in PHA-stimulated cells/ ^{3}H-Tdr uptake in unstimulated cells.

[b] HVT vaccination of 1-day-old chicks.

[c] MDV injection at 21 days after hatching.

interpreted as a B cell defect, more currently available data
emphasize the importance of a transient but profound T cell
deficiency in Cy-treated chickens (50). The absence of vaccine protection in the Cy-chickens may relate to loss of T
cells as both targets for virus replication and as reactive
immunocytes, responsive to viral and tumor antigens. Conversely, vaccination protects T cell reactivity, which is
otherwise regularly depressed after the infection of susceptible
chickens with virulent virus (Table IV). Theis et al. (34)
showed that HVT vaccination protected T cell mitogen responsiveness in spleen cells cultured from chickens infected subsequently with MDV. Allograft reactivity also remained intact in vaccinated birds (33). Persistence of the functional
integrity of cell-mediated immunity in vaccinated chickens indicates the nature of lymphocytes spared by such procedures,
and reinforces the concept that T cell-mediated immunity is
critical in immunosurveillance and prevention of viral oncogenesis in MD.

SUMMARY

MD is a model system in which cellular events in both viral oncogenesis and protective vaccination can be studied.
The T lymphocyte apparently acts as both target cell for neoplastic transformation and effector cell in immunosurveillance.
After exposure to virus, cells become nonlytically infected
with MDV for in vivo dissemination of virus. B cell-mediated

immunity does not appear to be a critical determinant in the
early stages of MD pathogenesis, while T cell-mediated responses are affected soon after exposure to virulent virus.
Cytotoxic T cell appear early after infection and are reactive
against MD tumor antigens.

The development of live attenuated and antigenically cross-
reactive vaccines, which can prevent acute disease symptoms
despite superinfection with ubiquitous virulent virus, can be
of importance to studies of all oncogenic herpesviruses. Es-
tablishing the cellular basis for vaccine protection is the
project of the future. The mechanisms that result in natural
or acquired resistance to viral neoplastic transformation may
be the same. Effects of immunosuppression of T cell responses
have been increased susceptibility to MDV. Most recent evidence (21) would suggest that rapid activation of certain subpopulations of T cells to unknown antigens associated with MD
may act to contain potentially oncogenic virus transmission
in MDV-infected chickens. The generation of suppressor T
cells as a protective mechanism in acquired and inherited resistance to MD oncogenesis has been suggested(51). Although
factors suppressive of T cell proliferation have been generated in MDS (35), the role of specific suppressor cells in
either MD pathogenesis or prophylaxis has yet to be confirmed
in experimental systems.

References

1. Churchill, A. E., and Biggs, P. M. *Nature 215*, 528, 1967.
2. Nazerian, K., Solomon, J. J., Witter, R. L., *et al*. *Proc.
   Soc. Exp. Biol. Med. 127*, 177, 1968.
3. Calnek, B. W., Calbertini, T., and Addinger, H. *J. Nat.
   Cancer Inst. 45*, 341, 1970.
4. Biggs, P. M. *In* "The Herpesviruses" (A. S. Kaplan, ed.),
   p. 557. Academic Press, New York, 1973.
5. Purchase, H. G. *Progr. Med. Virol. 18*, 178, 1974.
6. Witter, R. L., Solomon, J. J., Champion, L. R., *et al*.
   Avian Dis. 15, 346, 1971.
7. Lozanek, H. *J. Gen. Virol. 9*, 45, 1970.
8. Purchase, H. G. *J. Virol. 3*, 557, 1970.
9. Nazerian, K., and Purchase, H. G. *J. Virol. 5*, 79, 1970.
10. Hudson, L., and Payne, L. N. *Nature 241*, 52, 1973.
11. Rouse, B. T., Wells, R. H., and Warner, N. L. *J. Immunol.
    110*, 534, 1973.
12. Powell, P. C., Payne, L. N., and Frazier, J. A. *Nature
    251*, 79, 1975.
13. Matsuda, H., Ikuta, K., and Kato, S. *Biken J. 19*, 29,
    1976.

14. Hahn, E. C., Ramos, L., and Kenyon, A. J. *J. Nat. Cancer Inst. 59*, 267, 1977.
15. Kenyon, A. J., Sevoian, M., Horwitz, N. D., *et al. Avian Dis. 13*, 585, 1969.
16. Theis, G. A., Schierman, L. W., and McBride, R. A. *J. Immunol. 113*, 1710, 1974.
17. Akiyama, Y., and Kato, S. *Biken J. 17*, 105, 1974.
18. Nazerian, K., and Lee, L. *J. Gen. Virol. 25*, 317, 1974.
19. Nazerian, K., Lindahl, T., Klein, G., *et al. J. Virol. 12*, 841, 1973.
20. Stephens, E. A., Witter, R. L., Lee, L. F., *et al. J. Nat. Cancer Inst. 57*, 865, 1976.
21. Sharma, J. M. *In* "Avior Immunology" (A. A. Benedict, ed.), p. 345. 1977.
22. Witter, R. L., Stephens, E. A., Sharma, J. M., *et al. J. Immunol. 115*, 177, 1975.
23. Nazerian, K., and Sharma, J. M. *J. Nat. Cancer Inst. 54*, 277, 1975.
24. Higgins, D. A., and Calnek, B. W. *Infect. Immun. 11*, 33, 1975.
25. Sharma, J. M., and Witter, R. L. *Cancer Res. 35*, 711, 1975.
26. Sharma, J. M. *Nature (London) 247*, 117, 1974.
27. Payne, L. N., and Rennie, M. *J. Nat. Cancer Inst. 51*, 1159, 1973.
28. Payne, L. N. *In* "Oncogenesis and Herpesviruses" (Biggs, P. M., de Thé, G., and Payne, L. N., eds.), p. 31. Int. Agency for Research on Cancer, Lyons, 1972.
29. Sharma, J. N., Nazerian, K., and Witter, R. L. *J. Nat. Cancer Inst. 58*, 689, 1977.
30. Trainin, N. *Physiol. Rev. 54*, 272, 1974.
31. Goldstein, G. *Nature 267*, 11, 1974.
32. Sharma, J. M. *Infect. Immun. 18*, 46, 1977.
33. Shierman, L. W., Theis, G. A., and McBride, R. A. *J. Immunol. 116*, 1497, 1976.
34. Theis, G. A., McBride, R. A., and Schierman, L. W. *J. Immunol. 115*, 848, 1975.
35. Theis, G. A. *J. Immunol. 118*, 887, 1977.
36. Theis, G. A., and Hapoineu, B. *In* "Oncogenesis and Herpesviruses," *3rd Int. Symp., Boston, July 25-29, 1977*. In press.
37. Mochizuki, D., Hedrick, S., Watson, J., and Kingsbury, D. *J. Exp. Med. 146*, 1500, 1977.
38. Ross, L. J. N. *Nature 268*, 644, 1977.
39. Calnek, B. W. *J. Nat. Cancer Inst. 51*, 929, 1973.
40. Pazderka, F., Longenecker, B. M., Low, G. R. J., *et al. Immunogenetics 2*, 93, 1975.
41. Purchase, H. G., Witter, R. L., Okazaki, W., *et al. Perspect. Virol. 7*, 91, 1971.

42. Kunn, K., and Nazerian, K. J. *Gen. Virol. 34*, 413, 1977.
43. Sharma, J. M., Witter, R. L., and Purchase, H. G. *Nature 253*, 477, 1975.
44. Kaaden, O. R., Dietzschold, B., and Ueberschar, S. *Med. Microbiol. 159*, 261, 1974.
45. Kaaden, O. R., and Dietzschold, B. *J. Gen. Virol. 25*, 1, 1974.
46. Witter, R. L. *In* "Oncogenesis and Herpesviruses," *3rd Int. Symp., Boston, July 25-29, 1977.* In press.
47. Ross, L. N., Powell, P. C., Walker, D. J., *et al. J. Gen. Virol. 35*, 219, 1977.
48. Ross, L. J. N., Biggs, P. M., and Newton, A. A. *J. Gen. Virol. 8*, 291, 1973.
49. Purchase, H. G., and Sharma, J. M. *Nature (London), 248*, 419, 1974.
50. Sharma, J. N., and Lee, L. F. *Infect. Immun. 17*, 227, 1977.
51. Rouse, B. T., and Warner, N. L. *J. Immunol. 113*, 904, 1974.

DISCUSSION

DR. PREHN: Yesterday during the discussion we heard from
Dr. Schwartz a concise and elegant, but totally inadmissible
definition of neoplasia, namely, that a neoplasm is a monoclonal hyperplasia. My question is whether or not the lesion in
Marek's disease is monoclonal.

DR. THEIS: This is difficult to answer since Marek's disease lymphomas have been examined only *in vivo*. There are no
markers at present other than MATSA and T cell markers on the
lymphoma cells of Marek's disease and these give no information
on monoclonality.

DR. WELSH: Do the tumor cells express cell surface antigens in the presence of an antibody response directed against
them?

DR. THEIS: I am not aware that experiments along these
lines have been done.

DR. WELSH: Antibody-mediated cell cytotoxicity against
herpes viruses has been detected in the mouse. Is it known
whether this also occurs against Marek's disease virus in the
chicken during the acute or chronic stages of disease and,
if so, why is the infection not controlled?

DR. THEIS: There does not seem to be any significant antibody-mediated cell cytotoxicity in Marek's disease; at least
none has been detected to date.

DR. ESSEX: Numerous mechanisms have been considered by
which the nononcogenic turkey virus might interfere with the
action of the oncogenic chicken Marek's disease virus. Among
these are immune effector mechanisms that might cross-react
and possibly compete for membrane adsorption and/or penetration sites. One common feature of oncogenic viruses, be they
popova, herpes, or RNA tumor viruses, is that they must have
a DNA stage that integrates into the genome of the host cell.
Has the possibility that the nononcogenic virus might interfere with the oncogenic virus by competing for integration
sites in the DNA of the cell been considered? Have nucleic
acid hybridization studies progressed far enough in this system to address that question?

DR. THEIS: Viral interference at some stage of the virus-
cell interaction is a possible explanation for the effects of
vaccine interference with viral oncogenesis. Perhaps nucleic
acid hybridization studies will provide a means to approach the
problem of competitive integration of vaccine viral genome vs.
Marek's disease virus genome into a particular site in cellular DNA. I cannot evaluate the availability of experimental
systems for these studies.

DR. BRITTON: You said that thymectomy of newborns abol-

ished the protective effect of vaccination in Marek's disease.
As I see it, such treatment would abolish Marek's disease, at
least the lymphomatous form, because the target cells for the
virus have been eliminated.

DR. THEIS: This is true. I neglected to emphasize that
neonatal thymectomy does indeed diminish the development of
visceral lymphomas very markedly in Marek's disease. This
is recent work by the Sharma-Artter group.

INFECTION DUE TO TREPONEMA PALLIDUM:
ESCAPE FROM IMMUNE SURVEILLANCE*

Daniel M. Musher
Robert E. Baughn
John M. Knox

Departments of Medicine, Microbiology
Immunology, and Dermatology
Baylor College of Medicine
and
Veterans Administration Hospital
Houston, Texas

Abundant evidence suggests that *Treponema pallidum* escapes normal immune surveillance mechanisms as it acts in the mammalian host to cause syphilis. The fact that a tiny inoculum (about 50 viable organisms) of this slowly replicating organism regularly produces a lesion already indicates that everything is not as it should be. Other infecting organisms, for example, *Streptococcus pneumoniae* or influenza virus, may initially grow unchecked in the nonimmune host, but a race between proliferation of the organism on the one hand and the immune response on the other determines, to a great extent, the clinical outcome. During an average three-week incubation in syphilis the human host has time to mount an effective immune response, yet obviously does not do so, at least to a degree sufficient to prevent infection. As the initial lesion (the syphilitic chancre) evolves into a clinically recognizable entity, antibodies of various kinds become detectable, indicating that the host does recognize something foreign about *T. pallidum*. Nevertheless, the infection continues to progress. When, after 4 to 6 weeks the chancre finally does regress, the disseminated skin lesions of secondary syphilis begin to appear. At the time of appearance of the skin lesions

*This work was supported by NIH grant # USPH AI 12618 PI 03/05 and research funds from the Veterans Administration Hospital.

of secondary syphilis the individual, whether human or experimental animal, is resistant to reinfection; this phenomenon is called concomitant immunity. The development of concomitant immunity suggests that whatever local factors enable the host to suppress *T. pallidum* at the primary site of infection are apparently not operative systemically. The secondary eruption may remain for weeks; when, in the absence of treatment, it finally disappears, relapses occur in up to one-fifth of cases (1).

The failure of the individual to develop immunity between the time of exposure and the appearance of a chancre, the later failure of the host to halt the progression from primary to secondary disease (despite clear evidence of immune responsiveness), and the relapse of some but not all untreated subjects are but a few of the intriguing and unsolved puzzles. Some of the unknown factors can best be highlighted by a series of questions:

(1)   Why are *T. pallidum* not phagocytized at the initial time of inoculation?

(2)   Why do opsonizing or bactericidal antibodies fail to develop, leading subsequently to eradication of infection?

(3)   If immunosuppression is partly responsible for the failure to develop antibodies that eradicate *T. pallidum*, why are so many other antibodies produced and what role do they play in the course of infection?

(4)   Is the acquisition of nonspecific cellular resistance during syphilis important in helping control infection or is nature, usually so economical, wasting an immune response in this disease?

(5)   What factor(s) ultimately lead to latency?

(6)   Why are most nonprimates naturally resistant to *T. pallidum*, whereas rabbits and primates are regularly infected by a few organisms?

(7)   What is the pathogenesis of late (tertiary) syphilis?

The present discussion will stress areas that relate to escape from immune surveillance. Accordingly, we shall not deal with question 7; this is perhaps just as well, because we are unable to present clinical or experimental data that help to answer it. The others will be considered in turn; for each, we shall try to indicate the present state of knowledge as well as problems that remain unsolved.

The interaction between *T. pallidum* and phagocytic cells appears to have several unique features. Phagocytes, whether polymorphonuclear or monocytic, make surprisingly little attempt to ingest *T. pallidum*. Electron-microscopic studies of syphilitic tissue have shown that the overwhelming majority

of treponemal forms are lying in the collagenous framework,
outside phagocytic cells (2-5). A careful search of many
fields has, in the opinion of some investigators, revealed
treponemes inside cells. Others suggest that these may be
artifactual, reflecting the association of treponemes with
invaginations of the cytoplasm (6). Support for the belief
that these observations are based on artifact comes from the
fact that treponemes have been found in lymphocytes, plasma
cells, and fibroblasts as well as within macrophages and polymorphonuclear leukocytes (PMN) (4-5); this kind of indiscri-
minate habitation opposes the concept of a specific role for
phagocytosis. Based on observations in our laboratory, as
well as on those of other investigators, we believe that phagocytic cells *in vivo* do not readily ingest intact treponemes,
and may not ingest them at all. This does not result from
some unusual adverse effect in the phagocytic cells. In collaboration with R. La Pushin, we have injected *Staphylococcus
aureus* into syphilitic chancres and observed these organisms
to be rapidly ingested by PMN and macrophages; similar experiments have also been carried out *in vitro*.

Dark-field microscopic examination of wet preparations *in
vitro* has also shown that macrophages and PMN fail to ingest
treponemes. Electron-microscopic examination of these preparations consistently fails to reveal *T, pallidum* inside cells.
However, a second striking observation is made under these conditions. Just as *T. pallidum* has been observed *in vitro* to
attach to epithelial cell cultures in a process that requires
active metabolism by the treponeme (7,8), this organism also
appears to attach to macrophages and, to a lesser extent, to
PMN. Killed treponemes do not attach, and when *T. pallidum*
and macrophages are maintained *in vitro*, loss of treponemal
motility is associated with detachment from macrophages (B.
Brause, unpublished observations). For an infecting organism
to actively attach to phagocytic cells and still not be ingested by them is, in our opinion, a unique situation. A further anomaly is that the presence of antibody (specifically,
serum from a chancre-immune rabbit) inhibits the interaction
between *T. pallidum* and phagocytes rather than facilitating
it. Based on these morphologic observations it is not possible to answer the important question of whether phagocytosis
has been attempted and has failed; studies utilizing histo-
chemical techniques have been initiated in our laboratory to
gain further insight into this phenomenon.

How *T. pallidum* escapes phagocytosis is unknown. If a
rich slime layer that repels ingesting cells were responsible,
one would imagine that there would also be no attachment. If
attachment were to occur, there still should be attempts to
phagocytize. As noted above, macrophages and PMN do not even

seem to try to ingest treponemes. Another possibility is that the foreign nature of the treponeme is not apparent. If the slime were derived from mammalian host substance then failure to ingest might result from nonrecognition. However, when *T. pallidum* has been obtained from rabbit testis and incubated *in vitro* with mouse macrophages, the same lack of interaction occurs. It is conceivable that the phagocyte simply lacks a receptor for the virulent treponemes, although this would represent a most unusual situation.

Other observations support the possibility of nonrecognition of treponemes at levels other than capsular. The presence of Wasserman antibody in treponemal and autoimmune disease suggests that there is substantial cross-reactivity between treponemal and human antigens. However, the nature of the antigen that stimulates Wasserman antibody is unknown, and it is not even certain whether the treponeme itself contains this antigen or whether infected tissue somehow generates it. Cross-reactivity between human and treponemal DNA is seen in the FTA-ABS test in which serum from patients with autoimmune diseases reacts with DNA that has extruded through the outermost treponemal layer (9).

We know that the host ultimately recognizes the foreign nature of *T. pallidum* because a variety of antibodies are produced in the course of infection. Since phagocytosis is not operative, the processing of antigen probably depends upon spontaneous death and disruption of some of the organisms. It is possible that large amounts of antibody--for example, Wasserman antibody--block the interaction between phagocytic cells and *T. pallidum* although no direct evidence for this possibility has been presented.

In summary, then, we have ample evidence that *T. pallidum* is not easily phagocytized, yet we have no good explanation for this. Possibilities include the presence of an unusual outer coat that inhibits phagocytosis, the failure of the mammalian host to recognize *T. pallidum* as foreign matter, the absence of receptor sites on phagocytic cells, and/or the presence of antibody that inhibits the interaction with phagocytic cells.

The failure of the host to produce opsonizing or treponemacidal antibodies might also be related to immune suppression. Suggestive evidence for suppressed immune responsiveness during syphilis has been found in several previous studies:

(1) Infected newborn rabbits develop thymic involution and depression of thymic-dependent areas of lymph nodes, in association with progressive, fatal infection (10)

(2) Thymic-dependent areas of lymph node and spleen are depressed during active syphilis in adult patients (11).

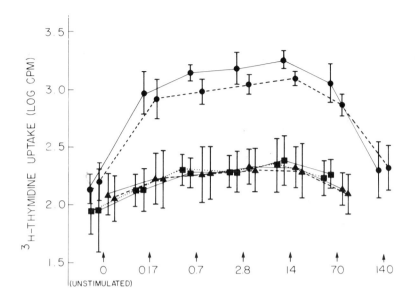

FIGURE 1. *Responses of lymphocytes from normal subjects*
(●━● *), patients with primary (* □ *) and secondary (* △ *)*
syphilis, and syphilitic patients 6 to 10 weeks after treat-
ment (●--● *) to* T. refringens. *Results of untreated syph-*
ilitic subjects are presented based on incubation of lympho-
cytes in the patient's own serum (broken line) or in normal
serum (solid line). Data are reported as mean $\log_{10}$ *counts/*
minute after correction for background. The variance is in-
dicated by brackets. The difference between normal and syphi-
litic lymphocytes is significant at every point from 0.17 to
70 μg *of treponemal protein per ml (*p < *0.001).*

    (3) The lymphocyte response *in vitro* to a variety of an-
tigens is suppressed during active syphilis (12-14a). Figure
1 shows the response to treponemal antigen of lymphocytes obtained from subjects with primary or secondary syphilis before
and after treatment. These studies, carried out in our laboratory, suggested that this suppression was unrelated to serum
factors; other studies in human beings and rabbits, have
suggested that serum factors are responsible (14,14b).
    (4) Lymphokine production appears later than might be ex-
pected in syphilis.

We believe that perturbations in immunoregulation occur during

infection and that increased numbers of suppressor cells may
contribute to the observed decrease in lymphocyte response.
It should be noted that in none of the aforementioned studies
were T, B, and K cells characterized prior to *in vitro* incubation.

Because of our interest in immunoregulation we have recently carried out a series of studies of the effect of syphilis on
the immunoglobulin response to sheep red blood cells (SRBC)
(R. E. Baughn and D. M. Musher, *J. Immunol.*, 121, 1691,1978).
Rabbits were infected with *T. pallidum* and, at various intervals thereafter, challenged with SRBC. Seven days later
spleens were removed and the presence of cells secreting IgG
or IgM was studied by Jerne plaque technique. Control animals
were those which were sensitized with SRBC and did not have
syphilis. Background plaque formation in rabbits that had
not been sensitized, whether infected or uninfected, was minimal. As shown in Fig. 2, the IgG response to SRBC was significantly reduced from 1 to 9 weeks after infection, being
nearly abolished at 3-6 weeks. An interesting contrast was
seen in IgM production, which was increased (Fig. 3). Similar

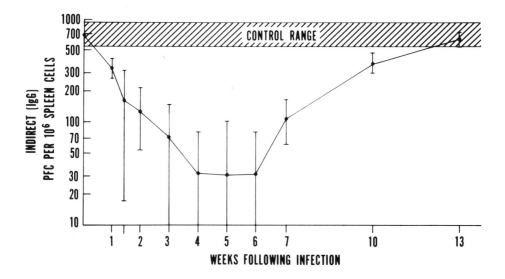

FIGURE 2. *Altered IgG responsiveness of rabbits to SRBC*
expressed as plaque-forming counts (pfc) per 10^6 spleen cells,
at various time intervals following intravenous infection with
T. pallidum. 2 × 10^9 SRBC were administered intravenously 7
days before the assay. Each point is the arithmetic mean ±
standard deviation of the PFCs per spleen in three rabbits.

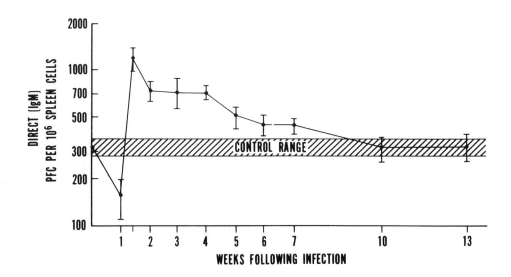

FIGURE 3. *Altered IgM responsiveness of rabbits to SRBC expressed as plaque-forming counts (PFC) per 10^6 spleen cells, at various time intervals following intravenous infection with T. pallidum.* *2×10^9 SRBC were administered intravenously 7 days before the assay.* *Each point is the arithmetic mean ± standard deviation of the PFCs per spleen in three rabbits.*

results were obtained in the secondary response to SRBC. Daily studies of the immune response from 4 to 9 days after SRBC challenge showed that a simple alteration in the kinetics of the response was not responsible. Although a full understanding of these observations awaits further studies, the data obtained to date give strong support to the concept that syphilis produces abnormalities in immunoregulation. One of these abnormalities could be the suppression of an IgG response with consequent failure to produce the "right" opsonizing or treponemacidal antibody.

The relation between immunosuppression and overproduction of other antibodies requires explanation. Certainly some antibodies are produced in profusion. Figure 4 shows a lymph node obtained from a syphilitic rabbit 7 days after intradermal challenge at several sites on the back. Many plasma cells are present, and one might presume that they are busily producing antibody. Wasserman antibody, which is called nontreponemal because it is directed against cardiolipin rather than specifically against treponemes, is detectable clinically in most patients with primary, and in all patients with secondary sy-

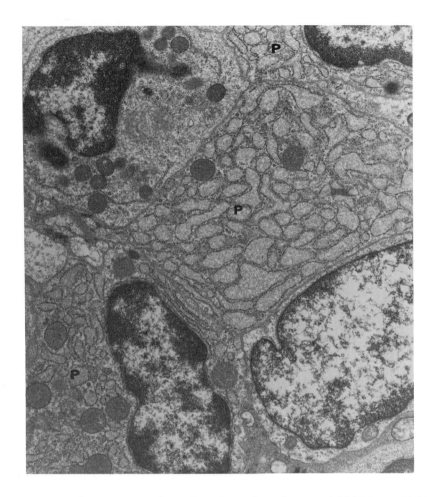

FIGURE 4. *Cortex from lymph node of a syphilitic rabbit,*
obtained 7 days after infection had been induced by injection
of 10[7] T. pallidum at several intradermal sites. Several
plasma cells (P) are seen; they have dilated endoplasmic re-
ticulum, indicating active protein synthesis. The finding of
plasma cells in germinal centers is distinctly unusual. (Elec-
tron-microscopic view 10,500× kindly provided by R. W. LaPushin.)

philis. IgM is the major component, although IgG is also present. It is interesting to note that Wasserman antibody is
associated with lesions; titers decline in latent syphilis,
and animals that do not develop syphilitic lesions also do
not produce Wasserman antibody. Also of great interest is the
presence of Wasserman antibody in autoimmune diseases (e.g.,

systemic lupus erythematosus) and other infections discussed
in this symposium (infectious mononucleosis and malaria),
especially when coupled with the observation that cultivatable
treponemes do not synthesize their own lipids, but rather in-
corporate fatty acids from the medium in which they are growing. As shown above, IgM responsiveness to antigens is increased during syphilis (Fig. 3). Other antibodies, which are
classified as treponemal, include those responsible for fluorescent labeling of *T. pallidum* or for hemagglutination when
tanned turkey cells have been coated with treponemal antigen.
None of these antibodies is known to serve a protective role(6).

An antibody that, in the presence of complement, inactivates *T. pallidum in vitro* (TPI antibody) is detectable in
virtually all patients who have late primary syphilis (15);
nonetheless, the infection is still not eradicated. We do
not understand why this reaction should take place *in vitro*,
yet fail to occur *in vivo*. The absence of complement is not
responsible, because complement is not suppressed in syphilis.
Whether high-affinity, nonprotective antibodies occupy sites
on the treponeme thereby blocking the interaction with TPI
antibodies is purely conjectural. Humoral factors confer some
degree of immunity in experimental syphilis as shown by suppression of chancre development when treponemal challenge is
followed by multiple infusions of serum from chancre-immune
animals (16,17). However, chancre suppression is incomplete,
and small, atypical lesions eventually appear. Certainly, this
is an unusual situation; the classical examples of humoral
protection would be associated either with opsonization of infecting organisms, ingestion by phagocytes, and eradication or
with bactericidal activity with or without a role for phagocytosis. Neither mechanism seems to operate normally in syphilis.

The apparent failure of TPI antibody to eradicate *T. pal-*
lidum early in natural syphilis, together with the observation that delayed hypersensitivity to treponemal antigen develops late in secondary syphilis (18,19), stimulated our laboratory to look more closely at the role of cell-mediated immunity (CMI) in syphilitic infection. It seemed logical to believe that cellular immune mechanisms might somehow be responsible for bringing about latency. We showed that infection
with *T. pallidum* stimulates acquired cellular resistance to
Listeria monocytogenes (20), a reliable index of CMI. This
resistance was transferable using thymus-dependent lymphocytes
and was abolished by specific antithymocyte serum (21). However, stimulation of acquired cellular resistance with other
agents such as BCG, *Propionibacterium acnes*, or Freund's
complete adjuvant did not protect against syphilitic infection
(22-24) even if small amounts of immune serum were administered at the time of challenge. In a recent series of experi-

ments (25), transfer of splenic lymphocytes from syphilis-
immune inbred rabbits to normal inbred recipients did not confer resistance. These observations suggest that CMI does not
play a protective role. Thus, the application of classical
immunologic techniques to the study of syphilis has led to an
unusual result: infection with *T. pallidum* stimulates both
humoral and cellular responses, yet both mechanisms together
fail to eradicate the infecting organisms.

We can not explain the onset of latency by citing any
specific event that appears to be responsible for it. Certainly, by the time latency develops, TPI antibodies have long
been present. Delayed hypersensitivity to treponemal antigens
is said to appear late in secondary syphilis and is uniformly
present in latency (19). It is possible that these two reactions work together to suppress *T. pallidum*. Against this
argument is the relatively frequent occurrence of relapses in
latent syphilis. Of course, antigenic shift, such as is seen
in borreliosis (relapsing fever) could be responsible for relapses, but our understanding of antigenic structure of *T.
pallidum* is so rudimentary that it does not appear possible
to approach this problem at the present time.

Natural resistance of animal species to infection is a
fascinating phenomenon, which has not attracted as much attention as it deserves. With most bacteria, use of a sufficiently large bacterial inoculum usually overcomes natural resistance. Despite the very low infective dose of *T. pallidum*
for rabbits and man, infection cannot be produced in mice by
ten million times as many organisms (26,27). *In vitro* studies
suggest that this is not due to the ability of mouse leukocytes
to ingest *T. pallidum*. Even in naturally resistant animals,
the absence of overt disease does not indicate that the host
has easily eradicated the organisms, because treponemes can
be recovered from mice months after challenge. The failure
to recognize the foreign nature of *T. pallidum* is not responsible, because FTA-ABS antibody develops in mice (28).

Tertiary syphilis of skin, bones, and viscera has generally been thought to represent a delayed hypersensitivity reaction. This reasoning is based on the presence of granu-
lomas that are characteristic of tertiary lesions. However,
the antigen that leads to granuloma formation is not easily
detectable, as is the case, e.g., in tuberculosis. If persistence of antigen following infection were responsible for
the later development of tertiary lesions, one wonders why
they follow the distribution pattern that they do, with frequent involvement of extremities. Silver impregnation stains
have been used to identify treponemes in tertiary lesions; but
these stains also react with cell membranes causing false posi-
tives, and, in the opinion of one authority (T. B. Turner,

personal communication), overreading may have been responsible for those instances in which treponemes have been said to be present in syphilitic gummas.

In conclusion, despite years of interest in clinical and immunologic aspects of syphilis, the major questions relating to the interaction between *T. pallidum* and the mammalian host are unanswered. We know that humoral and cellular responses are observed during infection, but phagocytosis by PMN or macrophages does not seem to occur. Although antibody which inactivates the infecting organism *in vitro* is regularly present, the infection is not eradicated. The unusual situation in which an infecting organism actively attaches to phagocytic cells is all the more difficult to understand in light of the failure to be ingested and destroyed. Syphilis causes a number of aberrations in immunoregulation, but it is unclear how these might contribute to the progression of the illness. Acquired cellular resistance is stimulated early in experimental infection and delayed hypersensitivity appears later in human syphilis, but a number of experimental studies suggest that CMI may not be playing a role in eliminating *T. pallidum*. Finally, the natural resistance of most animal species to infection by this organism is not understood. Just as in the early part of this century it was said of a clinician that he who understands syphilis knows clinical medicine, it might be said today that he who understands the immunology of syphilis understands immunology.

References

1. Kampmeier, R. H. *In* "Syphilis and Other Venereal Diseases" (J. B. Youmans, ed.), *Med. Clin. North Am. 48(3)*, 667, May, 1964.
2. Drusin, L. M., Rouiller, G. C., and Chapman, G. B. *J. Bacteriol. 97*, 951, 1969.
3. Lauderdale, V., and Goldman, J. N. *Br. J. Vener. Dis. 48*, 87, 1972.
4. Ovcinnikov, N. M., Korbut, S. E., Bednova, V. N., *et al. Br. J. Vener. Dis. 49*, 413, 1973.
5. Sykes, J. A., Miller, J. N., and Kalan, A. J. *Br. J. Vener. Dis. 50*, 40, 1974.
6. World Health Organization. Tech. rep. ser., No. 455, Switzerland, 1970.
7. Fitzgerald, T. J., Cleveland, P., Johnson, R. C., *et al. J. Bacteriol. 130*, 1333, 1977.
8. Hayes, N. S., Muse, K. E., Collier, A. M., *et al. Infect. Immun. 17*, 174, 1977.

9. Strobel, P. L., and Krause, S. J. *J. Immunol. 108*, 1152, 1972.

10. Festenstein, H. C., Abrahams, C., and Bokkenheuser, V. *Clin. Exp. Immun. 2*, 311, 1973.

11. Turner, D. R., and Wright, D. J. M. *J. Pathol. 110*, 305, 1973.

12. Musher, D. M., Schell, R. F., and Knox, J. M. *Infect. Immun. 9*, 654, 1974.

13. Musher, D. M., Schell, R. F., Jones, R. H., et al. *Infect. Immun. 11*, 1261, 1975.

14. Pavia, C. S., Folds, J. D., and Baseman, J. B. *Infect. Immun. 14*, 320, 1976.

14a.Wicher, V., and Wicher, K. *Clin. Exp. Immunol. 29*, 480, 1977.

14b.Wicher, V., and Wicher, K. *Clin. Exp. Immunol. 29*, 487, 1977.

15. Turner, T. B., and Hollander, D. H. Monogr. Ser. No. 35, World Health Organization, Geneva, Switzerland, 1957.

16. Perine, P. L., Weiser, R. S., and Klebanoff, S. J. *Infect. Immun. 8*, 787, 1973.

17. Bishop, N. H., and Miller, J. N. *J. Immunol. 117*, 191, 1976.

18. Marshak, L. C., and Rothman, S. *Am. J. Syph. 35*, 35, 1951.

19. Thivolet, J., Simeray, A., Rolland, M., et al. *Ann. Inst. Pasteur 85*, 23, 1953.

20. Schell, R. F., and Musher, D. M. *Infect. Immun. 9*, 658, 1974.

21. Schell, R., Musher, D., Jacobson, K., et al. *Infect. Immun. 12*, 505, 1975.

23. Graves, S. R., and Johnson, R. C. *Infect. Immun. 12*, 1029, 1975.

24. Baughn, R. E., Musher, D. M., and Knox, J. M. *J. Immunol. 118*, 109, 1977.

25. Baughn, R. E., Musher, D. M., and Simmons, C. B. *Infect. Immun. 17*, 535, 1977.

26. Gueft, B., and Rosahn, P. D. *Am. J. Syphilol. Gon. Vener. Dis. 32*, 59, 1948.

27. Schell, R. F., Musher, D. M., Jacobson, K., et al. *Br. J. Vener. Dis. 51*, 19, 1975.

28. Ohta, Y. *J. Immunol. 108*, 921, 1972.

DISCUSSION

    DR. DOHERTY: Have you attempted to determine whether the
organism will multiply in immunologically compromised mice,
for instance the nu/nu? Also, have a number of different
mouse strains been tested?
    DR. MUSHER: We have studied *T. pallidum* infections in a
number of mouse strains including hairless and nude (nu/nu)
mice but have been unable to produce active lesions. There
was no apparent difference between nude mice and any of the
other strains studied.
    DR. PREHN: I have a comment. If no strain of mouse will
support treponemal infection, perhaps one should transplant
rabbit testis to the nude mouse and use that as a substrate
for treponemal growth. The same principle could be applied
to the investigation of a large number of difficult diseases,
for example, Hansen's bacillus might be induced to grow in
human skin transplanted in the nude mouse.
    DR. WALDMANN: In considering the role of immune responses
in disease, it has been helpful to study patients with the
primary and secondary immunodeficiency diseases of humoral or
cellular immunity. Do they develop classical secondary syphilis? If the secondary reactions are reduced in immunodeficient
patients, this would imply that these reactions are due in part
to host immune responses.
    DR. MUSHER: Although administration of steroids to rab-
bits with latent infection is said to reactivate infection,
there has been, to my knowledge, no such information presented
in human subjects. I once asked an epidemiologist at the M.D.
Anderson Hospital whether there was anything to suggest enhanced rate of infection and/or reactivation in cancer patients undergoing chemotherapy and he felt there was not.
    DR. KIRKPATRICK: I have two questions. (1) Is there
any evidence that the lesions of secondary syphilis are due
to hypersensitivity to treponemal antigens rather than infection? (2) It would be interesting to study maturation of
IgG- and IgM-bearing lymphoid cells in animals with congenital
syphilis. It could be that there is normal maturation of μ-
bearing cells, but impaired maturation of γ-bearing cells.
This would be compatible with your observation of IgM plaques,
but poor IgG plaque formation, to sheep cells in infected rabbits. Another possibility derives from your report of thymic
atrophy and atrophy of thymus dependent areas of lymphoid tissues. Could the rabbits that do not produce IgG plaques be
deficient in necessary help?
    DR. MUSHER: (1) Histologically, the lesions of secondary
syphilis closely resemble those of primary syphilis, and they

are not characteristic of any typical hypersensitivity reaction. No direct evidence has been advanced to support the possibility that these lesions are any more a manifestation of hypersensitivity than lesions in other infectious diseases, although this possibility is frequently mentioned in the form of speculation.

(2) Either mechanism may be responsible for altered immunoglobulin synthesis in experimental syphilis in adult rabbits. Congenital syphilis is even less well-understood, and different mechanisms may be responsible. This certainly needs to be studied further.

DR. ROSEN: Is there C_3 deposition on *T. pallidum in vivo*? If there isn't it might explain the lack of phagocytosis and treponemal killing. For example, IgM antibody to Hemophilus and Neisseria is not, in most cases, complement fixing and therefore not opsonophagocytic or bactericidal.

DR. MUSHER: *In vitro*, complement certainly appears to be bound during the interaction between *T. pallidum* and antibody. Some evidence has been obtained for complement fixation in the unusual situation of glomerulonephritis associated with secondary syphilis, but complement has not been found in secondary lesions by British investigators who have looked for it. I would have imagined that the antigen-antibody reaction does bind complement *in vivo*. At the same time, neither syphilitic rabbits nor syphilitic humans are complement deficient, and the question of why *T. pallidum* is not killed by exposure to immune serum remains unanswered.

DR. WYLER: There is a report in the literature stating that serum from syphilitic patients contain an inhibitor of *in vitro* lymphoproliferation. Has this observation been confirmed, and is this factor characterized?

DR. MUSHER: There was one early study in the English literature indicating that serum factors inhibit transformation of syphilitic lymphocytes but I am told that there were difficulties in confirming this work. We found no significant effect of serum from syphilitic patients on lymphocyte transformation. However, our criteria were quite stringent. More recently, several investigators have found that serum factors do suppress the *in vitro* transformation of lymphocytes from syphilitic rabbits, and similar results in humans have been reported.

DR. SISKIND: (1) What happens if you allow treponemes to adhere to polys or macrophages and then add antibody and complement? (2) Also, what happens if you couple a hapten to the surface of a treponeme and then expose it to antihapten antibody and complement? Can it then be phagocytized?

DR. MUSHER: (1) Prior exposure to antibody blocks the attachment of treponemes to phagocytic cells and fibroblasts and, in fact, causes them to drop off if they have already attached. (2) I know of no such experiment; this might be very interesting to do.

DR. SCHWARTZ: Your comments about resistance to reinfection by *T. pallidum* indicate that there is, in fact, immunity to the organism. Thus, the situation in syphilis is directly comparable to that in the case of many parasitic infections and tumors in which there is clear evidence of concomitant immunity and inability to protect against the organism or the tumor.

DR. MUSHER: This is entirely true and is one of the great enigmas in syphilis research.

DR. LEVY: Have you tried extracts of *T. pallidum* in *in vitro* studies. For instance, do the extracts cause inhibition of the Jerne assay or get phagocytosed?

DR. MUSHER: Dr. Baughn and I have already planned these studies.

DR. WEINSTEIN: What causes the treponemes to disappear in untreated patients? What are the mechanisms involved in the "biological cure" of syphilis?

DR. MUSHER: One might think that the appearance of circulating antibodies is responsible for the great decline in treponemes in late chancres. However, secondary lesions then appear, and antibody levels must certainly still be as high, so I can not be sure of the mechanism for the reduction of treponemes. Disappearance of a "biological cure" in the sense of a complete cure probably does not occur in syphilis, since the host continues to house *T. pallidum* indefinitely after infection.

DR. PLATE: I wonder whether the findings of Dr. Sher of host antigens on schistosomula is a more general phenomenon common to parasitism. Have you looked for host antigens on the treponemes?

DR. MUSHER: This is a very important question; we have not yet done any studies along these lines.

Session VI
Workshop
Collated by Charles H. Kirkpatric and Göran Möller

INTRODUCTION

Göran Möller

This meeting has dealt with the relationship between immune mechanisms and diseases and particularly with various forms of escape from immune surveillance. In order to outline the themes for the general discussion I think we ought to separate diseases caused by immune reactions from those caused by escape from immunity (Table I).

Immune reactions constitute the major barrier to the successful use of organ transplantation. In addition, autoimmune reactions certainly cause several diseases. It may be useful to distinguish between autoimmune diseases, which are caused by a specific immune reaction, from those we may refer to as generalized autoimmune reactions. A typical candidate in the former category is myasthenia gravis, where specific antibodies to the acetylcholine receptor cause the symptoms of the disease. Allergy is another example of a disease where antibodies are considered to be responsible. It should be pointed out, however, that only a few individuals actually get these diseases, although there is no reason to doubt that every individual could produce antibodies to the acetylcholine receptor or that most individuals produce IgE antibodies. Obviously the profound cause of the disease is to be found at another level, possibly genetic, even though the symptoms are precipitated by immune reactions. In the groups of more general autoimmune diseases, systemic lupus disseminatus being an example, it is still unclear whether the autoimmune manifestations constitute symptoms or actually cause the disease.

In situations where we definitely know that the symptoms are caused by a specific immune reaction, the aims are obviously to induce specific unresponsiveness. In principle this can be achieved in four ways:

1. Classical induction of immunological tolerance by high doses of antigen. This possibility has been complicated by recent findings concerning the mechanism of tolerance at the

TABLE 1. Diseases (Conditions) Caused by

	Immune reactions		Escape from immune reaction			
Condition or disease	Transplant rejection	Specific autoimmune diseases (e.g., myasthenia gravis)	General auto-immune diseases (e.g., LED)	Virus infections	Parasite infections	Cancer
Aims	Specific immuno-suppression	Specific immuno-suppression	To distinguish between immunity as a symptom or a cause of the disease	To understand mechanisms of T cell activation and effector functions	To ananlyze mechanisms of parasite escape; to develop vaccines	To show whether immune surveillance exists; to study possible role of immunity in cancer treatment
Means	Tolerance induction Antigenic suicide	Anti-idiotype suppression	Induction of specific suppressor cells			

Genetic predisposition

Linkage between HLA and disease; role of genes; possibility of genetic engineering by, e.g., killing sperms

B cell level. It seems likely that tolerance to thymus-dependent antigens does not affect B cells in adult animals, and
tolerance to thymus-independent antigens only affects a subpopulation of B cells. Thus, B cell tolerance is not caused
by clonal elimination in any situation, and therefore it is
easy to break tolerance by the encounter of cross-reacting
antigens.

   2. The possibility of inducing antigen-mediated suicide
by treating individuals with antigen labeled with radioactive
isotopes or other toxic materials has been achieved in experimental situations. Also this method may be more complicated
than simple binding of antigen to B and T cell antigen binding
receptors, since macrophages seem to be required for suicide
to occur.

   3. Suppression of a specific immune response by treatment
with anti-idiotypic antibodies may turn out to be a promising
way. It has been shown that this treatment can induce immunological memory during certain--as yet undefined--conditions.
However, it has been found that an animal can be made to produce antibodies against its own idiotype, which results in a
prolonged suppression of the ability to express immunity to
antigens against which the suppressed idiotype is directed.
This suppression allowed skin grafts of the correct antigenic
constitution to persist for prolonged periods, whereas other
grafts were rejected normally. Although the mechanism is unknown, it seems that it may involve clonal deletion or possibly clonal suppression.

   4. The possibility of inducing specific suppressor cells
should be kept in mind. This has turned out to be possible
in certain situations, not the least with regard to suppression
of the IgE response.

The diseases that are due to escape from immune surveillance
are primarily infectious diseases caused by viruses in one
group and parasite and bacterial diseases in another. The
spontaneous cures of virus-induced diseases are most likely
caused by activation of T cells, which specifically interact
with the virus-infected cells and kill them, rather than T
cells directly interacting with and neutralizing virus particles. One important aspect of T cell recognition of infected
cells is the nature of the virus-host cell complex that is
recognized, e.g., virus in combination with cell surface
structures such as MHC products of various types. The nature
of the T cell receptor obviously deserves some further discussion. An equally important aspect is the mechanism of T
cell activation and what receptors the T cells possess to receive activating signals after they have interacted with the
antigens on the target cell.

The remarkable efficiency with which various parasites can escape attack from the immune system has constituted an important aspect of this meeting. We should discuss various mechanisms by which parasites have the ability to change their surface coat in different hosts, the role of antigenic variation, and other possible routes by which the parasites evade immune destruction. Equally important is the study of the immune response against parasites, the role of T cells and B cells, the possible participation of other killing mechanisms, such as antibody-mediated cell-mediated cytotoxicity and possibly the function of natural killer cells.

The final category of diseases in which escape from surveillance has been implied as an important mechanism is cancer. The famous concept of immune surveillance against spontaneously appearing tumor cells is considered to be fundamental for tumor immunology, although I do not think it has to be. The concept has also come under intensive criticism during the last years and consequently we should analyze whether there is sufficient scientific support to continue to regard immunological surveillance against tumors as live and well.

An overriding mechanism for the expression and control of diseases is the genetic determination of susceptibility or resistance to all the types of disease discussed above. I would suspect all diseases in Table I to have an important element of genetic control determining disease penetrance and severity. The striking linkage between HLA and disease, the discovery of Ir genes in the MHC complex, the role of genetic factors in certain cancer diseases, the family inheritance of HLA-linked genes for disease susceptibility also in cases where the particular disease does not associate with a particular HLA antigen in the general population, all argue for the important role of genetic factors. The interesting possibility to be discussed is whether we can manipulate the genetic predisposition by, e.g., removing sperms carrying Y chromosomes in the case of sex-linked diseases or by removing a certain haplotype associated with a particular disease in the case of HLA-linked diseases with high penetrance. These manipulations can be practically executed today, but what unexpected negative consequences can we expect by such manipulations?

It is a wide area we shall attempt to cover, and probably only a few aspects will be dealt with in some detail.

TRANSFER FACTOR AND DEFENSE AGAINST INFECTIOUS DISEASES

Charles H. Kirkpatrick

Transfer factor has been with us for many years. The absence of adequate animal models and *in vitro* assays have severely impeded isolation and identification of the active components and determination of its mechanism of action.

Recently, there has been a resurgence of interest in transfer factor, and this derives both from improved methods of isolation and characterization of small molecules and the possibility that it may be a useful therapeutic agent in immunodeficient patients with neoplastic or infectious disease. My comments will be limited to our experience with one disorder, chronic mucocutaneous candidiasis.

The subjects of this study were referred to the NIH Clinical Center for investigation. Each subject failed to develop a delayed cutaneous response to candida antigen; the majority of patients were unresponsive to all of the antigens in the test panel. In addition, peripheral lymphocytes from the patients did not respond to stimulation with candida by releasing lymphokines (MIF or LMIF).

The first stage of the study was directed toward answering two questions. Could the patients receive a passively transferred cellular immune response and, if so, would restoration of cellular immunity have clinical benefits? Seven subjects participated in this study. In each case the patients received the transfer factor from 6×10^8 lymphocytes. The cells came from donors with strong cellular immunity to candida. Injections were given monthly and the patients were followed up to 8 months. All patients developed positive cell-mediated responses (skin tests and lymphokine production) to candida and other sensitivities possessed by the transfer factor donors. In only two patients was there even equivocal evidence of clinical benefit; in no case did the infection clear.

This study showed that the patients could be passively sensitized with transfer factor, suggesting that they did not have a significant inhibitory or suppressive component to their

ISBN 0-12-055850-5

immunodeficiency. It also showed that correction of the immune defect alone was not adequate therapy.

A new protocol was then introduced. Patients were first treated with intravenous amphotericin B, an agent that regularly produces remissions that last for 4-6 months or less. Transfer factor was used as a form of consolidation therapy to see if we could prolong antibiotic-induced remissions. Treatment with transfer factor was begun near the end of the course of amphotericin.

Two preparations of transfer factor are being used: one from candida-sensitive donors and another from candida-insensitive donors. The seven recipients of the candida-sensitive transfer factor have become skin test-positive, although three of the patients have reverted back to a candida-negative state even though they still receive transfer factor. None of the five recipients of the candida-insensitive transfer factor has become skin test-positive to candida although they have become reactive to other antigens that caused positive skin tests in the donors.

At the time of this report there are eight skin test-negative patients (the five recipients of candida-insensitive transfer factor and the three recipients of candida-sensitive transfer factor who reverted their skin tests from positive to negative). The other four recipients of candida-sensitive transfer factor still have positive skin tests.

All of the skin tests-positive recipients are in remission at 6, 16, 72, and 75 months after the last amphotericin B. They still receive transfer factor three times a year. Five (62%) of the skin test-negative recipients have relapsed, although in four instances the remissions were for seven months or longer.

The study is still underway, but at this point two points are suggested. Transfer factor from sensitive or insensitive donors may prolong amphotericin B-induced remissions. The longest remissions, however, are seen in those patients who receive and maintain cellular immunity to candida.

NATURAL KILLING

Hans Wigzell

Natural killer cells in the mouse and man represent a promising cell type for providing resistance to the outgrowth of
autologous tumor. Such cells arise spontaneously, and levels
of activity have been shown in the mouse to be under genetic
control. In the murine system they are not conventional B, T,
or macrophages; they function via contactual lysis and they
display certain specificity insofar as they preferentially
kill certain tumor types in short-term cytolytic assays *in
vitro*. Their *in vivo* relevance is suggested by the striking
positive correlation between NK levels in an individual mouse
and the *in vivo* resistance of the same animal to syngeneic tumors. It is possible to enhance the NK levels *in vivo* by several agents such as BCG, *Corynebacterium parvum*, and several
viruses. Lately, data have been obtained suggesting that interferon is a major inducing agent functioning via the above
agents in recruiting NK cells *in vivo*. It is interesting to
note that interferon as well as the above agents have all been
considered of potential importance in tumor therapy in mouse
and man. Other facts in the murine NK system are the correlation between NK cells and age, since very young and very old
mice display virtual absence of NK activity. When tested for
correlation with age and NK levels in relation to tumor resistance, again a clear-cut positive correlation was found.
The specificity of NK cells is unknown although they would not
seem to normally function via conventional antigen-specific
receptors of their own or passively acquired. It is suggested,
however, that NK cells may also function via Fc receptors to
act as K cells in ADCC, although this would not seem their
normal way of functioning as NK cells in the mouse. In conclusion, NK cells may represent an "old" system endowed with
ability to act as a primitive resistance-providing mechanism
against aberrant cells.

IMMUNITY AND SURVEILLANCE

Robert S. Schwartz

The increased incidence of malignancy in patients with congenital immunodeficiency disease has been widely cited as support for an immune surveillance mechanism. However, in many
of these cases there are other defects that can equally explain the susceptibility to neoplasms. The most striking example of this is *Ataxia telangiectasia*, a disorder in which
virtually all patients have an important abnormality of chromosomes (14 q). This abnormality of the fourteenth chromosome,
interestingly, is the same as that reported in many cases of
malignant lymphoproliferative diseases that arise independently of ataxia telangiectasia, including Burkitt's lymphoma,
Hodgkin's disease, and histiocytic lymphoma. Another important
fact is the increased incidence of neoplasms in the immunologically normal first-degree relatives of patients with ataxia
telangiectasia. Bloom's syndrome is another condition associated with immunodeficiency and neoplasms, especially those
of the lymphoid system. Here again there is a characteristic
disturbance of chromosomes. In view of these findings and
the widespread nature of the defects in *Ataxia telangiectasia*
and Bloom's syndrome, it would appear that immunodeficiency
is only part of the story. The conclusion that these patients
develop cancer because of defective immune surveillance may be
an oversimplification.

As for malignancies in patients treated with immunosuppressive drugs, there is now growing evidence that these agents,
in particular, alkylating drugs such as cyclophosphamide and
chlorambucil, are carcinogenic compounds. These drugs may produce genetic lesions that greatly increase the risk of acute
myelogenous leukemia (AML), as we see now in patients with
Hodgkin's disease, multiple myeloma, and ovarian cancer. In
these cases, the risk of AML is increased 70-200 times in patients treated with cyclophosphamide, melphalan, or nitrogen
mustard, especially when combined with radiotherapy. Although
there is still debate as to whether untreated patients with

myeloma are unusually susceptible to AML, the weight of the
evidence indicates that treatment with alkylating drugs is
strongly associated with AML. This, incidently, is not the
case of azathioprine. This drug may be associated with bizarre
lymphomas (immunoblastic sarcoma) through different mechanisms,
especially in recipients of kidney transplants. One possibility to consider here is that certain herpesviruses may be
oncogenic. The EBV is virtually established as an oncogenic
herpesvirus. CMV, another herpesvirus, infects virtually every
recipient of a renal allograft; its oncogenic potential merits
considerable attention.

POSSIBLE ROLE OF TUMOR-SECRETED MEDIATORS
IN HELPING TUMORS ESCAPE FROM IMMUNOLOGIC SURVEILLANCE

Harold F. Dvorak

Little is known about the mechanisms by which tumors elude
immunologic surveillance but a large number of possible explanations have been considered. In searching for clues that could
better explain the success of some tumors in bypassing the immunologic defense mechanisms, we examined the morphologic events
associated with the growth of two well-characterized diethyl-
nitrosamine-induced tumors (lines 1 and 10) in the subcutaneous space of immunized syngeneic strain-2 guinea pigs.
Our findings demonstrated:

(1) A hitherto unsuspected fibrin-gel enveloping both
tumors.
(2) When abundant, as in the case of line 1 tumors, this
gel subsequently became organized and largely replaced by the
ingrowth of fibrous connective tissue, leading to a scirrhous
pattern of carcinoma growth.
(3) The fibrin-gel itself, or soluble molecules associated
with the clotting/fibrinolytic systems, may contribute to the
induction of angiogenesis and fibroplasia.
(4) The spontaneous regression of line 1 tumors is the result of tumor infarction that is associated with widespread
microvascular damage.
(5) The vessel damage and infarction of line 1 tumors
probably results from an expression of cellular immunity.
(6) The more malignant line 10 tumor retained an intact
investment of fibrin-gel throughout growth and, although it
also provoked an immunologic response, this proved ineffective in arresting tumor spread.

These observations clearly indicated that both tumors had
mechanisms for manipulating host inflammatory pathways so as
to provide themselves with an investment of fibrin-gel matrix,
a blood supply, and, in the case of line 1 tumors a fibrous

stroma. We hypothesized that tumors might accomplish these ends by secreting mediator substances capable of triggering host inflammatory systems such as the clotting cascade and fibrinolysis. To test this possibility, line 10 tumor cells along with several nonneoplastic control cells were cultured in serum-free medium for 4 hours and the culture supernatants were assayed for various mediator activities. Four distinct mediator activities were found in line 10 culture supernatants: a vascular permeability factor (VPF), a procoagulant (PC), a plasminogen activator (PA), and a macrophage migration inhibition factor (MIF). By contrast, control cells secreted none of these activities.

The four mediator activities described here can account for certain features of the growth of line 10 tumors including the induction and modulation of a fibrin-gel. Whether the induction of a vascular supply, and the replacement of the fibrin-gel with fibrous connective tissue in the case of line 1 tumors, requires additional mediators is open to question, but there is some evidence to suggest that triggering of clotting activity may be sufficient to induce both angiogenesis and fibroplasia. The coordinated secretion of mediators that trigger in proper sequence various host inflammatory pathways, including the clotting and fibrinolytic systems, provides tumors with a mechanism for stroma induction and growth in the hostile environment of a foreign host and may be an important factor in determining a tumor's histologic pattern and degree of malignancy.

RESPONSE TO SPONTANEOUS NEOPLASMS

Richmond T. Prehn

It is now quite apparent that, at least in rodents, the immunogenicity of a tumor, i.e., the capacity of a syngeneic tumor to immunize its host against the growth of that tumor, varies remarkably from tumor to tumor. These differences may reflect differences in the number of antigen moieties per cell, differences in the degree of antigen shedding into the environment, differences in the nature of the host response due to blocking factors or suppressor cells, or to various combinations of these possible factors. Most important is the repeated observation that "spontaneous" rodent tumors, i.e., tumors that arise sporadically for no overt cause, have little or no immunogenicity. I have presented evidence suggesting that the immunogenicity tends to vary directly with the concentration of inducing carcinogen. This relationship appears to hold for tumors induced in the immune-free environment of tissue culture, so I infer that the degree of immunogenicity of a tumor is a property conferred, at least in part, directly by the inducing agent. Lack of immunogenicity may be a direct result of a low concentration of inducing agent rather than the result of immunoselection.

The relative lack of immunogenicity of "spontaneous" rodent tumors should not be interpreted to mean that most human tumors would be nonimmunogenic if they could be tested by transplantation techniques. Many human neoplasms show a marked lymphocytic infiltrate at early stages of their evolution. This infiltrate certainly implies an immunological reaction and suggests that these tumors are more analogous to the rodent tumor induced with a low to moderate concentration of oncogenic chemical than they are to "spontaneous" rodent tumors. Perhaps the best model for many human tumors is the mouse tumor induced with low concentrations of oncogen.

Although the lymphocytic infiltrate seen in many human tumors implies an immunological reaction, it is by no means clear that this reaction is basically defensive. It is now

well established that an immunological reaction can, under certain circumstances, stimulate target cells to grow better; in
fact the argument over whether or not the lymphoid infiltrate
is aiding or inhibiting tumor growth goes back at least to 1918
and is still unresolved.

My own view is that the accumulated evidence suggests that
the early tumor is actually promoted by the lymphoid infiltrate,
a viewpoint that I expounded in an editorial in the October
1977 issue of the Journal of the National Cancer Institute.
If this view is correct, the relatively good prognosis associated with a lymphoid ilfiltrate would have to be interpreted
as being due, not to the lymphoid infiltrate, per se, but to
the early nature of the lesion with which a lymphoid infiltrate is characteristically associated. It is the early, relatively well-differentiated tumor that attracts a lymphoid infiltrate. The latter may therefore be a marker of a tumor
with a good prognosis rather than a cause of that behavior.
In fact, it is reasonable to view the early tumor as being
"dependent" upon the lymphoid infiltrate in the same way that
an early mammary tumor may be dependent upon estrogen.

There seems to be little doubt that immunological defenses
are very important in the prevention of certain viral tumors,
such as feline sarcoma and Marck's disease in chickens. In
contrast, as I have pointed out, there is reason to believe
that an immune reaction may aid the growth of tumors induced
by moderate levels of carcinogen. However, the most important an overriding consideration is that there usually is an
immune reaction--whether defensive or not--and there is thus
the possibility that with more knowledge it may be possible
to manipulate this reaction to therapeutic ends. Certainly,
the prospect is much more favorable than would be the case if
most human tumors were, like "spontaneous" rodent tumors, truly
nonimmunogenic.

INDEX